I N N E R
GURU

THE GUIDE TO MASTERING
YOUR HEALTH, WEALTH & RELATIONSHIPS
FROM THE INSIDE OUT

CHARLES D'ANGELO

Foreword by Larry King

Copyright © 2017
Charles D'Angelo

Published by
CDA Publishing
St Louis, MO

Library of Congress Control Number: 2017903849

10 9 8 7 6 5 4 3 2 1

Distributed in Canada by
NBN (National Book Network)

Distributed in USA by
NBN (National Book Network)
15200 NBN Way,
Blue Ridge Summit, PA
17214

Printed in Canada

Publishing Director: Wendy Morley

Interior Book Design: Sarina Joy Lamothe

Cover Design: Gabriella Caruso

Copy Editor: Syd Waters

Proofreaders: Richard Mason, Barbara Heise, Syd Waters

Editorial Assistant: Quincy Tejani

Photography: www.graphicstock.com, www.dreamstime.com, www.pixabay.com, www.pexels.com

Photographers: Randall Kahn, Sarah Pritt, Cate Jackson, Kyle Kabance, Tony Meoli

Cover photograph of Charles by Randall Kahn

Success Story images in Chapter 11 provided by each respective person

All other images provided by Charles D'Angelo

Praise for Charles D'Angelo

Marcos Rothstein, MD, Professor of Medicine

"His clear and knowledgable guidance makes it possible – and even exhilarating – for someone to establish new patterns and habits, which is key to his program's success. Charles helped me find the motivation to incorporate a well-balanced, consistent diet and program of physical fitness into my life without any feelings of deprivation. I am confident that he can do the same for you."

Maxine Clark, Founder of Build-A-Bear Workshop

"Charles' story and strategies can empower you to take charge of your life! Don't let where you start be where you finish!"

Richard Simmons

"You have heard of Cinderella, now meet Cinderfella. Charles is an amazing man who turned his life around and who now will dedicate his life to helping others and I know he will. Bless you Charles and all that you do!"

Angela Bassett, Golden Globe-winning Actress

"Charles knows how to help you get the best out of yourself – he'll get you excited and ready to take action, formulate a strategy that works for you, and see you through to your goals. He really cares that you succeed. Thanks Charles!"

Senator Claire McCaskill

"Charles is an uniquely talented individual who guides you to your best self. Like many, I could never figure out why I couldn't find the discipline to be healthy. Charles helped me find that discipline. He changed my life."

For Crystal, my "burning bush" and soul mate. You bring God's presence and love into my life each and every day. I love you.

For my mom, dad and Ms. Valerie White. You each live on through the lessons and examples you shared that are now forever captured within these pages.

CONTENTS

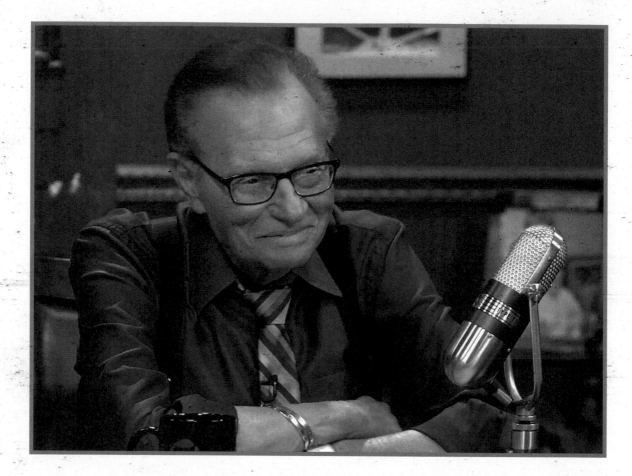

Larry King is an American television and radio show host, most known for his prolific career as host of the award-winning show, *Larry King Live*. He has appeared as himself in several movies and television shows.

FOREWORD

I met Charles D'Angelo when I interviewed him in 2015. I immediately recognized that there was something very special about Charles.

Yes, he accomplished something quite difficult, losing a massive amount of weight. That in itself was amazing. But what really stood out to me about Charles was that he seemed to have grasped life at a very young age, learning to truly transform himself from the inside out, and in so doing created a method of thinking and living that would help others to transform themselves as well.

I personally turned my life around after I had a heart attack; I quit smoking just like that, though I'd been a three-pack-a-day smoker, and started paying far more attention to my health in general by losing weight and starting a healthy diet. In my years of interviewing over 30,000 people, I have met many who have turned their own lives around as well, but it was apparent from the get-go that Charles had a very unique and different way of looking at things.

His focus was weight loss, and my interview with him was based on his first book about losing weight, called *Think and Grow Thin*. But our interview barely touched on diet or exercise. That's because, as Charles said in our interview, permanent success only comes when you change on the inside—changing your thought processes.

Once you change the way you think, anything is possible. You can and will achieve your goals whether that means finally achieving perfect health, financial freedom, escaping from substance abuse or transcending any other thing that's making your life anything less than you deserve it to be.

Like me and perhaps you too, Charles' life started out more difficult than most, but we both discovered and followed our calling. His book *Inner Guru* will help you to find yours, and help you to create your best and most fulfilling life.

Sincerely,

Larry King

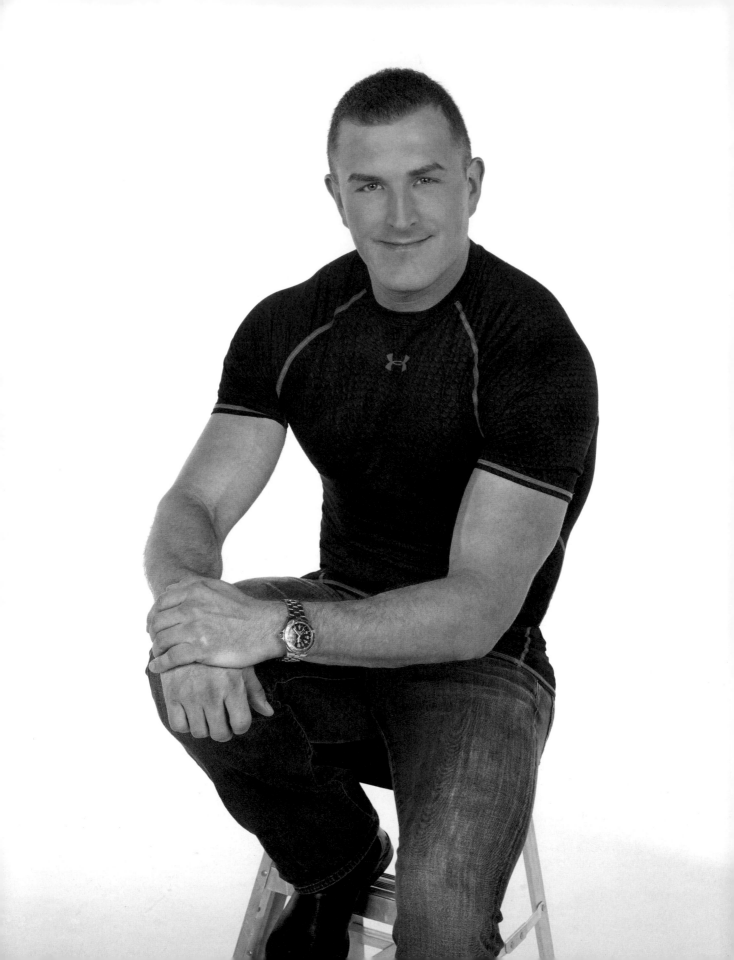

INTRODUCTION

You are holding this book at this moment for a reason.

You are dissatisfied with some part of your life, whether that's how you look, a feeling of emptiness and loneliness even when you are with other people, being unhappy with your job or relationship, feeling a sense of complete purposelessness or wondering why, since you've tried everything you could possibly think of, you're still not happy.

Am I right? If so, keep reading. The greatest gift I can give you, even if you don't read one more paragraph, is the knowledge that the following is true: You do not have to accept life as it is. Despite whatever you've been told before and whatever you've believed and whatever you think has been proven to you, you can create the very life you desire. I know this because I've seen it, over and over and over again, in my own life and the lives of my clients. You will read about many of these people throughout this book.

Many thousands of people know me as "The Weight-Loss Coach," and with good reason. I lost 160 pounds when I was still a teen, without any particular diet, guide or magical plan, despite a history that would not give the slightest hint of such a radical and rapid change being possible. I did not come from a supportive background. Most members of my family on both sides were either obese or using substances of all sorts just to deal with the drudgery of their daily life. Growing up this way gave me a tremendous appreciation for how people choose to deal with life's challenges. Sadly, I found most people accept their life

without question, feeling they have no ability to influence it for the better. As my grandparents, who had no more than an eighth-grade education, would say when an unexpected problem would arise, "Well, whatcha gonna do? That's too bad, but it's just how it is." This acceptance, which really bordered more on apathy, is the philosophy so many people subscribe to.

If an average person was given my biography, if they discovered the history of chaos in my childhood home, the abuse I faced and the lack of helpful role models in my world, they certainly would never have predicted my life would turn out as remarkably as it has. And yet it has. I know without doubt my success has not been coincidental, and I say that because many synchronies have occurred in my own journey—things that, while occurring in an unrelated manner, actually are related, affirming for me that I'm living my purpose. Grace had a whole lot to do with it, as did the strategies I developed. And both of these are available to you, right now.

More Than Weight Loss

With the success of my first book *Think and Grow Thin,* my office received stacks of letters, e-mails and even handwritten notes from people who had been overweight and who, after years of dieting, exercise programs, DVD's, therapy, coaching, and other efforts, were finally able to make the breakthrough they had always wanted after reading my book. But an interesting and unexpected thing happened. A huge group of others contacted me saying that they found my book called out to them even though they did not need to lose any weight. They said their lives had transformed completely, in ways that didn't have anything to do with their body's composition.

Perplexed, I responded to these letters, asking what they had found useful in my book since weight loss had been its focus. They said they found the strategies I designed for weight loss could be applied to define, achieve and ultimately maintain other goals they had almost abandoned because of their history or their frustration with their current life circumstances. They found the strategies effective to achieve things like financial independence, relationship mastery and overcoming addiction, as well as fostering a stronger connection with their Creator.

There was a common denominator among those who wrote to me. They all said what I was teaching and doing was different. It meant something to them that I had been where they now found themselves and was so open about it. These people said it was so simple but so profound. I've always found the trouble with "simple" is that the things that we find simple to do are also simple *not* to do. Go figure.

I kept hearing from people, asking if I would put together a program to help anyone who feels stuck in any place they can't seem to get out of regardless of their weight. They wanted a plan to help them break through years of limitations, just as they'd witnessed my personal coaching clients do, stepping into their God-given destinies.

We All Need Others

I lost my mother on my 30th birthday, of all days, after watching the decline of her health for nearly two decades, after years of trying to intervene in her poor choices, years of accompanying her on many doctor's visits, long hospital stays and in treatment centers, where the conversation was more focused on the symptoms she reported than the cause. Because of this experience, I realized something was missing in the larger sense in the world of personal development.

Before finally seeking help, my mom tried everything she could on her own, as intensely as possible. She didn't want people to even know she had a problem, much less see her suffering. What she failed to realize is that there is no shame in asking for help. We all need one another to help guide us to success. And

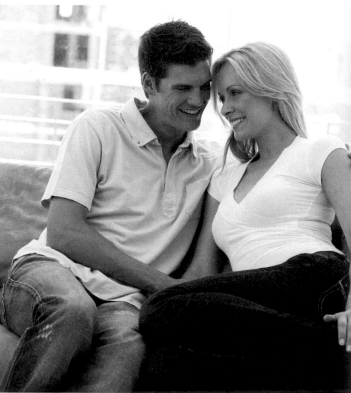

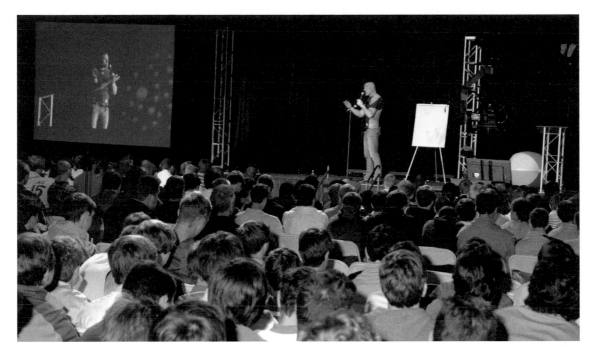

while this book is in the self-help section, that doesn't mean you don't *need* others. I'm at the place where I can help you because God put many people on my path along the way. This book will inspire you to open yourself to those around you for support along your journey.

I've realized that sometimes it's not another prescription or another diet a person needs to live the life they deserve and that God desires for them. Often just a curious, sincere, confident and loving listener can be the answer. When a person feels like someone else "gets" them, accepts them wherever they are, stands in their truth with them and offers the courage to step into a new unfamiliar healthy territory in faith, miraculous healings and life breakthroughs occur.

I have often wondered how different my mom's life would have been if she had sought out loving connection with others instead of the substances she used to try and fill the emptiness she felt in her life. Maybe she'd still be here today. What if a person like the professional me had come into her world, trying to understand her and help her understand

and accept herself and her feelings instead of numbing those feelings with the cocktail of prescriptions she took daily. Someone more interested in her spiritual and mental well-being and not just the physical. Someone who understood just how closely these are connected. What if my mother had seen all the pain from her history as a gift and something to learn from instead of being a curse or something to feel flawed by? What if she had grown enlightened instead of tormented? I know things would have been much better. Have you been trying to bury feelings you don't understand, perhaps throwing yourself into work, sex, food, alcohol or drugs? This book contains the map to escape this destructive pattern.

Considering this, I realized that while I had longed billed myself a weight loss coach, almost all of my time with clients over the years has been spent talking about their lives, their relationships, their feelings and their future, and very little about their weight. The bad habits like overindulgence, reaching for instantly gratifying junk, self abuse, negative self talk and doubt all seemed to miraculously stop when they felt heard, validated, and had a simple healthy strategy to follow. Almost everyone who came to me actually knew what to do—some of my clients were professional dieticians and nutritionists!—but were having trouble maintaining their resolve to keep at it. Once these clients began changing their perspective, they began improving their lives in a multitude of ways, from better relationships to more success in business.

If this is the case with my coaching, I asked myself, then could a book change a reader's entire life in a much more panoramic way? As I pondered this, synchrony after synchrony occurred that served as validation. I knew then that indeed this book needed to get to you. Inspiration rushed through, leading me to the realization that if my book were written with enough enthusiasm, focus, joy, purpose and sincerity, it would reach the hearts and souls of people like you, who need to hear it from a person who's lived it.

My goal, since realizing my own destiny, is to help as many people as I possibly can to realize their destinies and in doing so achieve success and happiness. With the help of technology, I've been blessed to coach people from all around the globe via Skype and Facetime who can't meet in person, but meeting one-on-one still is limiting. So I began lecturing to groups of thousands. Those whose lives I've had the blessing to touch have regained their sense of purpose and eliminated the distractions that had been stopping them from fulfilling their mission. With this book, you'll learn to take charge of your own mind. My strategies can help you begin to trust yourself and your Creator, becoming the ultimate guru on directing your life and achieving your dreams.

The time has come for me to pour out to you all God has poured into me in the years since writing *Think and Grow Thin*. Since that book was published, I've faced many more struggles, challenges and changes. I lost much of my emotional support and security in addition to the comfort of certainty within a short

timeframe. I lost three people very close to me. First my father lost his life to a massive heart attack at just 54 years old. Then my spiritual guide and adopted "grandma" died peacefully of old age. And then my mom was called to God on my 30th birthday. Ironically, after years of sobriety and being clean from drugs, she was found dead from an accidental drug reaction at only 51. But even in times of trouble, we can train ourselves to find meaning and joy. Grace is always operating; it's our challenge to see it. As this storm of events began, the woman of my dreams walked into my life. She has been and continues to be a source of ultimate joy, growth, and inspiration.

And so now the time has come to share everything I can with you, to help you take your life to the next level. If weight loss is your goal then of course I will help you with that, but that's definitely not this book's only focus. Regardless of your age or your history, despite the season of your life or any predicament you find yourself in life right now, I will teach you how to make the most of it and come through the other side with your feet firmly planted in the direction of the attainment of goals—ultimately fulfilling your unique destiny.

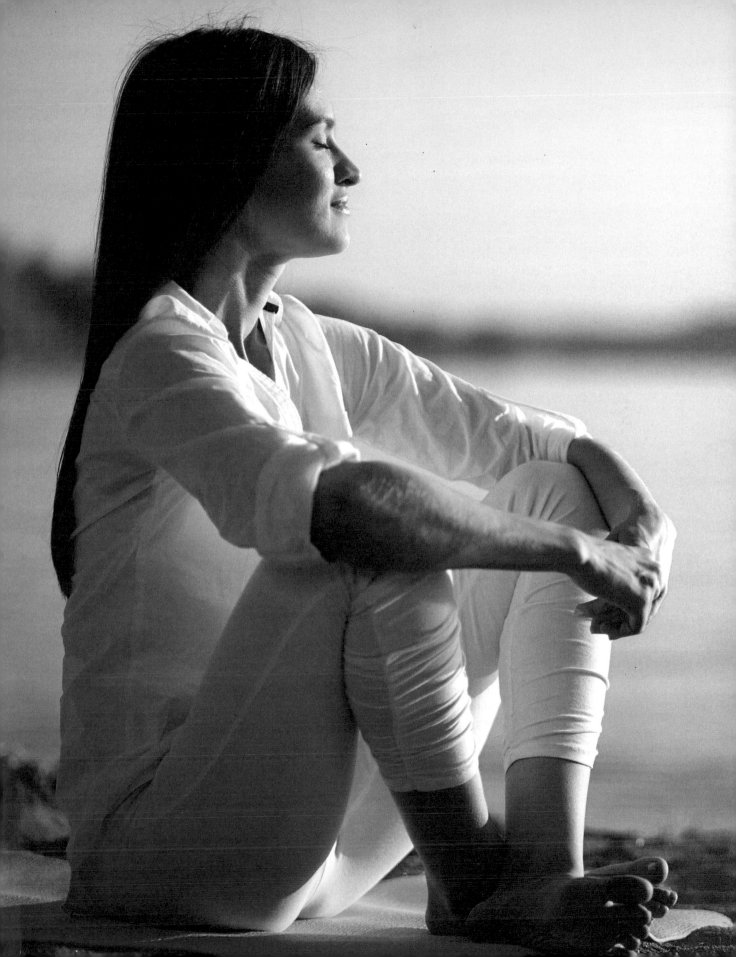

CHAPTER ONE
In the Beginning

Every single book available from a website or on the bookstore shelves started as a seed in someone's mind. The people who thought up and wrote those books—and this book too—aren't necessarily any smarter, more driven or even more disciplined than you are. The only thing different about us is we are not willing to live on this planet simply accepting the way it is, and instead we work to make it better. If we are unhappy with the status quo, we get to work on changing it.

People like me disturb the establishment, putting forth the question "Why?" to long-held belief structures. Asking this same question is the only way for you to continue to grow, and for our society to grow as well. In the face of police shootings, racially divided riots, ideologically divided elections, Middle-Eastern wars and terrorism, we are in a period of incredible social unrest and change right now. People have lost touch with their Creator and yearn for more than they see. We are all experiencing a hunger for more happiness, joy, peace, love and fulfillment, and independence from the societally enforced norms so many have bought into for the last hundreds of years.

We are moving toward a time in our society when love and peace can become more the norm than hatred and war, but to achieve this we must allow "difference" to take on a more positive meaning. The United States of America was based on the acceptance and rights of the individual. Greater acceptance of the individual differences that exist in each of us, integration of different faiths and understanding of atypical sexualities is the inevitable result. For the hatred and war outside of us to cease, we must end the war of self-hatred that occurs daily in our own body, heart and mind. We must become physically, emotionally, mentally and spiritually armored and skilled at waging and winning the internal battle that silently takes the lives of millions each day, cloaked in depression, obesity, drug abuse, war and terror. When you love yourself, you cannot help but have compassion and empathy for everyone you encounter. Judgment is immediately replaced with understanding, and hatred with acceptance. This book offers you an opportunity to do just that.

We are all born incredible learners. As babies we enter the world with only two fears—the fear of a loud noise and the fear of falling. This is a fact. That means everything else you tell yourself you fear along the way is something you learned to fear through conditioning. This is a fancy way of saying you got it from your own life experience or from listening to someone else. But even if this negative conditioning comes from the experience itself, this fear does not dictate your future. The lesson you take from experience or, better yet, the meaning you give to what has happened in your life is what serves as the GPS in your mind, and is not the only way to go.

Let me ask you a question. Does getting up and speaking in front of a group make you feel nervous? Since this is one of the most common fears in our society, you can probably make yourself feel scared by just thinking of getting up on stage, even if such an event is not actually happening. The simple thought generates a biochemical thunderstorm that sends your stress hormones through the roof, causing your heart to race. Isn't it true? Think of being in front of a group of people and you can make yourself sweat. This reaction is the result of a pattern you have habitually run, over and over and over, to get that same negative outcome. It has little to do with reality. Your mind is powerful, and you will learn to control it as you make your way through this book.

Patterns of Behaviour and Thought

Once I had the insight and understood that my fears were coming from within myself I was convinced, at a very young age, that anything I wanted to learn or do was possible.

Yes, of course, that isn't to say that there are no limitations in life. If you are only four feet tall you will most likely not be slam-dunking in the NBA, but you could still participate in the NBA serving in a different role. If you can't draw more than a stick figure you will probably not be the next Walt Disney, but you can develop the ideas and work with those who do have that gift, which is what Disney ultimately did!

Today, you can choose to take what you've got, which is quite a lot, improve on it and make it work for you, better than you might ever have thought possible. The great motivational speaker and philosopher Jim Rohn once said, "If you work hard enough on your gifts, they will make room for you."

I have certainly found this to be true. You are not doomed to a life of mediocrity because the world is too competitive or that all the good ones are gone, or because of your years of yo-yo dieting, overspending, or staying in a bad relationship. Far from it. You can learn to become aware of your patterns in this present moment, coming to terms with the ultimate spiritual truth that there is only the now, the past is an illusion and the future is without any guarantee. Stay present and channel all your energies into making the most out of this moment, starting now!

"If you work hard enough on your gifts, they will make room for you."

I remember teachers and counselors telling the obese teen I once was that maybe a nutritionist, dietician or counselor could change me. Before I continue this thought, let me say you do not *need* to change. You may *want* to, and only with that desire, *will* you. No one can change you but you. Our life won't change for the better unless we change our own thought and action patterns. When I was 160 pounds overweight and seriously in danger of losing my future, I personally had to learn how to change the disempowering pattern I had unconsciously constructed to get through life, one that had been playing out way past its efficacy. And I can help you learn to change your disempowering patterns. But it's you who must do it.

Good luck trying to make an impact on someone simply by telling them that they need to change, including yourself. The idea of change automatically conjures up pain, uncertainty, and ultimately fear. You do not need to change *yourself*, but today is your opportunity to look at the *patterns* you've been running in your life on all fronts—your health, your finances, your relationships, and whether or not you've been on mission and purpose with a force greater than yourself—and you will see there are more effective choices to make.

You need to consider the labels that were given to you about who you "are" before you could offer any objection, perhaps while you were a child. Maybe these labels came from inside yourself and not from others. Are these labels and your patterns of behavior serving you now? This question is not asked in judgment. It's meant just for you and only to be objective in helping you see where you truly are right now. I won't be upset if you decide you want to keep doing what you've always been doing. You just need to know it's naïve to think your life will be greatly improved on any level if this is the decision you make. If your patterns are not bringing you what you desire, then a shift is in order.

"You need to consider the labels that were given to you about who you 'are' before you could offer any objection, perhaps while you were a child. Maybe these labels came from inside yourself and not from others."

The Past is the Past

When you enter into any helping relationship, whether with a therapist, psychologist, psychiatrist, coach or anyone else, be careful that you don't get stuck in the mud of your history. It can be treacherous territory. Some will spend more time than needed on a problem's description and roots instead of it's resolution, digging in the soil of the past rather than reminding you of the joy of the present. I believe it can be great to take a quick trip into history in order to draw forth lessons you can use moving forward, but all too often people use it as a home to dwell in or as an excuse to relinquish the power they have today. In my experience this has never proven to be an effective strategy in helping people transform their lives. All too often, the story they harbor about their history becomes so familiar and comfy they lose sight of the promise of their future, or their helper becomes their new best friend and objectivity is lost along with the vision of their future. If you are using all your energies rehashing ancient history instead of constructing a magnificent vision of the next one, three, five or ten years of your life, then it's time for a new plan!

As for my own transformation, I didn't want to dwell in the past. I learned long ago that the best thing about the past is that it's *over*. Isn't that true? Drudging up pictures, sounds and movies of my worst experiences was not where I wanted to put my energies. I knew there had to be a better way. I had heard of and read about many people who were in a superior place in life—not just physically, but also in their relationships, spiritually and mentally—and their focus always seemed to be on the joy of their present life and an unbounded excitement that the best was yet to come, even though their "now" was really awesome! If they had found their way to that better place then that meant there had to be a road, and I was determined to discover it.

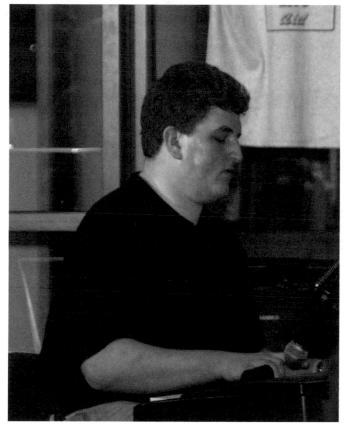

came up to me daily, sometimes hourly, to tell me just how "amazing" the change they saw was, and how "difficult" they "knew" it must have been for me. The funny thing was, it hadn't been difficult at all once I had figured things out on the inside. With the new inside, the new outside was inevitable. I didn't have to make all sorts of massive changes; I just had to replace the things that weren't working with what did work, and stay consistent with them.

With this newfound passion, it was as if I had found the secret recipe to designing and living a fulfilling life, and I knew that the reason God put me on this earth was to share that recipe, helping other people to live their own fulfilling lives. This led me to the realization that change can happen instantaneously for anyone in any area of life—they just need to be present, aware of their purpose and equipped with the right strategies and tools.

I figured that the best place to start was with my own health. For a long time I had tried to control what I saw as the unstable or harmful things around me, like my mom who was struggling with addiction to alcohol and drugs, or the bullying I suffered. Have you tried to create change by changing the things around you? The problematic kids, the way others think about you, how your partner doesn't respect or listen to you? If you have, you know where I'm coming from. At this point, however, I decided that the key to the change I was looking for had been within my grasp all along when I looked in the mirror, saw myself and knew any change had to begin right there.

I began studying the ways of the ultra fit and in just two years I was lean and confident after learning and implementing the way these fit people thought, acted, ate and moved. After I changed my life in such a visible way, people

Many people think of my work in terms of motivating and inspiring people. While both inspiration and motivation are two important ingredients in creating real lasting change, they alone are not enough. The focus of my work is helping people to remove, or find their way around, the barriers and obstacles keeping them from their own innate tendency toward growth and greatness. I am not as much a motivational speaker as I am an invitational one; asking people to apply timeless truths and disciplines to their daily lives.

Since my own transformation, I've coached thousands of people to liberate themselves from their excess weight, get control of their

"I didn't have to make all sorts of massive changes; I just had to replace the things that weren't working with what did work, and stay consistent with them."

lives and find joy, from A-list movie stars, CEOs and national politicians to high-school students and stay-at-home moms. I've helped some people lose 10 or 15 pounds and get their coveted flat stomach, but more often I've helped people who have really struggled with their weight and sometimes many other addictive habits.

One thing we all have in common is the unlimited, yes, unlimited capacity to learn new things. We start from the second we are born. How many musical instruments or languages can a child learn? As many as he or she is taught or exposed to, is the answer. Neuroscience now supports this fact, teaching us that are brains are plastic, or ever changeable. Somewhere along the path we call life we grow narrow minded, mostly because of fear or blind acceptance. We come to accept limitations imposed on us by those we see as authorities. We accept the negativity others tell us about ourselves—that we can never be a great singer, athlete, teacher, politician, actor or actress.

Whether our naysayers are authority figures such as parents, caretakers, teachers, religious leaders, coaches or politicians or our friends and classmates, we swallow whatever is fed to us and often short circuit our own future as a result. We subvert our own authority, replacing it with someone else's. It's easy to hand the authority over to someone else, because that means you don't have to feel as bad if things don't work out, right? After all, it was someone else who said it, not you! I believe this common error in thinking is the biggest mistake a person can make, and one I once almost fell prey to myself. That need not be the case for you. You do not have to accept yourself as powerless.

Does this mean I think the entire 12-Step Program philosophy is wrong? No. In fact, I believe giving up the idea that you can succeed alone is a critical step in personal growth, for all of us. I'm simply saying that labeling yourself in a disempowering way that forfeits your divine identity as a spiritual being on this planet having a human experience can really limit your life. Forgetting that you came into the world with only two fears—loud noises and falling—you can end up hypnotizing yourself into believing that you don't have power and influence over the things in your life you're dissatisfied with, leaving your existence less joyful than it could be and leaving the planet no better than you found it!

Reclaiming your Identity

Many of the people I have helped thought they'd tried everything and were on the brink of giving up, but ended up losing 50, 100 and sometimes over 200 pounds to regain their health and their entire life, both literally, by regaining health, and figuratively, by finding joy, love and pleasure in their daily lives again. They began to understand what they really had tried to do with food, which was meet their psychological needs, and they learned that food was not going to meet those needs. It's like trying to put out a fire with gasoline.

They accomplished these incredible goals by reclaiming their true identity and place on this planet, removing the pattern they'd long used to turn themselves off, to numb, to distract. They succeeded by eliminating the thing that

"This minute is the time to realize God has a plan for your life, and it begins with you."

was holding them back from being present and in the moment. In my case and with many of my clients this numbing mechanism was often choosing unhealthy foods, but it also manifests itself in the abuse of alcohol, drugs, sex, gambling or even work. Each of these people, however, decided that life was too precious to let it pass by unconsciously.

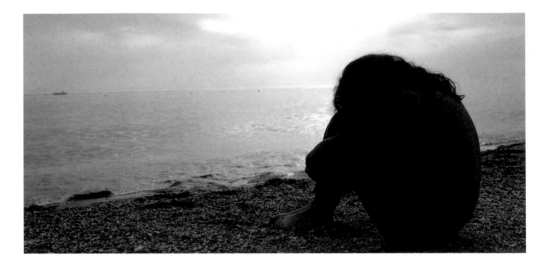

Are you feeling this way? Have you felt stuck in a pattern of disappointment, frustration, sadness or despair, replaying your history over and over, using something to numb that painful past? Or are you anticipating calamity and destruction in the future, constantly searching for ways to make yourself feel better in the moment in the wake of this horrific self-generated movie you're playing, totally missing out on the now and losing ground as we speak?

This minute is the time to realize God has a plan for your life, and it begins with you.

This is what I realized when I reached out to God as a desperately unhappy and morbidly obese teen, and it's what I've helped people to realize ever since that time, through my weight-loss coaching. As demand grew for my personal coaching and the strategies and tools I had developed, I wrote a book about it. *Think and Grow Thin* helped me reach thousands more people than I otherwise could have. I know it really did help change lives because I've heard from so many people who have said it changed theirs. Nothing makes me happier than when someone reaches out to me through email, Facebook or Twitter, or sometimes even in person.

When I transformed my own life I made a promise to God: If He helped me become

"I know you can make the changes and create the life you want not only because I've done it myself, but because I've helped hundreds of other people, both in my personal life and professional life, to do it too, regardless of where they've started from."

"normal" sized, I would do everything in my power to help others. At the time, I was desperate and willing to do anything, but ultimately, I wanted to be of service to more people. He did help me become "normal" sized. He did it by helping me understand my own power, resilience and abilities. He helped me see that all I needed was strategy, foresight, planning and consistency, and I would reach my goal. Boy, did I reach my goal! I reached it and surpassed it, becoming incredibly fit and healthy! Once I developed a reputation of helping those who felt there was no hope, I soon made a name for myself as a weight-loss coach, helping people across the country.

But as I've been hinting at, I'm not really a weight-loss coach. I'm a life consultant.

Because living a joyful, satisfying and purposeful life is not just about losing weight or giving up substances. Losing weight, being healthy and in great shape is all fantastic, but if your relationships are bad, or if you find yourself mentally replaying old videos of your most miserable moments, or if you're spiraling into out-of-control debt, then you're still not going to be very happy. I'm here to tell you that whatever it is that's making your life difficult, whatever it is that you feel trapped in or chained to, you can change. You can change it by recognizing we are all simply doing what we do to try to feel better.

Feeling better is fine, but are these negative choices really making you feel better, or are they just hiding what makes you feel bad? I want you to ask yourself if the things you are choosing to do each day are a deposit or withdrawal into the next 3, 5, 10 years of your life. Maybe you're vastly overweight. Maybe you've been using marijuana, alcohol, hard drugs like cocaine or heroin, prescription drugs, like my mom did, or even over-the-counter meds to change your emotional state. Maybe you're in a dead-end job where you feel you're not growing or accomplishing what you could. Maybe you dread going home because you're so bored with your relationship you feel like you're watching paint dry every evening. Maybe you love your spouse but find that the fiery passion is gone. Maybe you have achieved everything you thought would light you up and make you happy, only to ask yourself "Is this all there is to life?"

Many if not most of us feel there are some things in life we want to change. To put it another way, we want to enjoy certain aspects of life more and get more out of them. But few of us make the changes that will bring this about, at least permanently. How many DVDs, seminars, YouTube videos or books on motivation and personal development have you watched or picked up, finding you feel

excited and motivated for a few days, soon to sink back into the familiarity of your old ways? If you are like most us, you have probably had this experience more than once. What causes you to slip back? Why can't you seem to make the lasting changes you want?

You can.

I know you can make the changes and create the life you want not only because I've done it myself, but because I've helped hundreds of other people, both in my personal life and professional life, to do it too, regardless of where they've started from.

I've always found the best way to really learn and have that learning stay with us is through stories, because we become emotionally involved and connected. Which do you remember better: your statistics class or the Genie in *Aladdin?* Anything we can emotionally relate to we tend to remember better. Studies show that we retain how we feel about things much longer than we retain the actual data.

My Story

Since one of our mutual goals is that you actually leave this book with a plan you will act on

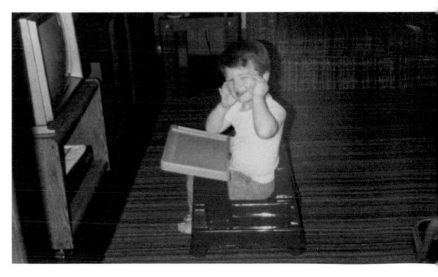

I'VE *ALWAYS* LOVED LEARNING! HERE I AM AT MY DESK WATCHING *MR. WIZARD* ON NICKELODEON.

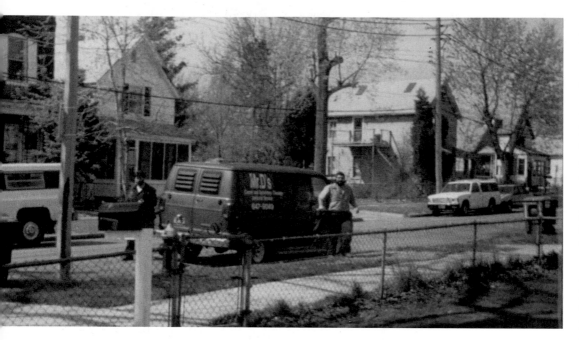

inordinate stress plagued his life in exchange for the "freedom" of entrepreneurship. He was lucky to steal away a few hours a week to be with my mom and me. (My siblings were not yet born.) My time in my early years was spent almost entirely with my mom.

My mom wasn't just my mom; she was my best friend. I was always very different as a kid.

MY DAD STARTED HIS OWN CLEANING BUSINESS WITH NOTHING BUT THIS VAN, A DREAM, AND INSANE DETERMINATION.

consistently, let me tell you a bit about my own story. While I had sincere parents, I certainly had a difficult time growing up. I know what you're saying: "Didn't we all?" and in a way, you're absolutely right. We all had our hidden family problems and secrets and issues with self-confidence. We can all filter our history through a lens to see what was wrong instead of what was right. Some kids have terrible things going on in their lives that others don't know anything about. If you're like me, you can think back to some pretty sad or even horrific moments from those early, important and impressionable years.

Neither of my parents had much formal schooling, but that did not mean they did not have life education, and they were very hard working. My dad went to work as a janitor, and when he recognized there was only so much room for his own financial development working for someone else, he took a huge leap of faith and opened his own cleaning company with a few hundred dollars and a van that he bought with borrowed money. It was then he, like all of us, learned that there is a cost to any opportunity. Long hours, hard labor and

I was always much bigger and taller than the other kids, and I was also very studious and polite. I was, and have always been, an insatiable learner, just like you. In my dad's absence, my wonderful mom would bring me to Walgreens every week to see if any new spelling or math workbooks were available, and we would spend hours on things I wanted to learn about as a toddler. She made learning so much fun. But this one positive aspect of my life was not to last, as you'll hear about shortly.

My family was very far from well off. We lived close to poverty, as my grandparents had. This in itself caused me to be different from the other kids. But because of my psychological and physical differences I really didn't fit in. I was bullied terribly. Children can be very cruel and most kids learn that different is bad. As an introverted kid, I would often spend my recess reading rather than playing. They would do things like kick a ball directly at my face with as much force as possible while I was minding my own business reading a book, as one small example. The bullying got so bad that I'd get my parents to drop me off before any other kid could arrive, and I'd wait in the bathroom or church until school started. I became well acquainted with the bathroom, as I would also eat lunch there to avoid the harassment.

As a young child I had my mom as my biggest cheerleader and best friend, there to support me throughout all this torment. She would tell me that the future held incredible promise for me. Daily, she affirmed that I had a destiny and purpose, and I would turn out much better off because of the things I suffered. She told me this over and over. Great hypnotic suggestions to plant in a young person's mind, by the way! Often we unconsciously move toward the things we hear often, making them true, so be careful what you are allowing to influence your thinking.

But once I reached about the age of 10, my best friend turned into my worst enemy. My mother, who had her own treacherous history she never dealt with emotionally, became addicted to prescription drugs and alcohol to numb her consciousness. The little joy and normalcy my life had held was gone like a puff of smoke.

I don't tell you this to gain sympathy; I'm saying it so you understand that I didn't come from a family like we all saw on TV sitcoms each day. We always think others are so much better off than we are, that their lives are like those lives on TV, but we are probably more alike than we are different.

I'll get into a little more detail about this later on when it's relevant to our discussions but what I need you to know is this: your past does not dictate your future any more than my past dictated my future. My poverty did not make me poor, my parents and grandparents with no education did not make me uneducated, my

my mom in 1992

mother's drug and alcohol problems did not make me a drug or alcohol addict. (In fact I've never touched the stuff.) My former life as an obese, despised, miserable kid all but disappeared as I became a fit, confident young man surrounded by people who love and respect me.

You can decide what you want to improve, and you can improve it. Labels, no matter when they were given or by whom, do not in any way need to limit what you contribute to this world or do with your life. I will offer you some important strategies that will enable you to make the dreams you have for your future really happen. I've made my own dreams come true, and continue to do so. I've helped many others make their dreams come true and I will help you make your dreams come true too.

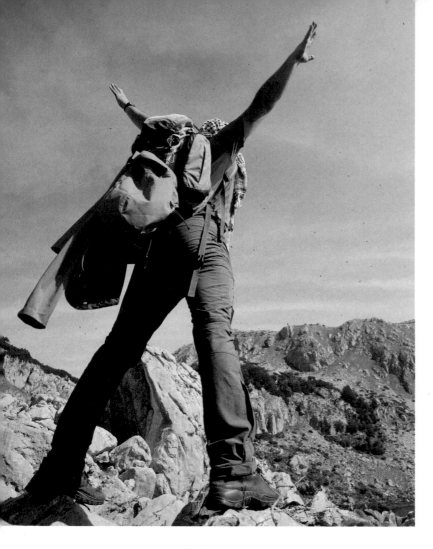

CHAPTER TWO

Energy: The Core of Lasting Change

Have you ever experienced this? You go to hear a motivational speaker and you get incredibly excited. You can't wait for the end of the talk so you can run to the back to buy the book or DVD. You're determined to really give this new plan everything you've got!

You're going to do it! You're going to change your life, lose weight, get ripped, start your business, find your soulmate, change careers and build your financial future—all in the

same week! You can see the checks coming in already. You repeat positive phrases to yourself. You've bought a huge vision board, downloaded a bunch of inspirational quotes to tape to it and watched *The Secret* for the fifth time. In a few years you'll be yachting on the Riviera and you can almost feel your gorgeous life partner on your arm. You fall asleep imagining your new life and you're excited to get this process started!

Your intentions are good, but when you get home you get comfortable again. Maybe someone you know—even someone close to you—derides your new plan and outlook on the future, telling you why it's not going to work. Despite the fact that you're not happy with where you are, you buy into their story, come to agree with their perspective and end up keeping yourself shackled to the way things have always been. As your cynical friend says, "If it were that easy, everyone would be happy." Why should you think you are any different? Your friends, family members and even your partner tell you that it's impossible to do what you are setting out to do, especially in the short time frame you've stated. I remember the voices of the people I thought would cheer me on when I made the decision to transform my life. Instead of being supportive, they pointed out to me that I was most likely setting myself up for huge disappointment. I didn't understand at that stage that "impossible" is an opinion. Impossible means nothing once you achieve the things you intend to!

Now what happens? Since you've allowed your environment to influence your core belief system with all that negative energy, maybe you don't start making the changes you had been so excited about. Or if you do, you do them half-hearted—what had seemed so exciting and attainable just moments before now really does seem impossible. You start to shift your focus from how great life will be when you've accomplished your goals to how hard the change will feel, and you give up before you've begun, falling back into that gray area of life where you are just trying to get through another day, waiting for the weekend. Or maybe you make a plan and start it, and you truly begin to see some success. But a few days later, you start slipping up. Instead of getting back on track you start falling back into old habits. Another week and that yacht has sailed away into the Mediterranean sunset without you, your soulmate gleefully waving from the rails. You're back to your normal daily life, all that fiery motivation you had just a few days ago totally forgotten. You're back to repeating that same pattern that is so comfortable, familiar and miserable until maybe some day in the future, you think.

Why does this pattern happen to so many of us? How can you be so excited and determined one day only to have that determination completely disappear so soon after?

The trick to breaking this silly disempowering pattern is to get fully associated to the new you. That means not only being cognitively aware, or just understanding it in your head, but also, and most importantly, feeling it in your heart! The reason most people don't change for long enough to bring about what they truly desire is that they compare their slightly better version of themselves with their pre-change self instead of keeping their eye on their goals. They tell themselves things like, "I've already saved $1,000! Sure my goal is $5,000, but I'm doing so much better now than I was! Why not go ahead and buy this expensive purse? I deserve it after being so good!" They constantly make withdrawals from the moment, rather than making investments into their future.

This is an incredibly common pattern in people who want to make changes. They conveniently forget the fact that they are breaking the agreement they made with themselves. Isn't that all change really is? Learning to keep an agreement with yourself? Holding yourself to a new standard or set of expectations? The people who find themselves falling short of

their dreams often fall prey to the habit of comparing the current better situation to the past worse situation in order to justify doing something stupid that leads them away from their goal! It's amazing how good humans are at rationalizing irrational behavior!

Here's another common way people bring about the end of their goals: They go back to their old habits but convince themselves it's just temporary. "It's just for tonight," they say, as they dig into pizza and margaritas, their healthy food plan forgotten. Or just for this week, they tell themselves as they go shopping and forget their savings. "I'll go back to saving after my next paycheck," they say.

"The key is that you have to burn the mental bridges to your excuses. You can no longer accept anything less than keeping the agreement you've made with yourself."

Have you been there? If you're like so many others and definitely the former me, you've mastered the art of bullshitting yourself. But a key to transformation in any domain of life is honesty. Honesty in this context means setting a standard for yourself superior to anyone else's standard for you, and holding yourself to that. Now, you can decide what you need to hold yourself accountable—whether that's recruiting a mentor or sponsor or utilizing a more private method, like using a journal or calendar—it is up to you. If you're being honest with yourself you will set up a way that works for you consistently. The key is that you have to burn the mental bridges to your excuses. You can no longer accept anything less than keeping the agreement you've made with yourself. You can never go back!

Your cynical friends might tell you your goals are unreasonable, but let me remind you that no one from time immemorial who we look upon with great awe and reverence for the impact they made was described as "reasonable." Being reasonable leads to mediocrity. When you think of the word mediocrity, understand it comes with the reality that the potential for greatness was always there but never fully tapped, because of lack of consistency or discipline. In other words, you settle.

You've got to be relentless with your future! It's the only one you have! No one cares as much about your future—your health, your wealth or your relationships—as you do! Time is subtle and moves fast. You spend your days as if you have forever when the truth is far from it. You tell yourself you will visit your friend out of state the next time you travel there, not thinking how few opportunities you will really have to do so. Figure out your age and how often you might get to travel there each year. Would it be once per year? Once every two years? You might only have a handful of opportunities to see that friend again, and that's how life is.

"While the past doesn't predict the future, it does if you don't change the present."

Whether or not you make changes in your life, pain is inevitable. To stay in the place you don't want to be is painful. To change can also be seen as painful, but only if you frame it as a loss rather than a gain. In order to make the change you seek, you must see the pain of staying the same as being greater than the pain of changing. Once the pain that motivated you to change decreases, it can be very easy for you to go back to your old habits and old ways

because they have been hardwired—conditioned through habit. They're familiar and for many of us, well practiced for decades. This is why it can be so easy to talk yourself out of your agreement. Once you've lost 10 or 20 of the 50 pounds you want to lose, your condition is no longer painful.

To emotionally connect to the pain of not sticking to your plan means going beyond the moment. Think about the ultimate cost of screwing it up yet again, the cost of not changing what you need to change. Ask yourself how you will feel when you're even more broke, overweight and alone than you are now, if that's the track you've been on the last two or three years. While the past doesn't predict the future, it does if you don't change the present. You will follow whatever trajectory you are on, so to not end up at the place you've been heading to, you have to change the trajectory.

How will you feel if you find the chance you have at this moment disappears at midnight, never to be given again? Jim Rohn, a great teacher who has influenced me, reminds us that we only have so many springtimes in life, and they always come after winter. The key is remembering that there are only so many. To have a bountiful harvest in the fall of our life, we must busily plant as much as we can in the spring, metaphorically speaking.

I learned this lesson the most personal way imaginable. As I mentioned, my mom was the most loving supportive person I could have ever asked for until I was about 10. She made every day a fun-filled adventure. While many

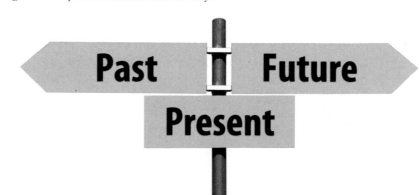

would later say we were poor, I would have never known it! Whether we were making toys out of things around the house, visiting relatives, having lunch and playing at the park or going to Blockbuster to pick out new releases for movie night together—it was the most joyful rich upbringing I could have wanted. While my dad was working his tail off to provide for his fledgling family, my mom more than filled his absence with her presence and love. I was able to get through the torment of being bullied by knowing I had my mom to come home to.

All this said, she tied a lot of her identity into her function as a "mom." As I grew up and she felt she was needed less, I suppose a sense of purposelessness came over her. A spirit of despair and loneliness permeated her existence and since she didn't think of creating a compelling future, her mind did what so many of our minds do—it reverted to the past. She started thinking about all the injustices she suffered as a young girl and the strained relationship between her, her mom and her sister, whom she pretty much parented. The reality is, she never had a childhood of her own. This discontent and lack of spiritual fulfillment led her to look outside herself for the answer.

My mother and father's relationship had withered since both of them had turned their focus toward things outside of each other, and so it was probably challenging coming back to just the two of them once their kids were no longer babies and didn't need them as much anymore.

I once coached a priest who did a lot of marital counseling. He told me after five decades of counseling couples contemplating divorce, he had learned where the loneliest place was on earth: the marriage bed. If you don't work as hard on your relationship as you do on other areas of your life, it can begin to die.

You'll never fill that emotional void for connection and love with a physical substance,

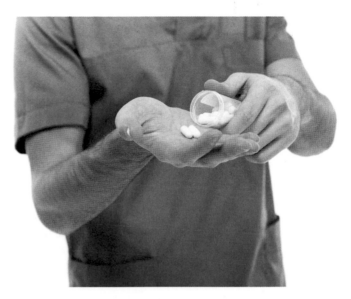

"You'll never fill that emotional void for connection and love with a physical substance."

but that's what my mother ended up trying to do, unwittingly. Feeling hopeless and unable to sleep, my mom visited a doctor who hastily diagnosed her with depression after a five-minute talk, scribbling a prescription for a mood-altering drug without a second thought and certainly with no consideration of the history of addictive behaviors in her family. Giving someone such a substance with that history is asking for trouble, in my opinion. She found that while the pills were helpful initially, she quickly built up tolerance, and spent the next few years going from doctor to doctor playing the game many addicted people play, getting the same prescription from different doctors. The side effects of these drugs messed with her sleep cycle, and the next thing she was drinking alcohol in an effort to relax. (She never exercised formally or learned anything about nutrition and its role in the body—two things I believe can tremendously benefit those suffering from such issues.)

It seemed like overnight she had been possessed by a demon. Chasing me through the

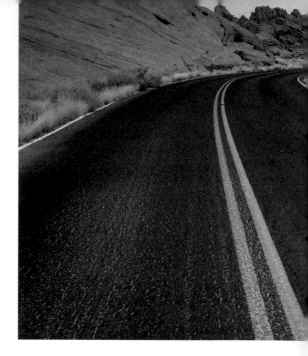

house, throwing glass jar candles at me with all of her might, literally slamming my head against walls, threatening to pull me out of school—and saying things she could never forgive herself for later. She would wake up the next day with only faint echoes of the day past, but ridden with tar-like guilt over what she felt she had done.

Why do I say all this to you? I'll refer to these times for various reasons throughout the book, but in this case I use it to illustrate the importance of making the change you need to make right now. My mom eventually got to a point where she really wanted to change, but by the time she made that choice, the possibility of true health and happiness had passed. Yes she chose to stop using drugs and alcohol, but the damage already incurred was so immense it was like trying to stop a freight train moving at 1,000 miles an hour. The engineer can take his foot off the pedal and apply the brake, but the momentum will keep the train moving in the direction it has been, and fast. My mother soon suffered acute pancreatitis, a condition brought on from her alcohol abuse. Her pancreas, the organ we all have that makes insulin to get rid of the sugar from our blood, stopped working. This meant she had to be on even more medicine, and this medicine required injections. It's name: insulin.

Imagine, if you will, a person who is having difficulty functioning, with tons of meds circulating in their bloodstream, some to simply counteract the negative impacts of the others, being told she has to learn to test her blood sugar regularly, give herself shots, and be responsible. I remember as a teen when I learned she needed this. My stomach churned and I think I had diarrhea for a week because I was so worried that she would accidentally end her life with the insulin or forget to test her blood or take the insulin at all. It soon became normal to find her passed out with a blood-sugar reading of 40 and we had to call the paramedics so many times that we knew them all on a first-name basis.

So while she'd stopped drinking and using mind-altering prescription drugs, these changes came too late for her to truly enjoy her life. The heat impacted her greatly; she would sweat easily and get out of breath with only slight exertion. She totally lost her sense of independence and personal power.

I don't say this to bring you down. I say this to you because you do not have to end up at a place where the momentum in the wrong direction is so great that damage is irreversible! Your spring is today. You can take advantage of this spring and plant seeds of good habits in every area of your life for a bountiful harvest!

The Change You Choose

I often have said "Change is possible!" but I have to recant that. Change is inevitable. You are going to change. Look at pictures of yourself at 2, 7, 13, 21, 30, 40, and beyond. While you didn't intend it to, change happened. And guess what, it will continue to happen whether you like it or not! The question is, will you choose to start directing that change so it begins to move you toward the things you want? I've done it and thousands of others have done it. How? How did we all get to that point? How did we continue on and make the

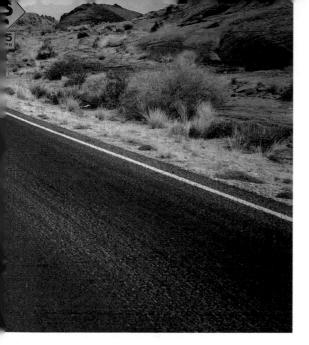

"It's energy that makes you go beyond motivation to action, and it's energy that inspires you to take continued action, enabling you to make those little choices each day that will bring you to your eventual goal despite any obstacles in the road."

changes and adjustments we wanted despite the pain of our condition decreasing? How did we escape going back into our familiar old habits and instead see it through and reach our goals? The answer is: Energy!

It's easy to get motivated. There are thousands of people who can get you motivated. But motivation is nothing without action. As the famous speaker Zig Ziglar said, it's like a bath: you need it at least once a day! You ever hear the phrase "All talk, no action"? That's what motivation can be if you don't follow through.

It's energy that makes you go beyond motivation to action, and it's energy that inspires you to take continued action, enabling you to make those little choices each day that will bring you to your eventual goal despite any obstacles in the road. Just like a car needs fuel to drive to its destination, you need energy to drive to your goal destination. Where does this energy come from? How do you harness it?

I bet sometimes when you run into someone and ask how they are, they say they're "tired." I bet you've said it yourself. Some people feel tired all the time. If you feel like you can't even function in your daily life then how will you get the energy to make the changes you want and reach your goals? And how will you keep that energy up every day for long enough to achieve and maintain your goals?

Feeling energized when you've just read the motivational book or listened to the speaker is easy. But where do you get the energy to help you stay on your path as you reach your goal and beyond? There are four keys that will help you to unlock this energy: The Physical, Mental, Emotional and Spiritual keys.

Physical key:
Food and Movement

The first thing to look at is the actual real energy that you are putting into your body: your food. If you're skipping meals or living on low-quality food—fast food, chips, soda, candy—you will not have anywhere near the energy you could have, and you may have a hard time keeping up your motivation. Is most of the food you're eating highly processed? When you look at the ingredients label, are there more things you can't pronounce than things you can? These are red flags. If you are spiking your blood sugar with high-glycemic foods (foods that are high in simple carbs but low in healthy fat or protein), you can expect a never-ending yo-yo of energy surges and

"The first thing to look at is the actual real energy that you are putting into your body: your food."

drains, perpetuating endless hunger. Eat a good diet that gives you nutrition. Remember, your body can only work with the building blocks that you give it! Those blocks come from the foods you eat.

While it seems like common sense when you really think about it, few people actually consider that the way the body heals, repairs, grows, and functions is, to a great degree, a result of those choices, but that's what eating is for! To provide your body with the nutrients it needs to function properly. Food is not meant to be used as a drug for filling emotional or spiritual voids in your life or to give you constant sweet, salty, fatty oral pleasure. I talk a lot more about this in my book *Think and Grow Thin*. When you remove your emotional connection with food and think of it as fuel, fuel that provides you with what you need to make the most of every day God has given you, you will begin to experience life in a much more vivid way.

Remember, He has a plan for you. Once you make this initial shift, transforming the inside to allow the outside to change, you no longer feel controlled or shackled by being dissatisfied with your body or health. The simple act of deciding has a mentally positive impact! Are you going to let your craving for nachos get in the way of that mission? You need to recognize that the core of any dissatisfaction comes from replacing our own power with something outside of ourselves.

You would be amazed at how little you actually need to eat to live healthfully. Studies have shown that longevity increases as intake decreases. (To a point!) Many people, like the former me, mistake the desire for more food as physically needing more food. This causes them to eat until they are over-full and feel uncomfortable—way beyond satisfied. Often once I help clients embrace a more mindful approach to food, they tell me they had forgotten what it felt like for their bodies to be actually ready for food, as they had been totally spontaneous in their habits, eating when they were not hungry and continuing to eat past satiety. They had conditioned themselves to think they needed much more food than they actually did, simply out of habit.

Can you relate? Have you plopped on the couch with a bag of Doritos intending to eat just a few with a can of Diet Coke, only to find the entire family-sized bag devoured by the end of an episode of *The Walking Dead*?!

> Maybe food isn't the issue for you. Which substances are you using to change how you feel? Are you turning toward caffeine throughout the day to get your body going, and then taking some kind of artificial depressant to get your body to wind down as a result come nighttime? Are these habits really adding value to your life, or in truth, subtracting from it? Are they moving you closer to the person you know you are meant to become, or are they giving you more ammunition for self-loathing, guilt, and hate? What you feed yourself, both physically and mentally, has monumental impact on how your life ultimately turns out.

Next, you have to move your body. No, I don't mean relocate and leave your negative family and neighbors, though that might be wise. And no, though it may be sounding a little like it right now, this is not a diet and exercise book. The fact remains: you need action. It's

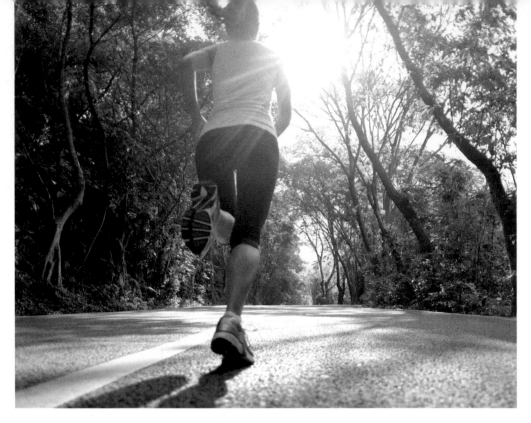

"Success is the result of almost unnoticeable small and practical disciplines practiced repeatedly, hour after hour, day after day, month after month, and year after year—until they are so unconscious you don't even think about them!"

not only the massive intention that brings real, lasting change to your life; it's coupling that with massive action. Making the decision and acting on it immediately. Success is not some grand moment. It's more procedural and processional. It's the repetitive practice of consistent habits every day. That is why it is subtle. No one arrives at their destination overnight, and those who do certainly don't stay there long! Think of the people you hear about who win the lottery only to be back in a trailer park a year later.

Success is the result of almost unnoticeable small and practical disciplines practiced repeatedly, hour after hour, day after day, month after month, and year after year—until they are so unconscious you don't even think about them! It's been said that habits are so light when being formed they are like thread, almost imperceptible, but once hard wired are like iron chains. Be mindful of what you do each day without thinking about it. Take great care to think about the momentum you're establishing from the things you are repeatedly doing. After making the choice to begin the practice of good habits, you wake up one day looking at all your achievements, in bed next to the partner of your dreams, money in the bank, purpose in your career, wondering how it all happened because it came so easily and gradually! Success comes through changing your day-to-day choices and staying true to the decision to do so for the long haul, even when the storms in life come that offer you an excuse to swerve away from your purpose.

Much like the principle of compounding in investing, there is a similar effect in personal growth and development. What we think about most of the time shapes how we feel, which determines what we choose to do or not do, and ultimately this decides our future. It's been said that you do not decide your future, your choices do. But you do get to decide your choices! That may not feel nearly as exciting, but I'm telling you it sure is when you realize that there are no limits to your life design and you've achieved it!

Sorry, I got excited there. Back to step two for energy. You have to move to get physical energy. If you're like most people you drive to work in the morning, sit all day in front of your computer, drive home and spend the evening sitting on your couch. Our society has devolved quite a bit— gym classes have even been removed from many schools! Kids used to play outside all day long, but how many children have you seen outside in the heat of the summer lately? If your neighborhood is anything like mine, probably not too many. Instead, Xbox , iPads and cell phones have replaced backyard trampolines, roller blades, tire swings and swimming pools.

Movement—exercise—is a strange thing. It takes energy to start doing it, but once you start moving regularly you end up with far more energy than you had before. What do I mean by movement? Anything you want! You can join a gym or start a walking or running program if you want, you could join a Barre or yoga class, you can swim or dance or ride a bike. Make sure whatever activity you choose, you do at a fast enough pace to get your heart rate up. Walking is a perfect start. Go for at least 30 minutes per day, five days per week. You will want to gradually challenge yourself: go a little further or a little faster, or go uphill. Try to move more in the rest of your life too. Take walk breaks at work and park farther away from stores. Many of my clients at a major corporation in St. Louis would walk across a skywalk that bridged across a highway during their lunch hour. Great thinkers like Steve Jobs, Darwin, Nietzsche, Dickens and Beethoven were all known for walking, and credited it as a source of their creativity! As your energy increases you can add the other exercise/movements I mentioned if you want:

do a lunchtime yoga class, a morning running club or a weekend hiking group.

Exercise begets energy, and this will help you immensely in accomplishing your goal, no matter what it is. You cannot feel bummed out when you're splashing around in a swimming pool or running alongside smiling people blasting your favorite music in your earbuds! When you are gritting your teeth, pushing weights,

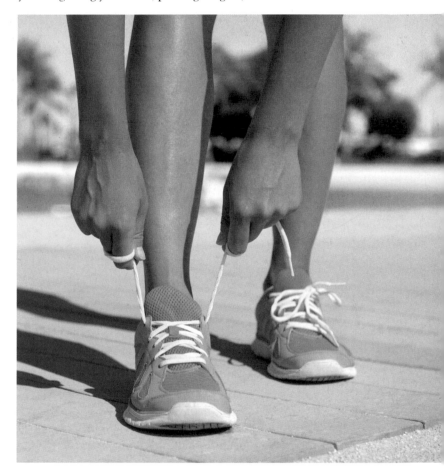

"Movement—exercise—is a strange thing. It takes energy to start doing it, but once you start moving regularly you end up with far more energy than you had before."

working muscles you forgot you had, you can't help but shift gears mentally and emotionally. Your emotional state is directly impacted by your nervous system. To test this, try feeling bad while smiling broadly. It's next to impossible, as your body tells your brain and its chemicals that you're happy. To test this, spend a morning or afternoon purposely making eye contact with every person you meet, and smile—you will find they will smile in return, which will amplify your own good feelings!

The unique thing about exercise is that it really is physiologically addictive. Afraid to start? If you get comfortable being in discomfort, you'll find fewer and fewer things cause discomfort over time. Consistent movement makes your nervous system recognize that you truly are alive, and brings consciousness and awareness to all parts of the human part of you!

Mental key part 1:
Your Thinking

Another facet of energy comes from the way we process our life's experiences. Perception is reality. Two people can go through the same experience and have entirely different interpretations. Here's an example. Let's say you are sitting in a restaurant across from a friend. When you look behind your friend, you can see a person with a handful of colorful balloons in hand. If you ask your friend what color the balloons are, he will think you are

crazy. Even though you are in the same restaurant sitting across from each other, he has a completely different perspective and can see only from his position.

To increase your daily energy, make sure you intentionally keep your goal in the forefront of your mind. You must also remember where you're coming from, so you are conscious of both what you need to do and need to avoid each day.

We are inundated and barraged with useless material that tries to influence us to make decisions that aren't part of our daily or weekly plans. Spend more, buy more, have sex more with whomever you find attractive, buy these clothes so you can be that attractive person … if you're not careful, you can lose your sense of self. Taking back control of your own thinking means learning how to filter your experiences in a way that gets you closer to your desired outcome rather than further away.

As in my example, you can always look at things from different perspectives. Look toward that which is true and empowering! Truth won't necessarily feel good, but it will stand strong in the face of anything you are going through, and truth presents an opportunity to learn and grow.

There really is no such thing as failure if you commit to taking a seed of equivalent benefit, or a learning experience, from everything

"These positive daily choices that bring success emanate from a worldview that offers empowerment, a worldview you can create even if the environment you were born into didn't offer it."

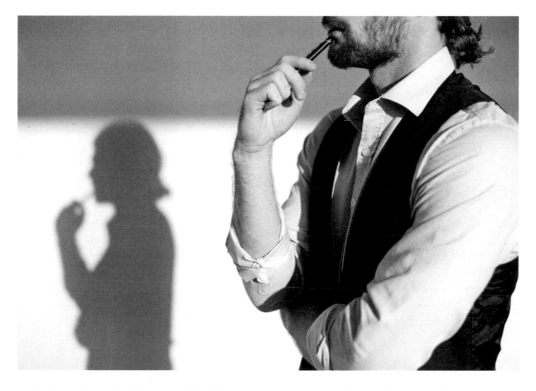

you've been through. Many people's definitions of success and failure are so limited they make it nearly impossible for themselves to enjoy their days.

The extremely influential woman I call my grandma taught me the most about this. She would find powerful and empowering meaning in anything that happened, even tragedy. My favorite example is when I went to tell her the news that my dad, who was only 54, had died unexpectedly in the middle of the night of a heart attack. She was 86 and had a wealth of wisdom. After her initial consolation of all of two minutes, she looked at me wistfully, put her hand on my shoulder and said, "Well, at least he wasn't murdered! Thank God he went now. Taking care of parents when you have children of your own is really a burden!" I couldn't help but laugh, in the midst of my tears. The speed at which she could reframe a situation that looked so bleak to a young man who was about to take the role as patriarch of a family was astounding, and Godly.

Here's a good way to figure out if you're thinking about things in a good, honest and effective way: Ask yourself if your interpretation helps you learn from the experience and provide useful information that you can apply to create a more positive future. For example, if you end a relationship in divorce, you can tell yourself you're a terrible human being who is meant to be alone forever. Stop, take a deep breath, and ask yourself, since we know life is all about growing, does that interpretation bring with it helpful constructive information to move your life forward in a positive direction? If the answer is no, then you must force yourself to come up with another interpretation until you find one or many that move you forward. Maybe the divorce was the greatest gift you could have given to your partner. Maybe you were able to free your husband or wife from a relationship that was just as unhappy as you found it, or maybe even if that were not true, you offered them a position in life where they might find someone to love them as you could not.

Life is not easy. We will all experience the inevitabilities of our humanity: death, sadness, sorrow, grief and loss. I have, and if you haven't yet, you will. We are all here to smooth out the rough edges of our souls, and it seems, as best as I can tell, the frustrations of life are just as important as the celebrations, and possibly more so.

You can make the choice to focus on what you consider to be losses. You can focus on the negative news stories of the day. You can get yourself so worked up that you never want to leave your home, fearing anyone of a different skin tone or belief system, thereby draining yourself of every thread of hope and energy.

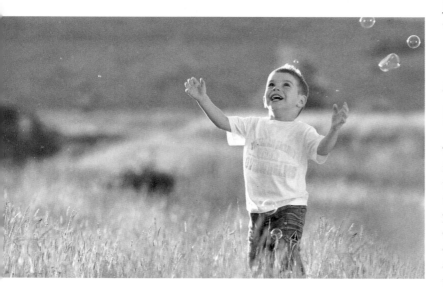

Or you can begin to reawaken the child inside who, even when he or she experienced loss, did not take it too seriously, whose insatiable curiosity and intuitive "knowing" (something I will come back to later in the book) gave peace that things would work out even if he or she didn't know how to make that happen. The little child who would walk up with a popsicle grin, excited to embrace a friendly looking stranger, wondering what lessons the person had to offer, regardless of their bank account, education, skin color or religion. Which way would you rather live?

These positive daily choices that bring success emanate from a worldview that offers empowerment, a worldview you can create even if the environment you were born into didn't offer it. If your goal is a better relationship, then stay conscious of the things you need to do to foster a better one, and do those small things each day. To get what you want, you must ask yourself who you must become to have it. One thing we know for certain, anyone you look to who is successful has a steady supply of emotional jet fuel to propel them toward the things they are after! They don't have too much drag. Like a jet, if there is more drag than lift, you can never get to cruising altitude. Remember, in any flight there will likely be turbulence. Just expect it and ride it through rather than complaining about it.

Mental key part 2:
Little Changes

There was a movement a few years ago for saving marriages. Created as a divorce prevention tactic, the movement was all about making the tiniest of positive changes in dealing with your spouse. Let's say as an example that it drives you crazy that your spouse leaves his dirty socks on the floor. He's done it for years and he knows it drives you crazy because every time he does it, you get angry with him. "Why can't you just put them in the laundry hamper? Is that so difficult?" you say, not even attempting to keep the irritation out of your voice. Serving its purpose, it gets under his skin and he quickly retorts: "Well if you'd stop leaving the cap off the toothpaste maybe I'd put my socks in the hamper!"

Every action has a reaction. Changing the action will change the reaction. You can't make another person do what you want but you do have control over your own actions, and can influence the outcome by changing what *you* are doing! Instead of yelling at him to put his socks in the hamper, how about this: you attach a little basketball net to the top of the hamper, so you make it fun for him to try to get his socks in each day. This will make him pause. It may even make him feel affectionately toward you as he tries for his first basket.

I know that when my significant other does sweet things for me, taking initiative without scolding me, I'm that much more likely to want to do something nice for her. If you do something like this for your special someone, it's likely he/she will be touched by the sweet idea and ultimately do something thoughtful for you, maybe give your shoulders a little rub when you're working at your desk or even wake up in your place to quiet the screaming newborn through the night!

Again, small changes in daily choices are what bring about success.

Mental key *part 3:*
Faking It

You've heard the term "fake it till you make it" before. There might be some areas where this is not a good idea. Practicing medicine, for example! But you will get the energy to achieve most goals by behaving as if you have already achieved them. This is known as the "act as if" principle. If every day you have to work to convince yourself to do what you've got to do in order to bring about the change you seek, then every day you will need that little bit of extra energy in order to jump into that way of thinking. When you "act as if" you are already there, you've won half the battle.

You do not have to cross a chasm you've already crossed!

Here's an example from my background working with people on fat loss. Let's say you are making a dietary and exercise change in your

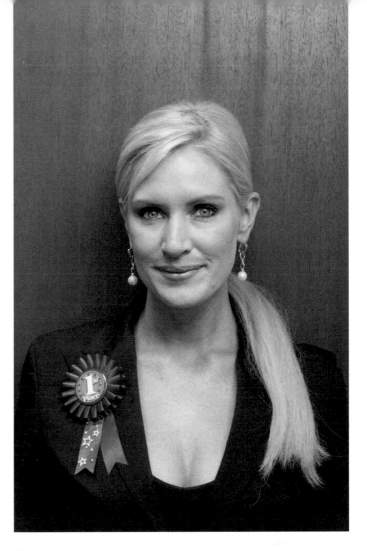

"You will get the energy to achieve most goals by behaving as if you have already achieved them."

life. Up until now your habit has been to skip breakfast, eat donuts during your morning break, have a fast-food lunch, eat a frozen dinner over your desk at home and then sit around on the couch watching TV and munching on chips. If you still maintain your old identity and self-concept as an overweight person, then every step of the way throughout the day you will have to fight against your old habits.

If instead you update your self-concept, recognize that all that remains of your history is the memory of it and live each day as the person you already are: healthy and thin, or non-

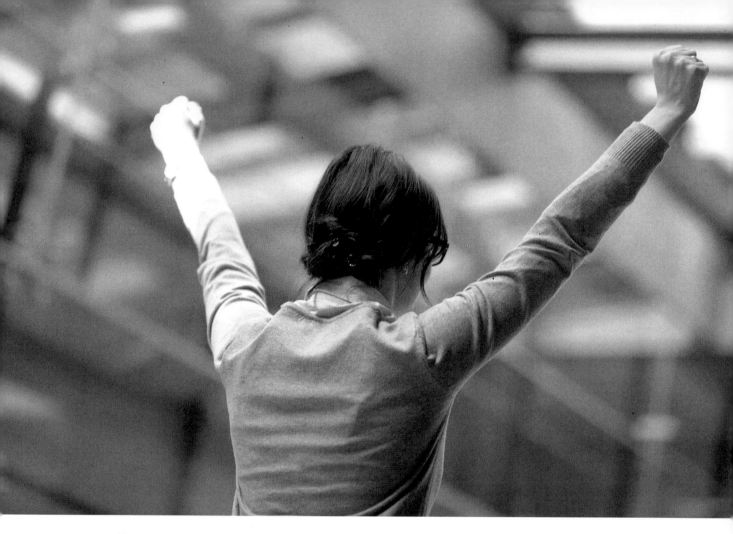

"When you 'act as if' you are already there, you've won half the battle. You do not have to cross a chasm you've already crossed!"

procrastinating, or financially responsible, or giving in your relationship, then your actions will ultimately begin to match your beliefs. Since you know healthy, thin people tend not to skip breakfast and that's who you have decided you are then it's no problem for you to be strategic and eat breakfast. A healthy, thin person would not eat donuts and so you don't eat donuts. A healthy, thin person eats healthy food for lunch and so that's what you do. You don't have to expend excess mental energy fighting every step of the way because you're already there.

It's very much the same no matter which life changes you're trying to make. If you have already made the leap, then you will make the right choices as part of your identity. This is very different and much less taxing than having to bridge a gap in your own self-perception before making every one of those daily choices. If you have a debt problem and need to stop using your credit card, for example, you need to change your identity to someone who already has total control over their credit cards and bank account. Then stopping yourself from purchasing things you don't have the money for will not be hard, because that behavior matches your identity. If, on the other hand, you still identify as someone ok with using your credit card to buy things you can't afford and who expects to be called by debt collectors every night, then you will have no issue with purchasing something else you can't afford and putting it on plastic. Doing so is congruent with how you see yourself. Saying no to purchasing the item is incongruent with your identity, and therefore takes more energy to get beyond.

If you view yourself as someone who has taken control of your debt and will soon be living debt free, then it will not be a problem to say no to the item you're itching to purchase. In fact, getting out that plastic will be hard, because it does not fit the new debt-free you, the you that you are meant to be, that God wants you to be. Once you accept that you are already the debt-free person, or the thin person, or the person who is prepared to do whatever is necessary to train for the career you've always wanted, then you will need less energy to stay the course and achieve your goals.

Mental key part 4:
Create a Compelling Goal

Most importantly, to gain and keep the energy you need to follow through and succeed, you need to have a compelling goal. This goal needs to be clear and exciting for you, and it needs to necessitate bringing that habit into check. Maybe it's that you realize by cutting your expenses, you and your kids will be able to enjoy a much-needed theme park vacation come summer! Some arbitrary goal about saving money might not be compelling enough to keep your spending in check. But when the promise of what you want is very clear and exciting, then taking the actions for its achievement is easy. Since we often do more for others than we do for ourselves, I encourage you to bring others you care about into the folds of your motivation strategy, reminding yourself that by being a better you, you have more to give to them. Imagine telling your kids they can't have that vacation you got them all excited about because you spent the money feeding your shoe addiction!

Emotional key:
Positive energy

Have you ever spent time with someone who just drains you? You meet up with that person and you're feeling fine, but 30 minutes in you feel a virtual black cloud hanging over your head. Everything is negative with this person, and he or she easily makes you question your idea that you can accomplish your goals. We all know someone like this. We say that person brings us down, and it's true.

You need to spend your time with people who help keep you charged up and excited, who are positive! People who will get as excited about your goals as you are, and who have goals of their own that they are working toward. Their goals don't have to be anything like yours; people who set goals and work to achieve them understand you and lift you up. A study I recently read about showed that there was one common denominator between successful people in business. Every single one avoids negative people. That's because negative people don't just cause their own failure, they rob others of their joy, faith, hope and motivation too. And positive people do the exact opposite, inspiring success!

"You need to spend your time with people who help keep you charged up and excited, who are positive!"

The people you surround yourself with will help keep you energized or they will drain your energy, but it's not just the people you have to think about, it's everything you encounter in your life. You have to keep as positive and inspirational an environment as possible. How can you possibly do that? "It's hard enough to control who I spend my time with—how can I control the rest of my environment?" you ask.

What do you watch on TV or on the Internet? What do you read? What do you listen to? How do you spend your spare time? There are amazingly motivational books, TV shows, documentaries and clips you can find easily that will help keep you energized. But you don't need to focus on motivation; you can also focus on learning! If your goal is fitness, then read everything you can get your hands on about fitness. Follow fit people on Twitter and Facebook. Find websites about health and fitness. Read about different exercise techniques and healthy recipes.

If your goal is to create a successful business, then take courses on business management, follow business leaders on LinkedIn and read books written on the subject.

No matter what your goal is, you will be able to find an enormous amount of helpful and even life-changing information. As a bonus, this can help you find your mentors. You can follow them on social networks and even interact with them! How exciting is that, when the person who has what you want takes time out of his or her life to converse with you! You can purchase or borrow their books and watch their videos. This will all help keep you energized, motivated and on track.

Spiritual key

Some of the least happy people in the world are the people considered the most successful by others. They are ultra rich, ultra beautiful, famous and hugely successful in their business, but something is missing for them.

The reality is, we are all human and that means we are all creatures of God. It's easy to get sidetracked by other things in life, especially when we are continually bombarded by marketing and advertising and TV shows

telling us what we should want. It's not very often that a spiritual organization or someone attempting to bring us closer to our own God and life's purpose purchases a 30-second ad spot during the Super Bowl.

"Somewhere in the core of your being is a belief system, and you cannot have the presence and energy necessary in your daily life unless you are living in a way that harmonizes with your beliefs."

This constant bombardment of things we "should" want can make us forget or neglect the most important thing of all, which is our own spirituality. You don't need to believe in God as I believe in God for you to receive the richness and the sense of peace, calm and intense satisfaction that comes with being in tune with your spirituality, but it's imperative that you find your own version and that you live your life in a way that's congruent with that.

Yes, there's that word again: congruent. If you believe in peace but are internally waging war then you will never be happy, and I mean that in a metaphorical way. Somewhere in the core of your being is a belief system, and you will not and cannot have the presence and energy necessary in your daily life unless you are living in a way that harmonizes with your beliefs, because you will always have something negative floating around with you. You will always have a feeling that something isn't quite right, that something is missing.

Does this sound familiar to you? I can't begin to tell you how many times I've heard it before, people telling me that something in their life doesn't feel quite right. If this is the case for you, then I suggest you look to your own spiritual existence and ask yourself, am I living my life the way I know to be right?

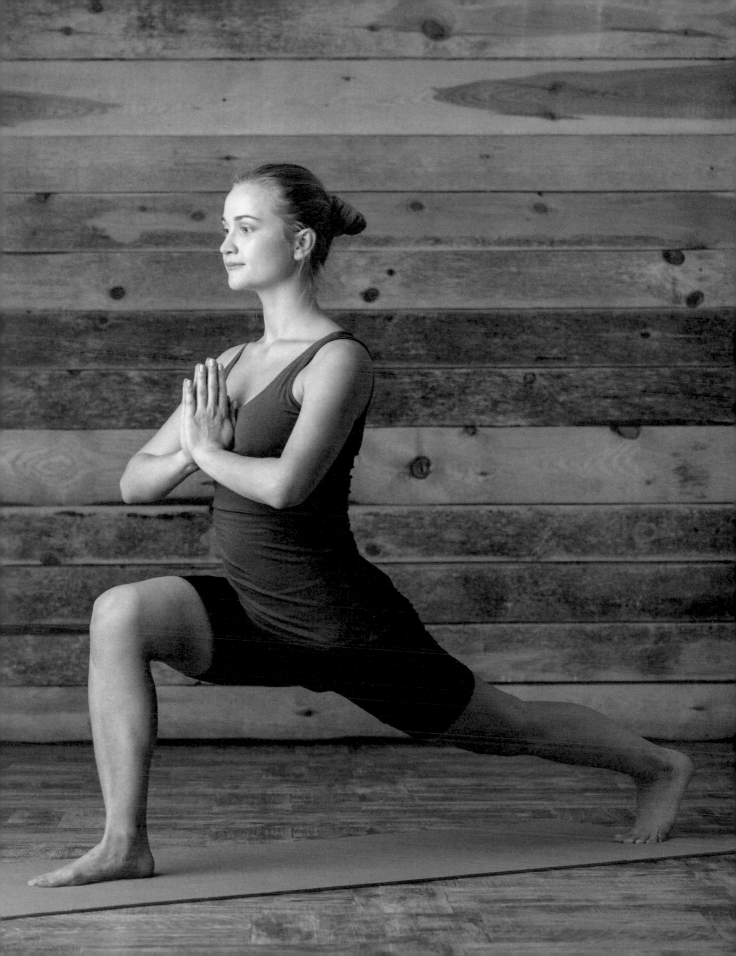

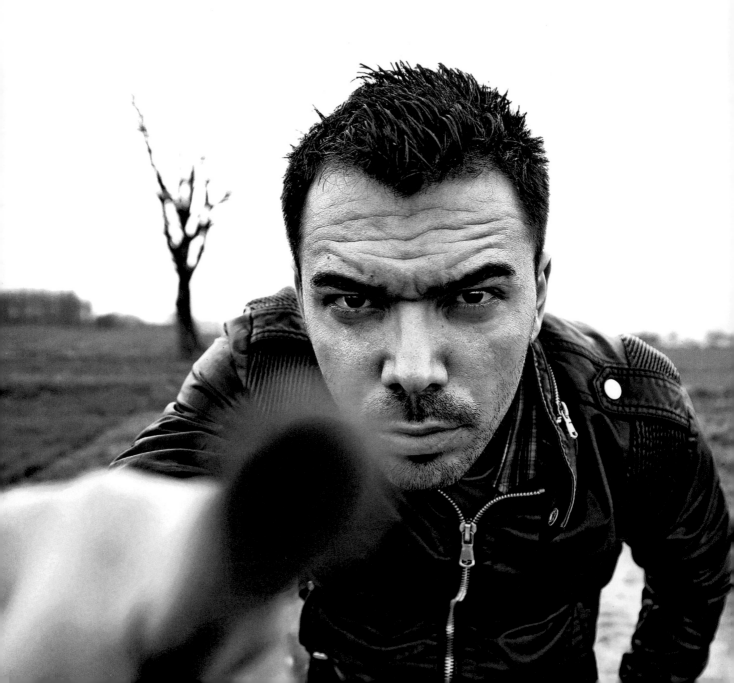

CHAPTER THREE

The Blame Game

Lately, people have been talking a lot about freedom. We want less government involvement; we want lower taxes and fewer rules. We want our friends and family members to stop trying to control us; we're looking for ever more freedom on a personal level. When we want more from life, however, we must ask what that increased freedom requires from us. Sadly, many people who say they want more personal freedom do not want to pay the price for it: personal responsibility. Unless severely mentally challenged or ill, you too must pay.

Personal responsibility means recognizing that the only reason you find yourself where you are right now, whether positive or negative, is because of one thing. That thing is not the family you came from, what happened to you or didn't happen to you, the money you do or don't have, the people you live with, your education or lack thereof. No, it's your choices. Your choices and only your choices have decided where you are right this second, and ultimately, where you will end up.

You might argue, "Charles, that's not true! You've never even met me. How dare you say it's my fault my life is screwed up?! I don't have a job, I've 'tried everything.' How could I possibly have time to take care of myself with the pressure I'm under, with a family like mine, with work, school, and the little time I get?!?" Was your response something like that? If you're anything like I once was before I gained control and lost 160 pounds, I'm sure similar words to those came to mind.

I'm all for appreciating the situation you might be in, and for argument's sake I'm willing to go along with you that outside situations have caused you to be where you are today. That said, where you end up from this point on is something you must take charge of and responsibility for, deal? We often stop at complaint and do not think through the options we each truly have.

If you ever have the luxury of experiencing great coaching, you will find it is really nothing more than helping you see more of the options you have at your disposal. You simply have to take the time away from being distracted by busy-ness to consider them. Coaching—which is what you are getting right now reading this book—comes from a philosophy of seeing people as magnificent Godly works under construction rather than as broken, diseased or mentally ill, dysfunctional people. We are all ultimately the same, under different levels of construction. I'm not any better than you. I've simply made my own personal development my life's focus, and so can you!

Your Poison Is Your Cure

I once read about how people are cured after being bitten by a venomous spider like the black widow. If you suffer such a painful experience, you are immediately given anti-venom. The funny thing about anti-venom, however, is that it is actually derived from the thing that infected you: the poisonous spider! Scientists extract the venom from the spider, inject it into a healthy animal, and that animal's body has an immune response, causing it to create the solution to your problem. The doctor injects that into you and you get better, so the cure comes from the poison.

Take that in for a moment: That which poisons you also cures you.

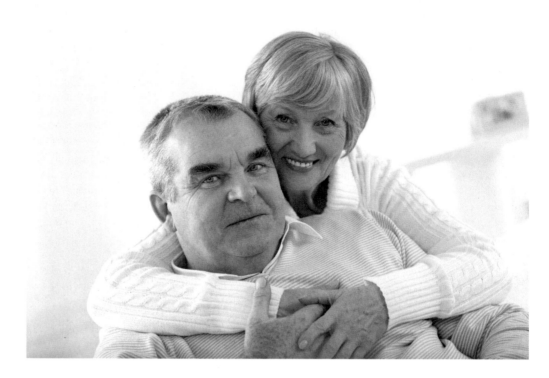

"Rather than blaming your past for the trouble you are currently experiencing, think what you can take from your own experience not only to move forward in your own life, but also to be of service to others."

When I realized that same truth but in a more general sense, my entire world changed. I've since always believed that you should seriously listen only to those people who have successfully overcome their obstacles and achieved the things you want to achieve. You can consider learning from people who have failed, too—so you don't end up doing what they did! But when it comes to getting constructive guidance, a surefire way to save yourself from years of trial and error is to find someone who's accomplished the goals you are reaching for.

Many business experts agree with me on this: People who have faced adversity and triumphed have a special understanding and empathy, and can use this experience to triumph further. To use the spider metaphor in another way, consider that your problems may actually be God's way of getting your body, heart, soul and mind prepared, forming the "antibodies" against your own future failure, and even other people's failure, because your influence and the sharing of your life experience might be someone else's cure!

In my own life, all the bullying, teasing and ridicule not only helped me overcome difficulties later in my own journey but also readied me to be able to be a source of strength for thousands, and I have found that many influential leaders grew similar ability out of the overcoming of their own misery. Destitute, broken, abused and at the end of their rope, they had to turn to the deepest part of themselves and faith in their Creator to get back on the road to success. These leaders often recount that experiences such as these were preparation for helping other people down the road. Living through my mom's addictions and her untimely death gave me a tremendous degree of empathy and compassion for those caught in their own negative patterns, also breeding in me an insatiable appetite to help others overcome what I had seen her overcome, but in their cases before it's too late.

What pain have you been through that God wants to transmute into a gift to others? Is it a marriage problem you're going through? When you do succeed, imagine how you'll be able to help others in a similar position. Rather than blaming your past for the trouble you are currently experiencing, think what you can take from your own experience not only to move forward in your own life, but also to be of service to others. Have you been cursing your situation, missing the truth that God will be using this difficulty of yours to be a force for good as your future unfolds? Are you abusing food or another substance, or are you allowing yourself to wallow in misery because you haven't considered the possibility of success?

When I was studying psychology and my mom was suffering from alcoholism, I wanted to find someone to learn from in order to help her. I sought advice from a psychology professor, thinking that after years of being in the field he would certainly know something I didn't. I was too embarrassed to admit it was my own mom who was struggling, so like most people, I did the next best thing: I lied. I told him I had a friend whose mom was in the darkest depths of addiction. But rather than getting personally involved, he suggested I call a 1-800 number, saying they might be able to help. Disappointed but still driven to get his direct advice on the matter, I e-mailed him persistently, intent on getting his advise. After some time, I finally was able to get a meeting scheduled with him.

Making my way to his office I thought about what I would say. Have you ever been too embarrassed about an issue to share it with someone, even a professional? That's how I felt. Finally I reached the office of a man decades my senior, sat down and poured my heart out with the truth that my mom was really, really sick. I spoke from my heart. At my first pause, he looked up and asked, "What are your plans for when your mother dies? I don't imagine she will live much longer considering what you've told me, Charles."

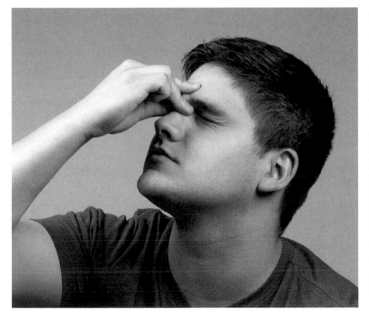

I was devastated and scared, for my mom and my family. I had never entertained this negative perspective. I left his office with tears streaming down my face. I was sad, but moreover, angry—not so much at him, as I'm sure his intentions were good, but rather at this myopic perspective. After the anger passed, I decided to interpret his message in an empowering way. He was trying to say in the best way he knew how that I couldn't leave my life up to the

Coaching	Both	Therapy
Acknowledges the pain of the past but focuses on the here and now, designing one's future	Strive to help people live life with more joy	Typically focuses heavily on healing trauma and wounds of the past that seem to hold a person back
Coaches see and market themselves as fellow travelers on life's road with a client, not medical professionals. Some choose to get accredited through a coaching organization	Provide a safe and helpful environment to improve	In most states, representing oneself as a therapist requires a both a college degree and license in Psychology and/or Medicine to practice
Focuses on current problem resolution and performance optimization in life issues and relationships	See people as capable of getting better	Looks at the relationship from a medical model perspective and can often incorporate medication as a means of 'treatment'
Directed, goal oriented, and often period-specific (relationship ends when goals are attained), with clients being held accountable for the goals they set		Often the relationship is open-ended and non-directed
Coaches do not label or diagnose, but see each client as a unique creation who has the ability to change habit patterns, and with limitless potential		Often clinicians diagnose and label patterns of behavior they see in a patient

outcome of my mom's choices. That said, it didn't inoculate me from the intense love I had for her and my commitment to do all I could to help. I had hoped that the meeting would have reminded me of my personal power to take charge of what I could control, offering an optimistic perspective on the outcomes of those things outside of me. Rather, my empathy informed me that this man didn't see much promise in her. I realized I couldn't let his doubt influence what God had put in my heart, that there was hope for my mom. We don't have the time or the need to convince others of what's possible with God; they'll realize it in time. Since I had already begun to take charge of everything I could control, starting with my health habits, I was that much better equipped to help my mom climb out of the despair she was in. With our innate spiritual drive for self-actualization, hunger for solutions, and God, all things are possible.

I left that meeting with more resolve than ever to find a solution to help my mom, and I am proud to say that alcoholism did not take her life. My mom was blessed with more than another decade with us beyond that meeting, I believe in great part thanks to my perpetual support, which eventually resulted in her freedom from drug use. Would she have had that extra time on this planet if I had shifted my focus from solution to the discouraging data this expert presented? If rather than acting on my faith, I had allowed his opinion about her "inevitable" demise to distract me? Probably not. I never give up on anyone, including you! This experience turned out to be pivotal, as it set my life ablaze seeking answers to achieve the impossible, defying the norms. Focus energizes things. Problems get bigger and bigger if you focus on them. So do solutions. Stay oriented toward where you want to go, not what you fear might occur.

Whose authority are you allowing to subjugate your own? Did a doctor, counselor, therapist, lawyer, parent or some other expert or authority figure you look up to tell you something that's keeping you from doing all you can with all you've got in order to go after what God's put in your heart? Are you letting their stance take precedence over the reality that with God all is possible? Are you letting past disappointments short circuit your destiny? If so, now is the time to drop that story and take action in faith, divorcing your fear.

Instead of blindly following the path of self pity and surrender, I turned to the people who taught that change can always happen when a person is really committed to a goal. It was shortly after this ominous meeting that I—a poor kid just scraping by and running low on hope—found a link to a Tony Robbins talk. In the talk, Tony spoke about how your past and circumstances did not have to define your future. It resonated with me and started me

"While education is incredibly important, sometimes our education can become a hindrance if it emboldens pride."

on my own journey of personal development, leading me to you today. As God would have it, a decade later Tony would personally call me after hearing of my success and invite me to one of his events as his guest! Talk about a synchronicity proving that I had found my calling!

Many people are not sure whether to seek out a life coach or therapist. The fact that you're looking for help is awesome! I've made a chart for you on the opposite page so you can see what they share in common and how they differ. When you find a passionate helper with either title, they can help you make dramatic changes in your life. One word of personal caution: I have learned classically trained psychologists are sometimes taught that a blank slate approach is most effective. I disagree and think it's important you find someone you feel a strong alliance with. The more rapport

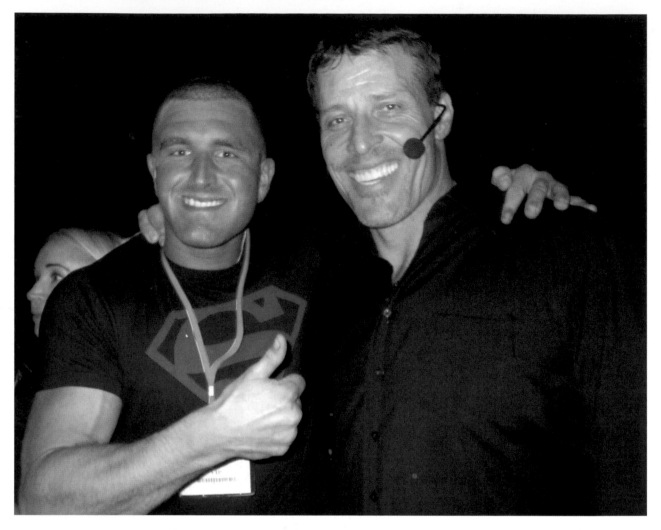

"I believe the more authentic you can be, the more influence you can have on feeling fulfilled in your own life and helping others to do the same."

and connection, the better. While I'm not a therapist, I believe that the more human the helper is, the better! The best coaching relationships are founded upon empathy, authenticity, transparency and honesty.

I'll let you in on a secret: not one of us is perfect! And personally, I believe the more authentic you can be, the more transparent, honest and sincere, the more influence you

can have on feeling fulfilled in your own life and helping others to do the same. You silently give permission to all those around you to live their truth as you live yours.

You will likely find that you accept help more readily when it's coming from someone who's been where you are, is where you want to be or has achieved the outcome you are after despite experiencing something similar to what you're going through right now. Empathy goes a long way. When you can see beyond your current situation and into your future by seeing the life of another, you can transcend what's been holding you back. When you know that the person offering you wisdom wants for you precisely what you want for yourself, that they are aligned with your values and needs, that they believe you know what is best for yourself when you are centered spiritually, and they truly get what you're going through because they've been in a similar situation themselves, you are more apt to take their advice to heart.

Growing from Challenges

God uses your past suffering as a blessing to help during a time when you might need it most. Don't regret the things you may have felt ashamed of—you can ultimately use them for the greater good if you'll think creatively. Can you think of a time when you were upset but happened upon someone who had gone through a traumatic event themselves and their sharing of it helped you deeply? I sure can. I'm laboring on this point because you can often see the direction of your life's purpose by examining what God has built into your life already, by looking back on it.

Rather than laying blame or asking "Why me?" when life's experiences don't match the blueprint you had, ask instead: "What could be the spiritual lesson I'm meant to learn from what I'm experiencing as difficult right now?" All achievers plan for failure moments—they just label them as events rather than taking them on as their identity. Don't let anyone, or yourself for that matter, blow out the fire. You have to continue to forge ahead in spite of setbacks. Maybe some expert told you what you're after is "impossible," like that expert who implied my mom wouldn't get better. A professional helper may have talent, skill and more degrees than a thermometer, but if they are not deeply connected to their own heart, if you don't feel you can open up and trust them completely with the most vulnerable parts of yourself, if you don't feel they're "safe," then their effect on the healing of your wounds will be minimal at best.

Be wary of advice from people who haven't achieved the goal you're after. A person's example of how they live their own life speaks louder than a framed degree on the wall, though that's not to say a degree cannot be helpful, as all learning can be. Why would you trust the advice of someone who isn't successful in the areas you're trying to improve? Or if they themselves aren't, be sure they've coached others who are! For example, I'm sure Tiger Wood's coach is not nearly as gifted as Tiger is at golf, but is still very effective. Evaluate the person you're considering asking to accompany you on your journey of self-improvement by how they lead their life, the relationships they have and the fruits of their labor— in other words, the results of their clients. If you don't do your due diligence in this regard, you might find someone who is often speaking from the same perspective that keeps them where they do not want to be, and their perspective is often negative. Ask yourself how they will feel when they see you begin to make the breakthroughs they've never been able to! At some level even if they care about you this can raise envy, jealousy, and the fear that they'll lose their relationship with you as you climb higher, and they stay where they've always been.

"Don't let anyone quiet the person you are or the qualities God put in to you, even if you don't understand why they are there right now."

Don't let anyone quiet the person you are or the qualities God put in to you, even if you don't understand why they are there right now. The sensitivity, empathy, tenacity, intense focus and curiosity that caused me to be misunderstood and bullied as a child ended up being some of my greatest blessings, which God put in me to help provoke massive breakthroughs in others' lives, like yours! What are some things that you don't particularly like or even understand about yourself right now,

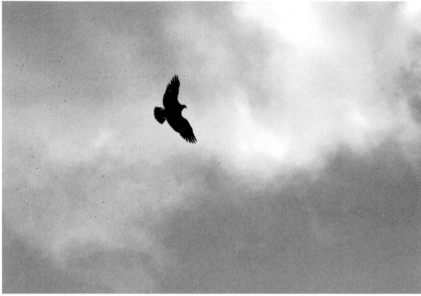

"Considering that your memory is just your perception of what happened, how much freer will you feel when you let it float off?"

results. Judge people by the fruits of their efforts. If they're making things happen positively, it would be worth it to pull up a chair and learn how they do what they do. If they're not, move on.

Who are you holding up as an authority figure, circumventing your own personal power by doing so? Have you or has someone else given you a label that puts the control and power to change outside of yourself? The most important question to ask in this case is what's the cost of the label or story you've put on yourself, or accepted from another? What will that limit cost you for the rest of your life? Rather than take steps to change, are you using the label as a way of shirking your responsibility to make a life you deserve? While discipline in the present may feel challenging, regret in the future is far worse. Knowing they should and could have done things differently often leaves people bitter in old age.

but ultimately could turn out to be a gift for others? If people say you're impatient, then perhaps you're meant to in a role that requires fast-paced decision making with a high degree of decisiveness and efficiency.

I think the greatest cures for life's ailments are brought forth from our greatest challenges. Each of us needs all of us and all of us need each of us, and sometimes the person who is the biggest thorn in your side can be the best teacher. I learned what not to do from people who spent their lives hiding behind titles, masking their own insecurities and fear. I learned what doesn't work in creating lasting change in people's lives, without having to go through that lesson myself. Life gives us the opportunity to learn from those around us, letting us draw examples from those who are successful in the endeavors we wish to pursue and warning us away from the practices of those who are all talk but no substance or

Because of my mom's illness, I had to develop a tremendous resolve and hunger for wellness and justice. If you have someone in your life who is a challenge to you, consider how much you are growing from the experience and the blessing that growth will have on your future and the lives of all you those you care about! Even Alcoholics Anonymous says "each one teach one," asserting that the best addiction counselor is often a former addict. While you might not have had the best helper or model around you growing up, you now have the awareness that the only thing that matters is this very moment, because it decides the next. You can use your history as a classroom to draw lessons from, or as a tragedy to excuse your own power. There is always an empowering way of looking at what happens, and a disempowering way. Both of these ways of looking at events—stories, if you will—will have seeds of truth. Don't be swayed in the wrong direction. Choose the story that moves your life forward, not backward.

Another strategy I use to help my clients free themselves from the past they feel is hindering them is asking that they imagine how their choices will instantly change when they accept that the past is an illusion—it is nowhere to be found! Remember in the previous chapter, where your friend can't see the balloons in the restaurant because of the different perspective? This is the same. When remembering any event you shared with another person you will find your respective memories will be totally different based upon your individual focuses. Considering that your memory is just your perception of what happened, how much freer will you feel when you let it float off? If you can forget simple things like where you put your sunglasses when you're trying to run out the door in the morning, why not choose to forget the things you believe about yourself that are hindering your progress, and begin to massively act on the dreams that God has given you? I believe if God's put it in your heart, then there is no question that it is possible for you to achieve it.

Do you want to know a really good way to never get where you want to be? Easy: blame someone else and use that as a distraction from action. You can also blame your environment, your personal background, your family's history, illness, physical limitations or disability, the difficult things you have to deal with each day, a health crisis, errors in judgment you may have made in the past, the neighborhood you live in, the bad teachers you had who told you that you would never amount to anything, a relationship you've stayed in that should have ended long ago, and on and on and on.

Busyness VS Progress

People often get so caught up with being busy they stop being productive. It's like a gifted artist feeling inspired to paint, so she begins a painting. Soon, however, she grows preoccupied with other tasks and the painting gets forgotten. After some time another idea comes to her mind and she starts another painting. She has half-finished paintings all over the place, but never completes a full project. You might also feel held back if you are a working parent. While you are at work, you feel guilty for not being home, but when you go home, you are distracted by thinking of the work you need to get done. This kind of mental craziness is what dilutes your mind's powers of concentration needed to create the breakthroughs and make the progress you are longing for.

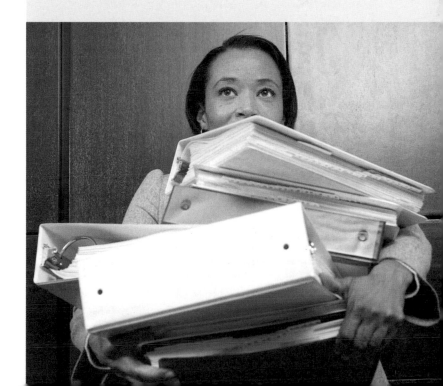

My Teenage Because List, aka "This is why my life is the way it is.":

1. I don't have the time to consistently work out.

2. I can't go to a place where all the fit people are, a gym! I'll be ridiculed.

3. I am not good looking so I can't find a girlfriend.

4. My family isn't like everyone else's. We have skeletons in our closet! [Like no one else does, right?!]

5. I can't buy clothes in the normal sized stores so why even try.

6. I never have been interested in sports anyway so it doesn't matter if I don't participate.

7. I can be happy being alone! In fact I hear some of the greatest teachers say you should be able to be happy by yourself.

8. I will make myself feel important by getting smarter since I "can't" get healthier. [Consider the contradiction there!]

9. My father has left home, leaving us kids to manage an adult struggling with chemical addiction.

10. I don't have a stable place to live. I don't even want to be at home anymore because my mom is abusing alcohol and prescription drugs so I cannot possibly focus on myself. To focus on myself instead of a person like her who isn't thinking clearly would mean I am a cold, heartless jerk!

Who could expect you to be any different than the way you are, considering how unfortunate your history was? It's not your fault.

As I write this I know I sound terribly harsh, and I don't mean to. After all, I was master of the blame game when I was younger. Why was I overweight? Because those kids in school picked on me. I ate poorly and too much because of a narrative that I constructed unconsciously, excusing my own responsibility and the power I had to change it all in an instant. Why didn't I exercise? Because people would make fun of me. Why had I never been on a date? Because girls were judgmental and superficial. I had a million reasons I was in that place I hated, but none of them included me! The only valid reason for being in that place was how I was interpreting the events in my life and the choices I was making about them. And this is extremely common. To change, we need to take responsibility and take control. Otherwise, our negative habits—both actions and thought processes—will continue. Have you, perhaps unintentionally, ever allowed bad habits to continue in your life because you've hypnotized yourself into believing it has to be this way for no other reason than that it has been for so long? Has something negative grown so familiar that you stick with it, even if you know without any doubt that it's bad for you?

I know that place well. To break the pattern, I will give you a simple mental exercise. Imagine your favorite superhero coming into your room right now. He says he's going to pick you up on

If your lack of success is someone else's fault or the fault of your environment or your upbringing then you never have to take responsibility. It's not your fault you have a job you hate and your relationship lacks passion and you're overweight. It's because your parents didn't pay for your education and your husband isn't as attractive as he used to be and everyone in your family is overweight.

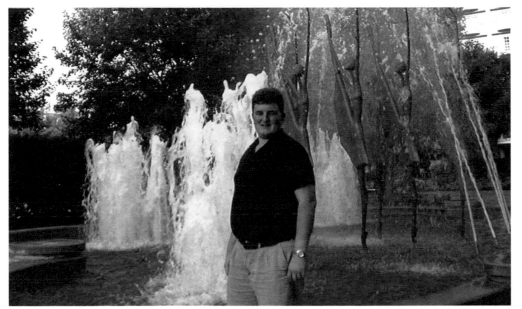

OBESITY MADE ME LOOK OLDER. HERE I'M ONLY ABOUT 15! IT WAS HARD FOR MANY PEOPLE TO BELIEVE I WAS A TEENAGER!

his back and fly you miles up into the sky, but you won't only be flying away from the earth, you will also be flying back in time. Close your eyes and picture yourself jumping on his back for this epic trip into history. Imagine flying up into the clouds, looking down on your house, your driveway, all the small cars that look like ants as you head back to where you were five years ago. Once there, put yourself back into that version of you and see if you had planned to be in the negative situation you currently find you want to change. If the answer is no, it's likely you're only where you are today because you did not take the time to plan for the future as well as you could have and are able to right now.

By the time I was 17 I weighed 360 pounds and couldn't manage to get up four steps without feeling like I was about to die. When other kids were out having their first kisses, hanging out with their friends, going to dances and going on dates, I had never been on a date and didn't really have friends to hang out with. On nights when all the other kids would be in an auditorium dancing and having fun, I'd be sitting in my house all alone watching TV, eating an entire large pizza and drinking a 2L bottle of soda, lamenting over my mom's alcohol problem and thinking about how I might be

able to change her, or at least manage her better. Some lucky evenings I might have enough money to go to a theater and escape into a movie, distracting myself from the dissatisfaction of my life.

"Take a moment and ask yourself, what are you currently focusing on that is a distraction from dealing with the issues that can bring you the life you deserve?"

Instead of putting my mind to work on how changing myself to become stronger and healthier would give me far more power and influence in managing these day-to-day difficulties, I was just a piece of the collateral damage we all can become when we have a loved one in the throes of an addictive habit. Moving closer to my own goals wasn't something I had even considered.

Even if you don't have someone who is ill or requiring your care, take a moment and ask yourself, what are you currently focusing on that is a distraction from dealing with the issues that can bring you the life you deserve? Sometimes we use the role of being a "rescuer" or "caregiver" as a way to avoid dealing with our own issues. It's much easier to feel good about yourself if all the people you're tending to are worse off than you are! This doesn't lead to resolving the core issue, however, developing strategies to raise your own self-esteem and sense of worth independent of whatever you're doing and who you are with. You want to get to a place where you are cool with just being, even when you're not in action. How much better will your life get when your focus improves? Will focusing on you, getting healthier, happier, more fulfilled and in control, help or hurt the situation or person you feel "needs" you? Be honest—the truth is, a better you means a better situation for others in your life. You show up more capable of effectively dealing with the challenging situation or challenging relationship when you are in a better state.

Being Congruent

Have you ever set your mind to doing something but for some reason you just can't seem to get going? You do what you think should work to start the engine and it just doesn't start. You focus on wealth, trying to attract it to you, but you're broke. You eat right and exercise and aren't getting the results you want. There is a problem if this is the case! I found my problems stemmed from being incongruent. My mind was saying one thing but my heart and soul were feeling another. The electrical cord between my head and heart somehow ended up unplugged. Emotionally I was exhausting myself on my environment, sacrificing my own future since I had depleted my resources on trying to change something that may never change.

This incongruity will never change while we make excuses or find reasons for it. Laying the blame for the state you're unhappy with may make you feel less responsible for it, but it does nothing to help get you out of that state.

When I was a 360-pound, miserable, lonely teen I had a huge list of reasons why I was in that lousy state. I call it The Because List. You can have a look at it on page 52.

Lists we create such as this, to make excuses and therefore halt our own personal change, do contain some truths, or at least half-truths, so they are very convincing. But spiritually we get sick when we fall into this disempowering thought pattern. You can look physically well but be emotionally and spiritually sick. The secret to joy is to get your mind, heart and body all in alignment.

One day, years after getting in shape, I was working in the yard. I bent over and felt a pull in my back. I didn't think much of it until I began walking and pain radiated down my leg like a laser beam of fire! I made an appointment with the chiropractor and he took a look, feeling my back. It turned out that one of my vertebrae had rotated slightly. Just a small misalignment had caused me massive pain! The same can happen with our life's alignment. What might be slightly out of alignment in your life right now that is causing you pain? Is it the way you are thinking about your past? Or maybe the present? Are you acting in a way that's incongruous with your beliefs? To make significant and consistent progress, you cannot accept that where you were or where you are is where you will ultimately be.

> To feel joy and to achieve your ultimate goals you must begin to speak faith over your life. Be congruent. Build a life where how you think, what you do, what you feel and how you treat both yourself and others all match.

What Are You Really Looking For?

I have coached so many people who are more concerned with how they look than how dissatisfied they feel with life. That simple error in thinking—focusing more energy and concentration on the outside rather than on the inside—is ironically all that needs to shift for their life to take the turn they've longed for. When you are more focused on your life purpose, how you are on the inside, in any context, whether health, wealth, relationship or career, the outside will take care of itself. I learned from years in the fitness world that there are great things you can do to get healthy on the inside and end up looking good on the outside, but also all sorts of unhealthy and even dangerous things you can do to achieve a certain look that might look healthy on the outside but are not: deprive yourself of food and water, take steroids or diuretics and over-exercise, just to name a few. It's the same

with wealth. You can get a high-interest-rate loan and drive a BMW or Mercedes on credit, but have nothing in your bank account! It's not long before the façade cracks. Yes, it's possible to consciously and wisely use the symbols of success to actively help yourself become more financially successful, but if you're just concerned with the outward appearance then you're actively holding yourself back from that financial success.

"What you've done, what you have or who you know is often used as a disguise for insecurity and internal dissatisfaction with the person you really are."

So the question is, what are you really after? One of the most empowering questions to ask yourself is "for what?" When you say you want that new watch, ask "For what?" I want to feel like I earned something valuable. "For what?" I want to be able to show I have resolve to follow through. "For what?" I want to prove I can do things I put my mind to. When you force yourself to examine the real reasons behind the things you think you want, you find often you're chasing a feeling. This is what marketers feed off of: getting you to buy things they've ingeniously conditioned you to believe will give you the feelings of joy, security, significance, connection and approval, the feelings all humans want. You're looking to recreate an emotional experience and have hooked up in your mind that the thing you want to buy or the way you want to behave is the mechanism that will give it to you. It's not. Why spend the money or indulge in the behavior when you can choose to feel that great feeling right now just by directing your own thoughts to all the things you have to be grateful for.

People often go for lofty ambitious goals in an effort to feel validated or loved. I met one young lady who was pursuing law school and working full-time. She shared with me that she felt totally dissatisfied and unfulfilled. Growing

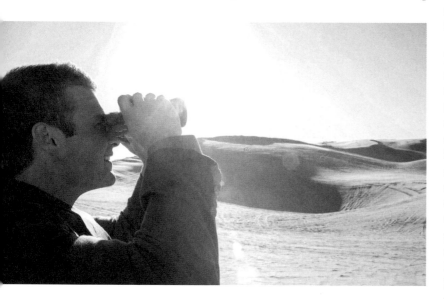

up, to get love from her parents she always had to compete and win. Now, decades later, she was continuing to live out this pattern without examining whether she actually wanted what she was aiming for. Are you still chasing the approval, validation or unconditional love from your parents, and so you spend your life trying to secure that elusive feeling through something tangible? Don't get caught up in the trap that keeps so many people dissatisfied, using the wardrobe of achievement and success. What you've done, what you have or who you know is often used as a disguise for insecurity and internal dissatisfaction with the person you really are.

When you learn to accept and love yourself, you will find others do too. You won't feel any need to impress them with what you have. You won't need the sportiest car, the flashiest jewelry, the biggest muscles, the elevated corporate title or to look like a runway model if that's not what really fulfills you. You can have all of these things if you want them, and if so I hope you get them, but please know that you don't need them. When you start to think you need them, they're controlling you and your life. You are still here today no matter what you believe you needed in the past and didn't have. You made it. That in and of itself is enough proof you did not need these things!

If you walk around with a spirit of fear that no one will like you because of your interpretation of the past and negative expectation of the future, that energy precedes you. We are all on an energy frequency. You attract people who are on that same level. Have you ever been in a bad mood and find the day gets worse and worse? It's not coincidental. Because you anticipate rejection you try to be impressive, and then other humans respond negatively to what they perceive as arrogance, when in truth you are simply protecting yourself. In trying to anticipate and prevent rejection you actually help to bring it about! You can never have a life of success and abundance if you focus on your appearance and controlling the opinion of others rather than working on how you really are.

Before she began abusing drugs and alcohol, my mom could always see through the outward me to the inside. I would come home from a bad day as a child, put on a face of confidence and joy, and she would penetrate it with her piercing blue eyes, asking me "What's bothering you, honey?" She could sense the real me. Who knows the real you? How can you get better if you don't let light into a dark

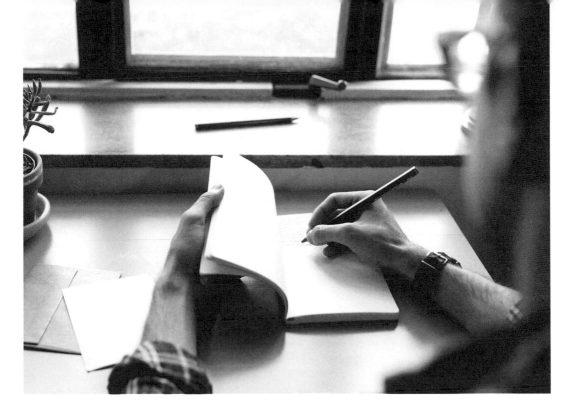

area that needs healing? While light can be painful at first, like when your parents threw on the switch to get you out of bed early for school, it's what we need to wake up and see our way out of where we are. What can ever grow or get better without light?

Effective Questions

Our internal negativity can really limit us if we allow it to. I never had an interest in playing sports, but if I had asked myself the question, "How can I possibly know I won't like sports if I have never tried to play?" My negative internal retort would be, "Well you were bullied when you did try, so don't go out there and suffer like that again!" Our brains are not hardwired for a legendary life and entrepreneurial success. They are hardwired to avoid threat, and with good reason: to keep us from being eaten alive by lions and tigers, moving quickly away from advancing real threats. The problem is this hardwiring kicks in when we don't need it, resulting in overgeneralizing and misinterpreting everyday life issues as threatening. It takes time and working on your

"Reframing the things you feel are permanent problems as the easily surmountable challenges they are and breaking them down into smaller digestible daily tasks can give you a better opportunity to grow."

own mindset to develop a more sophisticated framework where you develop the habit of courage—software, if you will—so the hardwired fight-or-flight response doesn't kick in unless it is truly needed.

Sometimes the only upgrade needed is to ask yourself more empowering questions. Reframing the things you feel are permanent problems as the easily surmountable challenges they are and breaking them down into smaller digestible daily tasks can give you a better opportunity to grow. For example in my own case a more effective line of questioning when thinking about getting involved in sports would have been, "Have you tried every possible activity and sport there is? Considering how many people are extraordinarily

"I encourage you to begin designing an ideal day in which you fulfill the disciplines necessary to achieve your desired outcomes."

passionate about so many different sports out there, can you be absolutely certain you won't find anything, nothing at all, to like about any of them? Even if the idea of playing a sport makes you feel limited and fearful like when you were a child, are you still the defenseless, unresourceful, dependent kid you once were, or are you now a capable, intelligent, resourceful, well-equipped adult who's handled many storms and is still standing despite it all? Can you take on the challenge of finding something to enjoy in a physical sport?"

A strong, well-developed question opens your mind up to the possibility of enjoying something you've not yet explored and have some trepidation about. I never understood this when I wouldn't eat vegetables and my parents would say: "You can't not like it if you've never tried it!" It wasn't until I was older and the pressure was off that I became curious and sampled broccoli. Much to my surprise, I did like it! I would never have known I could feel pleasure nourishing my body with this food if I had continued to live out the rebellious pattern I developed to demonstrate my free will in response to my parents' urging. Which behavioral patterns are you practicing that at an earlier time may have served a useful purpose but are no longer helpful? Are you rebelling against some former authority in your life and short-circuiting your own joy in the process?

See how powerful your internal questions can be? If you need help with this, a good coach will help steer your thinking away from the false, limiting beliefs of your history and on to the possibilities of creating your ideal future! What have you been holding yourself back from embracing because of this habit? What do you still feel that is robbing you of the energy you need to go where God is calling you: to that new relationship, that more fulfilling career, the life of service you've seen signs pointing you toward?

The truths from our history can act as stumbling blocks when we look at them a certain way, but when we look at those truths from a different perspective, those blocks can disappear. It's true that I left the house many times in fear for my well-being, like when my mom attacked me because I had found her alcohol and tossed it into the city street sewer. But it's also true that if I had been more fit and healthy because of my own habits, I may not have even been there to experience that. I may have been out with friends enjoying life more, and I definitely would have been able to run away from her much faster! That's hindsight. Good hindsight is not as important when you've planned your future well. Allowing the

"Planning your future starts with just planning your day. Days of successful habits are what lead to a fulfilling life of purpose in the future, yes, but also in the present!"

past to be the past can be an effective way of dealing with it. Planning your future starts with just planning your day. Days of successful habits are what lead to a fulfilling life of purpose in the future, yes, but also in the present! Just as living in the past prevents a positive future, if you live forever in the future, you miss the present. I encourage you to begin designing an ideal day in which you fulfill the disciplines necessary to achieve your desired outcomes. Following this habit will take the successful completion of your goals from "if" to "when."

Just as Tony Robbins taught me on that fateful day and as I've imparted to every one of my clients and the readers of my book, our past does not dictate our future. Incidents like the one I've mentioned when my mom attacked me were realities of my life. But were they a reason for me to stay in a place I hated mentally, emotionally and physically? Because my family's behavior was flawed, dysfunctional and unloving at that particular time, did that mean I had to make that dysfunction my identity? No, but I didn't realize that at the time. Psychology teaches that as children we often misinterpret the problems in our family as a reflection of ourselves. We take ownership of what's going on around us, thinking it's our fault things are screwed up. That was certainly the case for me as a teen. I took ownership of my mother's choices, thinking if only she would be better, so would my life, but ironically I did not take ownership of my own choices.

Many of my clients come to realize that their self harm, whether abusing food, drugs or alcohol or any other way they prevent themselves from having the life they want and deserve, started at a very early age when an error occurred in their interpretation of what was going on. For example, one woman remembered hearing her parents arguing at the top of their lungs night after night, then walking home from school at 12 and seeing her dad drive away in a pickup truck, never to be seen again. When she went in the house, her mom was sobbing and had baked cookies. She offered her some, telling her that her father didn't care about her or their family. This girl wondered what she'd done to drive her father away. Unfortunately, her narrative became: "Dad left because I wasn't good enough. If I can't trust my dad, who can I trust?" Years of half-hearted and ultimately failed attempts at intimate personal relationships confirmed this false belief in her mind until she reached out for my help. She learned to recognize that her path to happiness is connection and that she wasn't at fault for her father's departure. She learned to forgive her parents and also forgive herself for not seeing this truth at a younger age.

"I made the dysfunction in my environment part of my identity and also made it my responsibility, giving me even more guilt to carry around unknowingly."

My young mind had also connected that if my mom was "messed up" it meant I was too, and I was ashamed of that. I wouldn't tell anyone about what was happening at home. I made the dysfunction in my environment part of my identity and also made it my responsibility, giving me even more guilt to carry around unknowingly. Are you holding on to guilt? Now is the time to let it go!

You must recognize you shouldn't despise small beginnings or even difficult beginnings— it doesn't matter where you are starting from right now; it only matters where you are going to end up! Is it true that there are things in your life that are challenges and just plain out suck? Yes. Is it true that there are things in your life that can cause you to feel bad if you focus on them? Yes. Is it true you have things you can look back at and feel terrible about? Yes. Maybe you lost a loved one to cancer, or maybe someone you loved left you. Maybe you had this grand vision in your mind for how that person would be at your side forever and

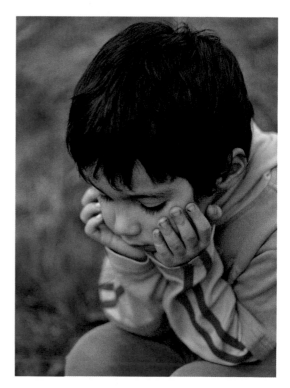

life took an unexpected turn, leaving your ideal vision in its wake. Maybe you feel it was your fault because you didn't appreciate that person enough or even treated them badly. Maybe you have an illness or disease that you are worried about. Or maybe you just look back with regret at things you didn't do, like finish school or take that job you were offered.

These things may be disappointing and they might even be true, but they are also part of our human condition. We all have disappointments we can focus on from our own personal history or from those we care about or in areas we care about. With enough practice focusing on these disappointments you might feel despondent, like life is no longer worth living. At the same time there are many positive things I'm sure you can consider, random acts of kindness you've seen personally, or perhaps read about—people going out of their way to help a stranger, a wealthy person giving everything away to those in need, a person who many might find undeserving of any care or love who is given a second chance—things that give you a warm feeling like you get at Christmas time!

Which is true? The bad or the good? The answer is, both are. However, what you choose to make your major focus becomes the filter through which you experience life, and ultimately plays a huge role in the choices you will make, which shapes the person you become. There are so many stories of people who experienced tragic beginnings and instead of using these tragedies as excuses for future problematic behavior, become hungry for success and use their gifts to improve the world. If you choose to focus on things in your life that make you feel bad or think about the way you feel life isn't being fair to you right now and you use these as an excuse to not create the future you want and deserve, then you are still making a choice, but your choice robs you of any chance of fulfillment.

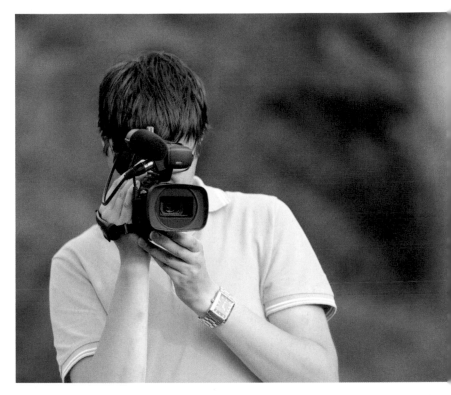

How are you using your story? Have you even thought of what your story is? If it were made into a movie and you are the lead character, what would you want to see happen next?

Are you ready to accept that you, with a little grace, are the only person who can alter the way your life will go? No one can force you to do anything. Even at gunpoint you have a choice: do whatever is being asked or get shot. While this example is dramatic and neither of these choices are enjoyable, you still have choice.

There's a little quiz going around on Facebook right now where you put X's next to things you've done. Every single time I've seen that list I've seen an X beside "I've done something

I'll regret all my life." Yet the people who have marked this X are often living happy and satisfied lives. To err is human. To lose is human. To hurt is human. But none of that means you need to choose a future that is less than it can be. Nor does it mean you have to continue to play out the drama you grew up with, or make choices that, while bad, are familiar and "safe."

Choose the life you desire and deserve. Leaving your future to happenstance is like getting in a taxi and saying: "Take me somewhere." What's the chance you're going to get to a place that you really would like to go? Since you want to greet every day with excitement, you've got to plan your activity for the coming day, week, month, and even decade! If you wake up dreading your days, that's a strong alert signal that action is required. Similar to the "Check Engine" light going off on your dash in the car, if you are waking up depressed or feeling down, this is a message from your unconscious telling you that the situation you have allowed yourself to be in or are choosing to focus on is not the way your mind knows it should be.

Blessings and Blame

I believe we all are given a spark of divinity and a "knowing"—some call it conscience, others a Guardian Angel—that we can listen to. An intuitive sense that we are on or off our correct path. Problems in life, which we all face, do not determine whether we stay on the correct path. Don't use problems to create a future that's less than it can be, whether those problems are substantial and possibly chronic, like my mom's illness, a bad relationship or getting fired from a job, or just something small and irritating, like a broken-down car. Doing so slowly paralyzes you and renders you unable to discern that voice so critical to good decision making. Use the problems of your past and present as

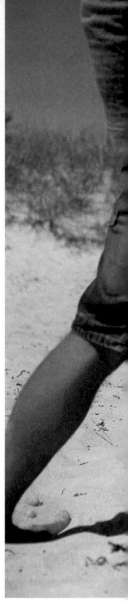

opportunities to learn from, reminders of all the good times to pull positive energy from, and catalysts to create a better future! Sometimes God allows horrible things (by our measure) to occur in our lives. In my opinion this is to give us contrast so we can recognize just how blessed our particular situation is. Sometimes I have clients who complain about having to wait at a stoplight longer than expected or perhaps being cut off by an angry driver, and they are allowing it to ruin their day. I help them get perspective, reminding them they truly don't know what a problem is if that's the worst experience they had that day. Think how many people every day are given a terrible notice about their loved one's health, or permanently lose someone to an unexpected accident. Take joy in the small blessings of your life. Maybe the longer-than-expected stoplight is God protecting you from an accident you would have been in if it had changed sooner! Sometimes our greatest frustrations are the biggest blessings unbeknownst to us at the time.

My grandma would tell me that every morning before getting out of bed she would thank God for the ability to see, hear, talk, smell, move her toes, walk, pay her bills, drive, eat, go to church and practice her faith. These were all things that, as a 16-year-old at the time, I had never considered. If you're broke in America you still have more than 99% of the world has. You have opportunity that few on this earth will ever imagine having. Don't waste it reliving your past, blaming it for where you

"Take joy in the small blessings of your life."

are. Your circumstances can only change by reinterpreting them in a way that empowers you, rather than preventing you from moving forward.

My grandma always told me: "Never look back with regret," meaning you can never go back in life, only forward, so worrying about what you should or shouldn't have done is useless. I've amended her statement to: "Make brave choices in the NOW so regret is something you never even have to consider!" Live life to the fullest and know that the best is ahead of you, no matter what your age. Learn from those times when you didn't reach out

for what you wanted. Often this happens in love, when people fear rejection, never reaching out to the person who may very well be just as interested.

To move forward without regret means you must have a vision, and know the first step you need to take to begin the journey. Remember, success, good health and meaningful relationships are not destinations; they are all processes! Sure there will be times you will need to pause for grief, recalibrate when life doesn't go exactly as planned, or just to vent. That's natural. But using that grief, anger or frustration as a distraction, keeping you from your purpose and preventing you from honoring those you may have lost or hurt will only stop you from living your life!

I, too, can still forget the blessings God has anointed my life with at times. Just recently while I was waiting in a lengthy line at a coffe shop an older woman was casually looking around near the checkout. People who know me may say I am virtuous, but patience is not one of my virtues! As I finally approached the counter to order my herbal tea, this woman decided it would be a good time to turn around and act as if she had been waiting in line too! I couldn't believe this sweet old lady would do such a thing. I was about to let her have it and tell her she could take her place in line like everyone else when I noticed that she was holding a book about Mother Teresa. Good thing she was! This reminded me, the guy who preaches to people about kindness, love and mercy, that we are all human and constantly have to check ourselves!

You see where I'm going here? It's so easy to find ways to blame other people, blame your circumstances or find excuses. Just the other day I heard a man telling a group of his co-workers why he couldn't complete a weekly assignment they had been relying on. I could tell without even knowing the situation that he was spewing out excuses, and I could tell by his co-worker's faces that they knew too. Excuse giving is a terrible illness that everyone else can see in a person except the one who has it!

I challenge you to embrace the reality that if you blame certain people for the poor quality of your life at this moment, you must also be fair and "blame" them for all the great things that have happened or qualities you have too. After all, your life is decided solely by them, right? All the bad in your life has nothing to do with you. In that case all the good you experience also has nothing to do with you. Would you accept that? Of course not, but it should awaken in you just how delusional a belief

system many of us construct to excuse away the power we have, and the pain of disappointment, and the fear of responsibility of running our own lives when things don't go exactly as we had planned.

You can find any excuse you look for. You can rationalize and you can blame. Go ahead! Rationalize and blame all you want, but you will still end up at the place you started—with yourself. You will likely lose even the ground you have. All that will happen is you will stay where you don't want to be.

> Time will continue to move on, whether you decide to move forward in a joyous state or a miserable one. At any given moment you can take charge of your thinking—this second right now, for example—and focus on all that you've done well and are proud of rather than the few things you're down about.

Find Empowerment

One thing is for sure: the high achievers of the world do not stress about their errors—they anchor themselves to their successes. Some call them grandiose or deluded, but many of the most successful people I've spent time with reinterpret their past "failures" in such a way that you would be hard pressed to get them to name a time they'd "failed." Rather, these important times helped them on the path to success. The achiever mindset is different, and much better to have if you're looking to get an edge in your life.

We all have times when things do not go the way we'd hoped and planned for them to. But these times have no bearing on the essential you and what you will achieve. You must know you are not the habits you have or the problems you face or what others say you are. The real you transcends all of that. I once heard Dr. Wayne Dyer lecture on this very subject. He reminded us that despite all the medical technology we have, no one has ever located the force that runs the thing we call "you." If they dissected your brain, they would find all the cells. They can get areas to light up on scans, they can even touch nerves to get you to move certain body parts, but they would never ever find the force, you, the soul, that is running the hardware.

Dr. Dyer talked about a study conducted years ago where they opened a man's skull while he was conscious. They found that part of the brain, when touched, would cause him to move his arm. They touched the area, and up went the arm. They touched it, and up it went again. Finally, they asked the person to resist the arm going up when they stimulated that part of the brain. Shockingly, despite the stimulation, he was able to! What was the force resisting the simulation? I challenge you to think of yourself as a spiritual being having a human experience, not vice versa.

You can find empowering, synchronous meanings in all of your life if you condition yourself to look for them. Rationalizing and making excuses will definitely not get you where you want to be. It's a temporary fix for a permanent issue. To get there, you have to follow your path despite what lies in your way, and let me tell you something: Giving up because you face a challenge is only going to make getting there more difficult, not less difficult. You need to change the picture mentally and not see the obstacle as something in your way, but rather, something you can use in your journey to becoming the person you were born to be. Build on your successes, not on your "failures." You might not need to even push

"The achiever mindset is different, and much better to have if you're looking to get an edge in your life."

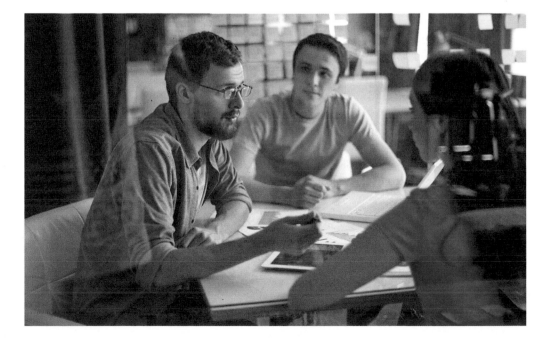

your perceived challenges out of the road, you might simply need to walk around them!

Fleeting or Lasting

Let's say your goal is to create a more fulfilling relationship. Your wife is an emergency room doctor with long tiring shifts where half the time the people whose lives she's saving or their family members are angry and ungrateful. She gets little appreciation for the mission she's on, but finds it tremendously rewarding—in fact, it's one of the reasons you fell for her. Now you certainly know she needs a little time to unwind after work because she comes home stressed and tense after a day of life-or-death situations and verbal abuse. You know that if you give her a little time to relax, then she will be a much more pleasant person

"We are all tempted throughout our lives and temptation is not the issue; it's your response to the temptation."

to be around, will be more responsive to you, and will gladly give you her attention, but you find it difficult to give her this time because you feel needy.

Now let's just imagine that you had an epic bad day. Maybe you were chewed out by your boss, lost a major client or got rear-ended, and you're not in the best mood yourself. You want to complain and vent about your day the second she walks through the door, but you know that's not really in your own best interest and certainly not in the interest of your goal. It's going to take effort on your part to give her that unwind time.

So what do you do? Do you tell yourself "I know I have to offer her some unwind time but gosh dang it I have to unload. I had a rotten day so I'm going to tell her all about it the second she walks in the door"? Or are you willing to be a bit more responsive, mature, less reactive, and more focused on your own desired outcome and future and say: "My ultimate goal isn't to have her tend to me right now. My goal is to build a strong relationship. By allowing her this unwind time it isn't just better for her, in the long run it's better for

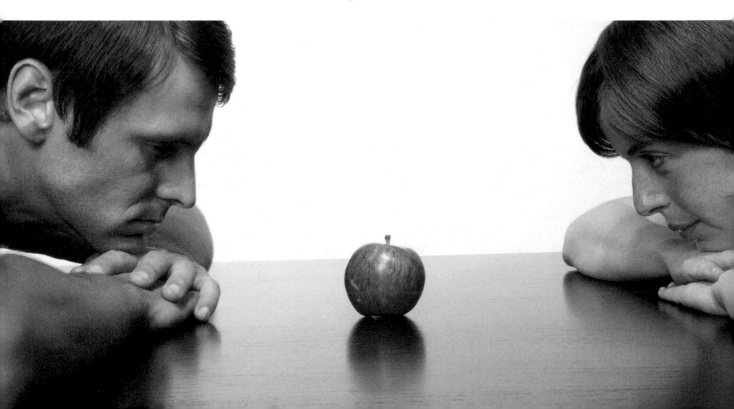

me too, because it helps me to achieve my ultimate goal. Besides, she will definitely give me the attention I need, but her heart will be more in it and she'll respond to my needs better once she's had the chance to remove herself from her work day." You can use your rotten day as an excuse to not follow through with your goals, or you can follow through with the everyday steps necessary to reach your goals despite your rotten day. Maybe it feels easier this second to make the excuse, but which choice is easier in the long run? Following through, of course!

Conflict in any relationship comes when you are more focused on your own needs than the other person's. You want to complain about what happened to you the second she walks in the door because you want her understanding. You do your share and you *deserve* her understanding, right? You're her partner and you're no less important than she is just because she has a stressful job. This might be true, but that line of thinking does not bring you what you truly desire. A major key to begin to train yourself to focus on is that a relationship—any type of relationship, whether business, personal or intimate—should be a place you primarily go to contribute to, not withdraw from. Give and ye shall receive is not just religious babble. By giving that which you want, you get to enjoy the feeling of it simply by sharing it, and in addition it psychologically induces reciprocation in the heart and mind of the other person, making them want to meet your needs too, since you so readily meet theirs.

Let me ask you a question. When you are pulled between doing what you feel like doing—maybe having a drink when you shouldn't, or being physically intimate with someone you know you shouldn't, or cheating on your diet, or procrastinating and not getting your paperwork done, then who ultimately gets to tell you that you can feel better after giving in to that temptation? Oscar Wilde said he could resist anything but temptation! Being tempted—even being tempted to blame oth-ers—is completely normal. We are all tempted throughout our lives and temptation is not the issue; it's your *response* to the temptation. If you give in and follow the same negative path you've been following, do you feel better or worse for it? How about if you don't give in and instead bring yourself closer to where you want to be?

What will that drink really do for you? Or that fleeting and meaningless sexual encounter? What will that 20 seconds of food enjoyment accomplish, or that extra hour watching TV instead of doing your paperwork? Will any of these bring you closer to a goal? When you stop to examine it, you begin to realize that you are the only person who gets to decide how you will feel about anything you choose to do. We can all justify our actions; the question is whether or not the justification we're giving is moving us in the direction of fulfilling our destiny. Sometimes we have been running a program or belief system for so long we have never examined if it even makes any sense!

> *"We can all justify our actions; the question is whether or not the justification we're giving is moving us in the direction of fulfilling our destiny."*

The word temptation itself conjures up dark and negative meanings, but temptation can be good. You could say you're tempted to do the right thing, to work out, to be more generous, to volunteer more often. See, you even get to decide your personal meaning of the words we all use! Think about how much power you have with just that insight alone! When you change the meaning of the words you choose to use, you can alter your entire experience. Instead of saying: "No one understands me," for example, ask yourself if it's true that really "no one" understands you. Could you be generalizing? When you say "understands" do you mean about a specific situation or in general?

Could it be your challenge to make things clearer for those who haven't had your experience, so they could see it from your perspective and understand you better? Could you find a support group for people in your situation and therefore find people who really do understand what you're going through? See, you always have choice, power, and control if you take time to think about it and look from a different perspective.

Just like how that sincere psychologist's bleak data-based opinion and doubt could have shifted my focus from the positive possibilities to a negative stance, if you subjugate your own thinking and let other's opinions hold more weight in your mind than your own, feeding it with all that's wrong in the world, it can be really challenging to gain speed on this new path you've chosen of taking responsibility. Most people would rather commiserate in misery than step into uncharted territory and harbor their resources to change themselves. Part of maintaining the power you've been given is creating good boundaries in your life so you don't feel pulled down, away from this new road you've chosen, and this can mean moving away from some people who do pull you down. As the world's most successful business people do, you should consider keeping only those who are honest, optimistic, faithful, nonjudgmental, genuine and kind around you. Break away from anyone who leaves you feeling down, drained, tired, cynical or pessimistic. If it's not feeding you and your spirit, it is not useful at this time. Taking up this practice won't keep all the negatives out of your life—life by nature requires both positive and negative forces, it seems—but it will free up far more space for good and decrease the probability of negativity thwarting your progress.

Is the substance or activity you've chosen to abuse, whether that's food, alcohol, street or prescription drugs, overworking, an affair, spending beyond your means, gambling, or any other activity you wish to break free from actually helping you get more from your life and invest in your future? For me, it certainly did not help in either of these ways. In fact, it probably made things much worse. I would bet whatever you are using to "help" is only exacerbating an already bad situation.

During this time of difficulty in my life, I isolated myself from others. I had felt I was protecting myself but this left me with no friends, no support, no places to go and nowhere to escape, meaning I didn't have any positive streams of energy flowing into my life. If a river loses all the streams that feed it, what happens to it? It becomes stagnant and all life dies. No man is an island. We were meant to

"Break away from anyone who leaves you feeling down, drained, tired, cynical or pessimistic. If it's not feeding you and your spirit, it is not useful at this time."

interact with our environment and with other people. God would have stopped with Adam if He didn't intend for us to be interdependent. If I'd created a positive way of dealing with my mom's addicted behavior instead of trying to escape by creating my own addiction to junk food, then my problems likely would have lessened, my outlook would had been better, and my situation would have rapidly improved.

Create a Legendary Life

The wonderful truth I came to appreciate about America is that we all can create whatever life we want. If you want more than you currently have in any area of your life, then you have to invest more in yourself. When you have more within yourself, then you have more to give to others. This is just a simple truth. Everyone in the world is not so lucky. Do you want better health? You can create it. Do you want to lose weight? You can. Do you want a better relationship with your spouse, your siblings or your kids? You can make that happen. Do you want unlimited wealth? You can have it. You are in the right place and reading the right book.

If you're questioning whether this is really true then I'll ask you a question. Do you know of anyone who has started with nothing and ended up with a legendary life? If you can't think of anyone, then you've found one without meaning to, because you're reading a book by one such guy. I have done it. My clients have done it. And other people completely unrelated to me have done it. You can join us in leading by example when you enact what I'm teaching. And there are many more examples. John Paul DeJoria, the man behind a hair-care empire and Patrón Tequila, with a net worth of over $4 billion, lived in a foster home and later a car in his early years. Oracle's Larry Ellison was raised by his aunt, and when she died he had to drop out of college and work odd jobs just to get by. Current net worth? Over $40 billion. Oprah, one of the most successful women the world has ever seen, was born to an unwed and unresponsive mother and was raped by numerous male relatives from the time she was nine years old. She is currently worth over $3 billion. These are just a few examples based on wealth, because those are the stories we hear. But there are plenty of people who make small choices every day that save their marriages, improve their friendships and give them a healthier, happier life.

And of course you know my story. My life improved in ways I would never have dreamed possible. I grew up poor, bullied, morbidly obese and lonely, with an addicted and abusive

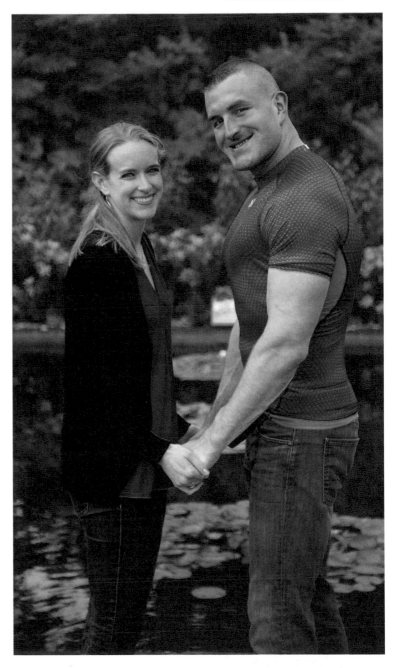

"If you want more than you currently have in any area of your life, then you have to invest more in yourself. When you have more within yourself, then you have more to give to others."

mother. I now have an incredibly good income, I am well respected and sought out for help by people around the world (including some of the very people who used to bully me!) I'm extremely fit and I have found an incredibly wonderful and beautiful woman who is the love of my life.

How did I do it?

The first step was to stop blaming others for being where I was. In fact, I'll go one step further. It's almost irrelevant what brought you to the place you are today, and it's almost irrelevant whatever challenges you have to face each day in order to get to where you want to be. The past's only relevance in your life is its service to your future goals. If it undermines your character, your vision and goals for the future, it's irrelevant. If you want it to serve you, ask what lessons it offered, take them, apply them, and move forward!

"It's almost irrelevant what brought you to the place you are today, and it's almost irrelevant whatever challenges you have to face each day in order to get to where you want to be. The past's only relevance in your life is its service to your future goals."

It's the choices you make every day, those seemingly insignificant ones, that create whatever your future will be for you. Not the place you live, the people you work for or even the person you marry. The time you wake up and go to sleep, where and what your focus is on day after day, how much you are mindlessly online surfing the web rather than being constructive with the hours each of us have, the food you are eating or skipping, the people you are associating with and allowing access to your innermost circle, the calls you are making or not making, the e-mails you do or do not send, the systems

you put in place and hold yourself to—these small daily choices compound, taking you higher and higher on the success ladder when you are consistent in your discipline. Success and failure, along with every little thing you have and everything you are, come from the small choices you make every day.

Begin to think of all these areas:

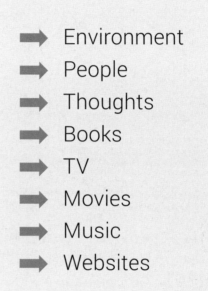

➡ Environment
➡ People
➡ Thoughts
➡ Books
➡ TV
➡ Movies
➡ Music
➡ Websites

Are the things that fall in these categories in your daily life in alignment with how you want your life to go, or are they filled with drama, despair and negativity? While you can't control the world, you can control *your* world and you can engineer your life. You get to be the choicemaker as to where you go, who you talk and listen to, which thoughts you focus on, whether or not you read empowering books and biographies. You choose if the shows you watch motivate and inspire you or activate fear and doubt; if the music you listen to cultivates creativity or depresses and angers you; if you are on websites that help you develop yourself or are mindless dribble or worse, bring up negativity and despair. It's all up to you!

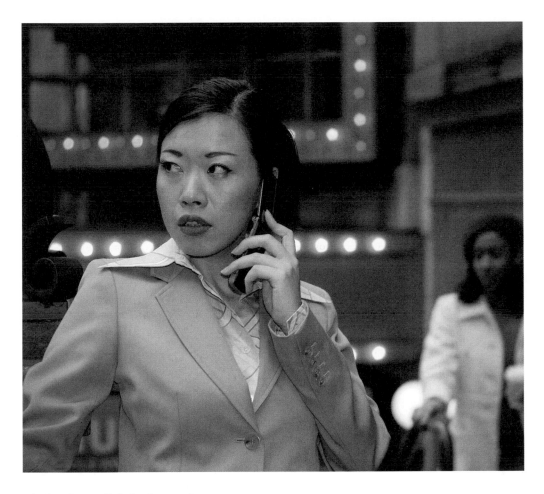

It's also the small daily choices that create your relationships. If you're at work all the time day in and day out and your kids always want to do things with you but you're never there, then a vacation to Disneyland is not going to make your relationship thrive. Taking a little bit of time each day to listen to them, help them with their homework and play with them? That will. We don't remember everything, but we remember special heart-felt emotion-filled, intimate moments, and as Maya Angelou famously said, we certainly remember the way a person makes us feel.

If you need to lose weight, then you can read a million books, you can plan, you can do some drastic fast and cleanse for a week, but none of those things are going to make you truly lose weight and be healthy. What will make

"While you can't control the world, you can control your world and you can engineer your life."

you lose weight and keep it off is choosing every day to eat the right foods in the right quantities, consistently and throughout your life. That is taking responsibility. You can define it as the willingness to pay the price for the desired outcome you're after, because one thing we all agree on is that everything has its price.

Are you waiting for a miracle? If you want to save money do you just say, either I win the lottery or I don't save? Heck no! The most effective strategy is to save a little out of each

"Forgiveness is the antidote to blame, and liberates you to move on with your life."

paycheck, intelligently invest it somewhere you cannot access it, and over time it will grow. You make small choices, consistently. My friend Tony Robbins has always taught, you'll never earn your way to being rich. That only comes from investing.

People who make these choices and who do succeed at their goals do not have perfect lives where nothing challenges them. In fact, I've found the ultra-successful have often had the highest highs and lowest lows. It's just the lows don't make the paper. Bankruptcies, failed marriages, even being disowned by family we were once close to—our lives are all riddled with difficulties. We gain experience, and experience is often the result of making bad choices earlier in life!

My poverty, losing my wonderful mother to addiction and abuse, losing my father because he left his abusive and addicted wife, being bullied, friendless and obese... all of these could be and were my excuses until I finally realized they could not continue to be my excuses if I wanted to succeed in life. I didn't want to keep finding reasons why I couldn't lose weight; I wanted to lose weight! I didn't want more excuses for failure; I wanted to succeed. And that meant accepting the responsibility for my future. If you want to create lasting change, then you have to be prepared to make changes, and you absolutely have to accept that you are the captain of your destiny.

To get to this place of taking full responsibility and moving forward toward a life you've designed for yourself you have to be ready to forgive. Forgiveness is the antidote to blame, and liberates you to move on with your life. It means realizing that all those in your life had their own needs they were trying to meet, and while your ego would love for you to believe you were the center of the entire universe, I'm sorry to break it to you, you weren't. The tragedy and abuse you suffered would have been thrust upon another person with another name if you hadn't been in that role.

You need to recognize all of us are working on ourselves on this planet called Earth. I look at this life as a spiritual training ground. We all come here with certain lessons we need to learn to develop more fully in the image of our Creator, and like Super Mario, we are bound to repeat the level over and over in our life until we learn the lesson. I think it's why you see people go from relationship to relationship, suffering the same type of disappointment with a partner of a different name. It's why we see people go from diet to diet, telling themselves they've tried everything. They've tried everything except the only thing that really works—personal responsibility for their own consistent actions.

Forgive yourself for past efforts that didn't turn out the way you'd have liked. You can be better for it. Forgive your parents for not giving you what you think you needed. Know they did the best with what they had, and were only human too, and they gave you a far greater gift, the gift of truth in the form of experience, teaching you that you never really needed what you thought you did. All you needed was within you all along. Here you are today in spite of it all, able to read this book and make the choice that your future is now yours for the making.

CHAPTER FOUR

Emotional Voids and How NOT to Fill Them

Chances are, you can easily think of a time when you attempted to fill an emotional void with something that could not possibly fill that void. Our pop culture is so replete with such anecdotes that this reaction is actually expected: your boyfriend or girlfriend breaks up with you and you sit on the couch watching an entire season of a TV show, tears streaming down your face, while devouring ice cream straight from the half-gallon container. You lose your job and you head to the bar to get plastered, hoping to forget why you're there in the first place.

These are negative attempts to try to numb the pain or make yourself feel better, a futile effort to fill an emptiness with a substance or activity that is incapable of filling it. Or maybe instead of consuming something that's not a great choice, you do something negative to get the feeling you're after. Perhaps after a particularly bad argument with your partner you vengefully flirt with others to make yourself feel more attractive and significant.

The emptiness you feel within is caused by your perception, whether conscious or unconscious, of the absence of a relationship. This absent relationship you sense might be with yourself, with another person or with your Creator. It can obviously not be filled or solved by something physical like ice cream, but this is a common and almost predictable response: You feel bad, and so you reach out blindly for something that you think will make you feel better.

That better feeling is short lived, however. Inevitably, after an experience like this, you actually end up feeling worse. Isn't

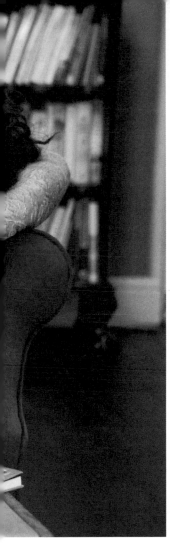

that true? A rush of regret and remorse floods you seconds after the taste leaves your mouth. Now you still have the circumstance that made you feel bad—the breakup, the loneliness you feel or the unexpected job loss—but you also have the sick feeling and lethargy that comes from whatever you did to delude yourself from the truth. You have a "hangover," whether in the traditional sense from drinking too much, in a physical sense, feeling horrible from overindulgence in junk food or another state-changing substance, or even in an emotional sense, feeling rotten because you flirted (or more) with a person other than your partner. The reality is, you're no better from this pattern and nor is the situation.

These are what you might refer to as acute versus chronic reactions. If the vast majority of time you respond constructively and make positive choices and this behavior on your part is limited to exceedingly rare times when something truly devastating has happened, then you probably will not be negatively affected by it moving forward, while it still isn't positive. If, however, you are relying on substances or actions outside of yourself on a regular basis, then this is a chronic situation and is definitely having a negative effect on your life and your goals.

"Weight loss is simple: eat less and do more. We all know this. To not choose it indicates something beneath the surface you must tend to if you are going to have a breakthrough."

Bear in mind that your life's chief aim is personal development. All things in nature grow to their fullest potential. Only we humans can interfere with that growth process in ourselves, since God made us in His image, creators in our own right. We can create extraordinary things that make life magical, or we can create terrible circumstances for ourselves and others, because we have the will and freedom to choose where we put our energy. Usually when you find yourself compulsively acting out in a destructive way, it's because you haven't been able to channel your energy constructively. Once you turn your creative energies in a positive direction, destruction will cease.

For those of us who do not limit destructive and painful behavior to rare occasions, making this shift back into being a creator of our life is as much a challenge as a blessing. In these cases, a person might continuously use ineffective substances or experiences to try to fill some sort of emptiness. You might be able to relate to this. It was definitely how I once felt. At an early stage of my life I used junk food to try and fill many needs. Junk food was my best friend, my comfort, my company, my reward, my celebration, my distraction and my consolation.

You've got to be honest and real with yourself. What are you not dealing with or not achieving by letting this behavior continue? Let's say you have more than a few pounds to lose. If you're honest with yourself, you come to the realization that you've undoubtedly been using food as more than just a way to provide nutrition for your body. Weight loss is simple: eat less and do more. We all know this. To not choose it indicates something beneath the surface you must tend to if you are going to have a breakthrough.

The same holds true no matter what habit or limiting behavior you're finding difficult to rein in control of right now. Maybe too many hours at work instead of at home. Maybe more time on your iPad than you spend with your kids. If you use drugs or alcohol on a regular basis, then you are probably using these things in a way you are not consciously intending and instead are using them to mask real feelings of loneliness, spiritual emptiness or other emotions that you find difficult to deal with in the moment.

The most challenging changes to make are those that have an emotional connection. They say that while quitting smoking is difficult for everyone, considering its strongly chemically addictive nature, for some people quitting is especially difficult because they don't only have the physiological component to handle, they have the emotional. To them, cigarettes feel like friends. This might be difficult for a non-smoker to understand, but maybe you can relate in other ways. Do you feel you are more real in your online life, or that your online "friends" know you better than your real friends do? Or maybe you feel an emotional connection to eating your favorite foods?

That's definitely how I used the unhealthy food I filled my life with, and I think most people who have an unhealthy relationship with food or anything else can relate. Logically, you know this emotional replacement cannot work, but your reaction to emotions isn't always logical. You have to look a bit deeper and be purposeful in committing yourself to bringing reason to the way you feel, challenging yourself, so you can be more clear in making choices for yourself moving forward. Clear thinking leads to a clear future.

Ineffective Solutions

Unhealthy foods, drugs and alcohol are common and even stereotypical choices for people trying to fill a void, like in the "acute" examples I gave above. Abusing junk food, alcohol and drugs are common long-term coping, void-filling mechanisms, but there are almost as many ineffective and negative ways of dealing with these voids as there are people feeling them. Here are some other examples:

- After a few years of marriage and having children, a couple begins to experience strains in their marriage. Rather than proactively dealing with the difficulties and finding a solution, one of the partners has an affair.

- An individual has a difficult time opening up enough for a long-term relationship but is hungry for love, and so engages in frequent sexual encounters with virtual strangers using apps to connect easily, risking not only their spiritual health but also their physical health, through the risk of STIs, and even life itself, through entering into potentially dangerous situations.

- Instead of doing the necessary work to complete a big project or study for an important exam, a person watches hour after hour of Internet porn.

- A person who struggles with interdependent relationships such as family begins to work more and longer hours, because at work he or she feels validated and in control in the workplace.

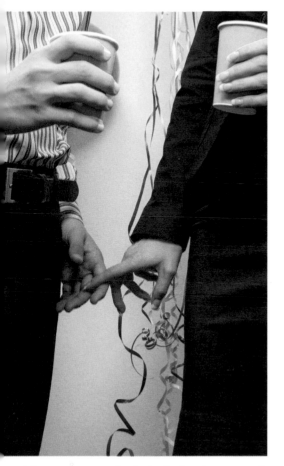

lives, and this can cause destructive behavior in even the most well-adjusted person, for short periods of time.

Dealing with emotional issues takes skill, but it is something many of us never learn to do properly. I've never seen a course in school on "emotional and relationship success." Perhaps if schools offered such courses our country would be more peaceful! Since these skills are incredibly important to your well-being and you did not learn them in school, you must begin to take it upon yourself to educate your feelings so the habits that are no longer serving you get replaced with those that will.

Time for an Upgrade

If you've ever taken music lessons or if you've been coached to play a sport or compete in another activity you may have heard something along these lines: "You're holding your hands incorrectly. You need to break this bad habit and learn how to hold them correctly before you can make any progress."

"To make any progress in life, we have to take a look at the things that might have served us well up until now, check whether or not they still are useful or if it's time for an upgrade."

The way we as individuals deal with emotional voids or negative situations depends on a number of factors, including our physiology, our self-confidence, our coping skills, our support of family and friends or the absence thereof, the circumstances that create those voids and how large the voids are. We all have things in life we must cope with and learn from. And while a person who had a healthy, strong and communicative family life growing up is generally better equipped to acquire healthy coping mechanisms, this is not always the case. Some of the most dysfunctional people come from supportive and wealthy upbringings. Some of the most well-adjusted come from the greatest dysfunction. I've discovered in my years of coaching that each person is unique and there isn't a rule of thumb. Some people have far more to cope with at certain times in their

If you're like I used to be, you might find yourself thinking: 'Hey that's the way I do it. It's worked well for me so far, so how bad can it be?' A part of you doesn't want to give up your way since it's so familiar and well practiced, and besides, you have improved tremendously since you began! But your coach or teacher sees that this habit is limiting and will allow you to go only so far. You may have progressed from the beginning, but later on when you are trying to get better at playing piano and you allow your wrists to fall, then you will not be able to reach the keys quickly enough to play a more complicated piece. If you're holding the guitar with the neck turned to the side, by the time you are learning to move quickly from one complicated chord to another, your fingers will not press the strings down properly.

Ineffective coping mechanisms are much like this. To make any progress in life, we have to take a look at the things that might have served us well up until now, check whether or not they still are useful or if it's time for an upgrade.

When you're young and your family is experiencing strife then you might get relief by hiding away in your room with your earphones on because it's the best you can do at that stage, but if later on in life your reaction to family strife is to hide away, you soon realize that the strategy that worked so well when you were dealing with your kid brother and parents doesn't work well with your partner or your children. You will start to notice you're having family relationship issues that can balloon to catastrophic proportions if they go on unchecked.

Optimally, we would grow up surrounded by people who deal with challenges in a positive and effective manner and who teach us to do the same, but most of us are not so lucky. Most people never get to learn from a good coach or helping professional. When we are young we see our parents deal with things negatively, we get tormented at school, we suffer from harm at the hands of others, people in our lives suffer from addictions or mental illness, and we deal with these things in whatever ways we figure out for ourselves. We come up with whatever story or reaction will help us survive in the now, and we never question it moving forward.

The person who escaped family strife by shutting himself away in his room listening to music might deal with family strife as an adult by shutting himself away still listening to music or watching YouTube but now adds a case of beer to the experience, escaping in two ways and causing even more of a problem. Typically, a person who uses these negative tools to try and fill (in reality, mask) the emptiness within will require more and more of them to achieve the same effect.

Such was the case with my mom. One sleeping pill turned into two, into five, into painkillers washed down with alcohol. This leads to an increased tolerance and even worse behavior, often ultimately costing the user's life, either literally, through death, or through living a life he or she does not want. The person who was given junk food to make himself feel better when being bullied at school—me—learns to use that habit as a way to get through anything unpleasant. A little here and there becomes more and more until the situation appears completely out of control. These habits can become so practiced that we equate them with who we are and begin to define ourselves with labels that take into account this pattern: addict, junk-food junkie, etc.

These unpleasant times and choices we make are often closely related to the emotional void I mentioned earlier. When everything is going your way—you've just got a new job in your field, you're in a program you like at school, you've begun seeing a new person and you're falling in love—you feel that all is right in the world. Your life is matching the way you think it should be for you. It's easy to avoid negative behaviors because you are feeling content and fulfilled. But life continually unfolds, and for growth to occur, there has to be trauma. Any breakthrough in life comes with pain. Look at childbirth—we call it labor for a reason!

Even if you are fortunate enough not to have to suffer through anything particularly tragic, it's divine and natural to want more because

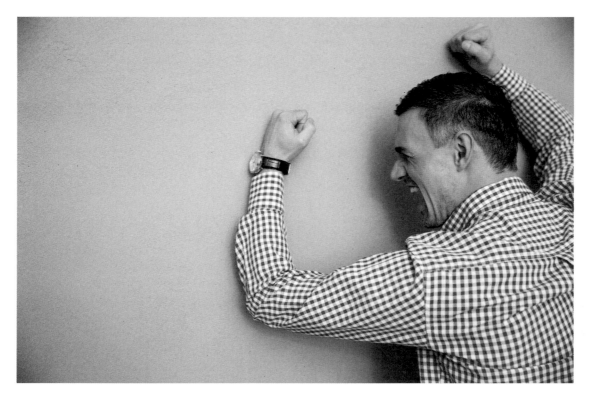

the desire itself leads us to becoming more of who God created us to be. It's what we were created to feel, so that we each could make this planet better. All parents want more for their children, and I think that's a good thing because that is how we create enriching experiences and leave the world better for those we love.

Feeling Emptiness

During this process of growth and creation, there will be times when you might feel something is missing. Instead of trying to fill that empty place, come to accept that this feeling is part of our human condition. It's not that something is missing, but rather, there is still more for you to achieve, have and do. We can be happy with where we are and what we currently have while still aiming for more in our own unique journey. When we come to this understanding, the pressure decreases im-

"You must destroy the enemy of self-doubt in your own mind. When you have, you will be free of needing anyone's approval. You will be a free thinker designing your life on your own terms."

mediately and peace comes in its place. If we don't learn to shift our awareness to a higher level in this way, we will continue to mistakenly feel an emptiness that we feel compelled to fill, and what we attempt to fill it with can often be very negative in its long-term effect on us and those around us.

As addiction counselors know well, addictions do not begin when a person starts taking drugs or drinking alcohol. Long before that fateful day, the person felt the need to fill an emptiness within. The truth is, there is no emptiness in you! It's all words! Be careful in your language. The word "emptiness" denotes that there is a void, which often stems from some kind of abuse or neglect. In extreme circumstances this might be severe physical or sexual abuse, which so often result in addiction issues. In an effort for those who suffered the abuse to numb the pain of their feelings, which they might find unbearable, they use something to try to stop the thinking that brings those feelings about. Really it's not the feeling that's numbed; it's the thought process that brings them there. Repeated use of this substance can lead right back to those feelings in an even more extreme way, which leads to greater substance abuse as they try harder and harder to reach that numbing point.

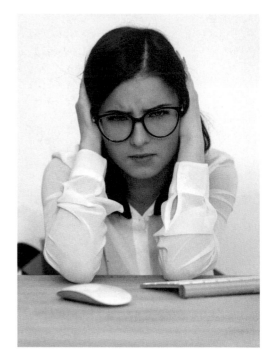

"You don't have to suffer the negative experiences of letting others define you."

There are many reasons a person might fall into destructive habits we call addictions. This empty, void feeling can result from neglect, when you do not receive the security and love necessary for healthy survival, or it can come from verbal abuse, people telling you through words or actions that you are not good enough or worthy enough. Children are open-minded, and often believe what those around them are saying. At that early point in our lives we do not feel we are the authority, since our life is literally dependent on whether or not another cares for us. I certainly accepted the opinion of others like it was gospel, never questioning its intent or validity. That is one disadvantage of being an unsophisticated learner—you find that you inadvertently take everything as fact, since you're so hungry to learn! It's easy to mistakenly consider everyone an authority. Companies take advantage of this in their marketing tactics, knowing that if their product looks prestigious or attractive, they will be more effective in influencing you to "buy into" whatever is being sold.

Despite this, being a learner ultimately serves you well, as I have a core belief that everyone you encounter is a teacher with a lesson to offer you that can add tremendous value to your life. Sometimes the lesson isn't to tell you who you are—it's to remind you of who you're not! I didn't learn that until much later in life. The names my classmates called me led me to question my own identity.

You don't have to suffer the negative experiences of letting others define you as I once did, doubting who you are at the deepest of levels. You can remember this valuable advice before accepting anyone's opinion: Consider the source. Would you take investment advice from a person living under a bridge? Would you get advice about a heart condition from your mechanic? Would you take nutrition advice from an unhealthy, obese person? Of course not! In life this is normally not so obvious, but still you must learn to discriminate when choosing what to accept from others into the storehouse of your own mind. Your most valuable treasure lies between your two ears—guard it with everything you have. A person might be financially successful but personally miserable, and you will find those who are truly successful throughout their lives will build you up, not tear you down.

Battling the Enemy Within

But destructive habits don't just come from someone cutting you down for their own messed-up purposes. The real problem, which is much more serious, is that the negative opinion resonates with something inside of you. If it didn't resonate, you wouldn't give it a second thought. The saying: "No enemy without will overtake you so long as there is no enemy within" comes to mind. So if an acquaintance says, "You're so stupid!" You're the one who chooses to give it any of your attention. The helpful question isn't "Why does he think I'm stupid?" It's "Why does that name trigger doubt in me?" You must destroy the enemy of self-doubt in your own mind. When you have, you will be free of needing anyone's approval. You will be a free thinker designing your life on your own terms.

The only opinion that matters on this planet in your life is your own. This doesn't mean you should never listen to others, but if you do allow something or someone external to influence you, be sure it's in accordance with what you truly believe to be right and good for you. If you find yourself doing things you don't want to do, buying things you don't need to own, reading, watching or listening to things that aren't adding value to your life, then you are probably listening more to what others think than you are to yourself. Let your true instinct be your guide. The more you tune out others and tune into yourself (which is, after all, listening to God, and whose opinion can be more important than that?) the more joy and peace you'll experience daily.

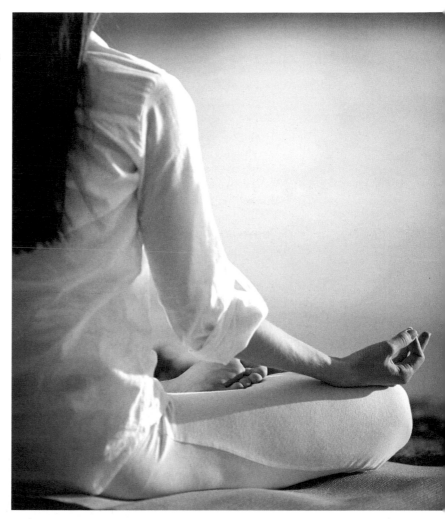

So many people spend their days feeling angry and don't know why. The reason is simple: they aren't being themselves. They are busy being someone or something for someone else at the cost of their own joy, and their spirit gets angry. To thine own self be true. Do what makes you feel good—sleep in, enjoy nature, go for a walk, turn your phone off, work out when it suits you, not when you "should" because someone told you it's more effective at that time. Answer your e-mails just one time each day. You don't have to explain your choices or justify them to anyone. See how much better you feel after a week of living in the way that is right for you. As long as these choices aren't hurting you or anyone else, start the practice today!

You can learn from my early errors internalizing the negative things my classmates said. Challenge the doubters. Believe in yourself. You are the architect of your life, and your worth does not depend on someone else's self-limiting beliefs—which are often just a reflection of their own perceived limitations. They don't know the real you and they definitely don't know what you're capable of. Don't substitute their opinion for God's promise in your life!

True Rewards

As I mentioned earlier, I can say most of the ways I was different from the average person ended up benefiting me later in life. I was different because of my size, but also I was mature and got along well with adults. I was a sponge for learning, and loved reading. Who wouldn't want their kid to read a lot, enjoy learning and have positive relationships with teachers? In fact, I'm sure many of my habits at that time set me on the road to my future success. But when I was young my differences did not seem so positive. I would have given anything to be like my schoolmates, to be "normal" sized and of "normal" inclinations. It would be a long time until I was to become comfortable with myself and thus develop into the confident person I am today.

Once I grew up and entered the business world, I found that difference from others was disproportionately rewarded! I quickly became very grateful for just how different I was, and so should you! Why is the tech company Apple so well liked? Because they "think different" and they are different! Colleges offer entire courses about differentiating your product and service from the competition. What a blessing that God gave me this gift! If you're "differ-

ent," you can feel just as content that He gave you the best gift as well!

But believe me, this confidence and positive outlook came much later. The troubled obese kid I once was felt a huge emptiness from evaluating myself in contrast to others. I replaced my judgment with theirs, forfeiting my own instincts and the intuitive sense that I was great the way I was. I was too scared to take the risk to just be myself in the midst of such hate, so instead I almost killed myself unintentionally by overeating. I let others direct my choices, buying into the way they had defined me. While it felt easier in the moment, those temporary good feelings were too high a price to pay, I soon found out.

If I had surrendered to external forces and others' opinions instead of learning to think for myself, I don't know that I would be here talking to you right now. I would have never claimed my birthright as a leader; I would have been another follower blindly walking through life, never really living. Sure I was Student of the Year several years in a row in high school, but my health was failing me. I could smile and tell everyone that nothing was wrong, but everything about me physically pointed to the truth. I was sad, lonely, and trying to cope. It wasn't until I finally began to build confidence in my own judgment as a junior in high school that I took charge of my life and my personhood, becoming congruent with who I was spiritually and doing what I had long known was right for me. I lost all my excess fat, earned my health back and developed the strategies I bring you today, strategies that have helped not only me but many thousands of others.

That hole I had been attempting to fill with junk food began way back in kindergarten. Maybe yours also started early. That deep pit sat dark and empty throughout my early childhood, and I never questioned it. Have you long felt something missing, like I did, but have never really chosen to look deeply at it?

Perhaps this is the moment you are beginning to understand it in the empowering way I did, and hopefully without all the years of suffering! But when and where it started isn't nearly as important as what you're going to start to do with the new perspective you now have.

I was lonely. I felt I didn't belong anywhere. School was torture. And like many people—maybe you—I attempted to fill that void with something that did nothing to help long term. I ate junk food in the morning for breakfast, on the way to school, had more junk food as snacks throughout the day, ate plate after plate of white pasta with butter at lunch, more junk food after school and all through the evening until bedtime. The problem was, of course, junk food did nothing to fill the emptiness. I just kept shoveling it in, trying subconsciously to fill that hole, but the hole just seemed to get bigger and bigger, creating a bigger chasm between who I really was and how I looked.

This is the same type of pattern we see with drug addicts, alcoholics and sex addicts. These people are trying to fill an emptiness they feel because of a lack of love in their lives or a lack of acceptance for who they truly are or some other thing they feel they are missing in the core of their being. The more we try to fill our emotional or spiritual voids with inappropriate things, the bigger those empty spaces become, and the more we shovel into them, and the farther we move from our true spiritual nature. The emptiness does not begin to be filled and we don't begin to feel fulfilled until we find the appropriate thing to fill it with. The devil wins a little more territory in your life every time you replace loving the divinity within yourself with seeking something outside. You need to realize that. At some level, even the person who's in the deepest throes of addiction hates the habit.

"Start to think more accurately and clearly. Clear headedness without erroneous emotion is essential to your success."

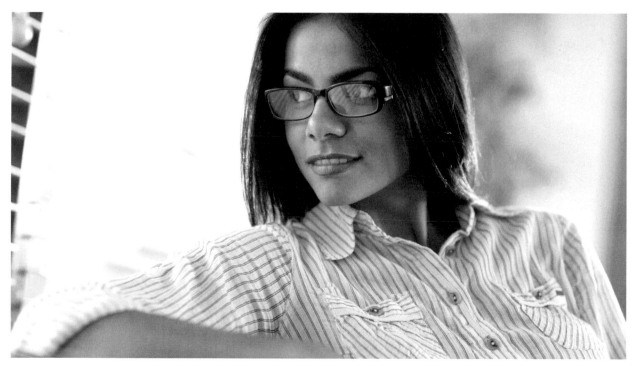

For me, that void I'd felt for so long began to be filled when I came to a number of realizations, mainly the following:

1. I am good enough as I am, other than the physical state I've put myself in because of being overfat.

2. My life and future are completely dependent on me and my choices from this second onward. Period.

3. I have complete control over what I do and think, regardless of what happens and what others say or do. Everything and everyone else is irrelevant to my future.

4. Where I end up tomorrow, how I feel about myself and my life and what I do or not do are all choices I must think about and make every day.

5. I have a purpose and mission in life that requires me to become more than I am right now. God intends that each and every one of us helps the community around us in some way.

Shifting Perception

As a teen, when I woke up the next morning after drifting off to sleep having just begged God for His help, telling Him I would spend the rest of my life helping others to become more if He would help me, I knew for certain that this had been God's intention for me all along. Something clicked. After that point, I didn't experience struggle in getting in shape, because I was no longer trying to fill a void. It was like the change from obese to fit had already occurred—I just needed the fat and muscle of my body to catch up.

The first step you can take in making such a shift is to change the way you perceive things. Start to think more accurately and clearly. Clear headedness without erroneous emotion is essential to your success. How you feel in the moment, if it's anything less than helpful, has to become irrelevant when it comes to designing your future. Instead of saying, "I feel so empty" say, "I am focusing on things that would make anyone feel like life is pointless. What can I focus on now that will immediately change the state I'm in to a much more resourceful and positive one?" That simple shift in how you are thinking changes everything.

When I was young, I hated Sundays. As soon as the sun began setting, a terrible mood would inevitably descend on me. When I started to examine my thinking I realized that an unconscious cascade of thoughts were in the background of my consciousness. Thoughts like, "This week is going to suck." "I wonder how many kids are going to make fun of me." "I know gym class is going to be embarrassing." "I wonder if Mom will be drunk tomorrow morning." "Will we even be able to get to school?" These were some of the statements that played continuously in the back of my mind. I wasn't consciously giving attention to them, but nonetheless they were operating and using up a lot of my mental RAM, like a window open on your computer that's hidden by the one you're typing on.

Think about the thoughts behind your feelings. They're there, even if you're not used to giving them your attention. Look for them and be sure they are not robbing you of vital energy that can be invested in your future! If you find yourself despondent about your job, thinking: "My boss hates me!" you can shift to "I wonder what could be going on in my boss' life that has her so upset all of the time." Rather than personalizing it, ask yourself about what else could be going on that is creating the turmoil you're picking up on. More often than not, it's not you!

A woman I know says she's afraid of heights. She isn't really afraid of heights; rather, she can make herself get extremely anxious when she focuses her thoughts in ways that promote fear. When she had to go to the top of a skyscraper for a business matter, she was able to do it by changing her focus, proving it's possible. She had just practiced the state of "fear" more than she had practiced the state of "confidence." These states are often the result of the inner dialogue that's going on in our heads 24/7, with the feelings that emerge coming from the way we are framing things in our minds and the way we are asking questions.

Sometimes the destructive things we do are in response to earlier influences. I helped a woman whose mom struggled with her weight all of her life and so put inordinate pressure on her teen daughter, who didn't have any weight issue. The mother made her attend Weight Watchers meetings, keep a food journal and weigh herself every day. If she was even ounces off what her mom thought she "should" weigh, she would be berated and often brought to tears. The mom would constantly whisper judgments about other women to her daughter when they were in malls or other public places and she saw someone she deemed as unfit. The mom had never taken charge of her own weight issues, but rather displaced them on her innocent daughter.

The daughter swore she would never be like her mom but found as she neared her 20s she began compulsively eating things that were not healthy. In an effort to control this new behavior, she became very strict. She soon started cycling between binging after long periods of deprivation, and starving herself, punishing herself for the choices she felt guilty for having indulged in. She would spend hours in the gym, not allowing even water, just so she could maintain some arbitrary and very unhealthy number on her scale.

"Every time you turn to food, a drug or other negative 'void-filling' behavior for an answer, you are silently telling yourself 'I have no power over this problem.'"

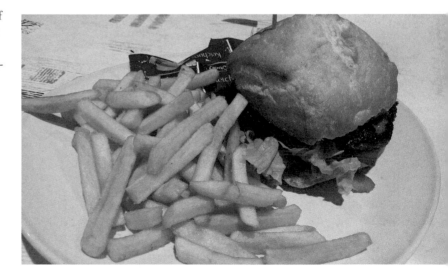

This self-loathing cycle continued until she sought therapy, but still wasn't fully resolved there. She substituted the therapist's relationship for the addictive behavior she'd engaged in, so when the therapist moved away, she was back to square one, eating so much food she found it difficult to go out in public. She would eat until she was beyond full, hating it so much she'd throw the junk food out in the garbage, later finding herself picking through the garbage to eat the remnants of half-eaten cookies. Her weight ballooned some 80 pounds. She was losing all confidence in herself and all purpose in her life.

A client referred her to me for a spiritual perspective. After some digging, she came to discover she was acting out against her mom. When she could see that she didn't need to prove to her mom that she was in charge of her weight and life, the self destructive choices left her, like a demon leaving a person after an exorcism. Her face, which had been tense, instantly relaxed with the realization this pattern was simply an effort to get back at her mom!

"First, you must recognize that your behavior, which may not even make sense to you, stems from the need to fill something you feel is missing inside you."

I asked her if being fat and unhealthy was the best way she could come up with to confront her mom for being so harsh and for projecting her own issues on her when she was a child. She said she'd never thought of it that way, and decided to call her mom and tell her just how much hatred she harbored. She told her mom she'd never felt good enough, that her mom had been too critical and that she never felt truly loved, but also that she forgave her, knew her mom did the best she could given the place she was making choices from, and hoped her mom would learn to love herself too. She wrote to me months after this breakthrough, saying she now enjoyed a healthy daily eating plan and exercised just enough to enjoy life, with no more excess or deprivation.

As kids, we have to do what we can to get by and survive with our limited life experience and, usually, lack of positive coping skills. But to have our best life we must learn to respond instead of react once we're no longer completely dependent on another person. Once you understand the directing role you have in your own life and the mission or purpose you have, making the daily choices necessary to bring you to the place you want to be becomes easy. And the choices you're making that are keeping you from realizing all you can be don't have to be extreme to be damaging. They can be as seemingly innocuous as watching too much TV or YouTube and not accomplishing the things you want to accomplish, spending too much time hanging out in bars or cafés wasting your time and spending your precious moments with people who are less than you are or could be. Any of these activities you choose will take away from the quality of your life and bring you to a place you don't want to be instead of adding to your life and bringing you to a place of fulfillment.

Every time you turn to food, a drug or other negative "void-filling" behavior for an answer, you are silently telling yourself "I have no power over this problem." Stop that pattern today. No one and nothing can give you the life you can give yourself. You need to begin to trust that all the power you need is within you at this very moment to take charge of anything you want to change about your life. There is not any void within you, there is a void only in your ability to understand the feeling you are having and use constructive language to grasp it. That's all. You can fill that gap by bringing your awareness to it. God equipped you with a mind to be able to do just that.

Focus on Giving

Relationships, or lack thereof, often bring about this feeling of emptiness. When you have a good relationship with yourself, rela-

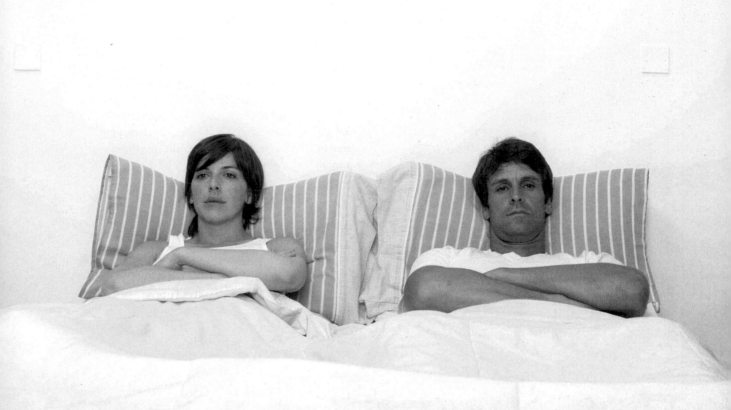

tionships with others are places you go to give, not to receive. Even in the most intimate of relationships, like a dating relationship or marriage, you and your spouse or partner might be having difficulties. You may have gotten to the point where you're openly hostile to one another, where you don't feel supported or that it's even a true partnership anymore. You may fight a lot or you may find your spouse antagonistic. You may find yourself reacting antagonistically as well.

If your relationship has devolved to this point, then it's extremely common for one or both partners to react to the negativity in an even more negative way — by drinking too much, eating gallons of ice cream, going shopping for "retail therapy" or even by secretly spending time with someone of the opposite sex instead

"The first step is to understand what your partner needs from you before trying to get what you feel you need. From that point, you can work on the relationship."

of your spouse, whether just flirting and talking or having a full-blown affair or anything in between. This happens. You are attempting to fill a void in your life with things that do not, will not and cannot fill that void, and in so doing you make the void even larger.

Maybe "this is as good as it can be" has become your mantra. It simply isn't true. This is a yet another challenge for you to grow from. You can lower your expectations like many do, trying to explain away the responsibility you have in either making the relationship better, or in truly doing everything possible, allowing you to leave guilt free so the person you love is liberated and can grow as well. Staying in an unhealthy relationship too long—something

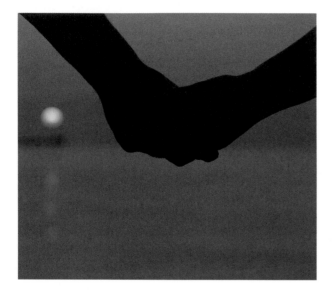

> *"We all feel conflicted when we make choices based around what we believe is best for others, but look at things rationally: when you do something that makes you unhappy, you are not adding value to any relationship you're in."*

we have all certainly been guilty of—is doing nobody any good, including your partner. Not only are you delaying the inevitable, but do you really think your partner doesn't notice that you haven't had sex in three months? Get real. If you're unhappy then your partner is too. Grow up and deal with it in a loving and mature way.

The first step is to understand what your partner needs from you before trying to get what you feel you need. From that point, you can work on the relationship. If you both deem

the relationship to be something you want to commit to, something bigger than the both of you are individually, then you have much hope. If not, then lovingly let each other go to move on and grow independently or into another relationship. The bottom line is that it all starts with you. Make the decision you will be happy with. We all feel conflicted when we make choices based around what we believe is best for others, but look at things rationally: when you do something that makes you unhappy, you are not adding value to any relationship you're in. Face the reality that you have to choose to do something you feel at peace with and you can walk away feeling good about. Own it.

You do not have to be in a truly antagonistic relationship to feel like something is missing. You and your spouse may have grown in different directions while distracted from the relationship raising kids or running a business, as was the case with my parents. Or you may just not feel a physical passion anymore. You are aching to feel the spark you once did. I wouldn't interpret this as the end of the relationship. If you're married long enough, it's not unusual to go through periods of wax and wane in passion. Something peeves you or resentment can stack up and erode attraction. Sometimes passion needs to be worked on, and this, in our world where we're so influenced by fictional romance and fictional sex, seems wrong somehow, but it's not. It's normal. Do things that make your partner feel attracted to you and you will get what you're looking for. Give what you want and you'll find it will come back, if you're patient and consistent.

Perhaps your situation is a bit different and you're not in a committed relationship right now at all. Your relationship ended a while back, you are having a hard time finding someone to be with and so are now trying to fill that emotional void with meaningless sex. Having a strong relationship and connection to others is important to our sense of contentment and well-being, and not having one can cause strong feelings of emptiness, whether you are in an unhappy relationship or not in one at all. Even if you go into these sexual encounters with the full awareness that they will not offer any connection, they can leave you feeling empty. This is stereotypically the case for women but can definitely be true for men as well. The best way to feel connection when you don't have a partner, especially if your friends are in relationships or have families and are not as available to you as they once might have been, is to get out and do something for others less fortunate. This does not replace the feeling of a partnership, but it really can be helpful, both by bringing you out around others and by making you feel good about the support you've offered them.

Relationships, whether with your peers, parents, siblings, friends or a spouse, are far from the only reason people can feel an emptiness or void in their lives. There are any number of reasons for experiencing this feeling, whether or not you are aware of it. You might choose detrimental behaviors in order to try to fill the void without being aware that you're doing so. You might not even describe your feeling as an emptiness or void. You might just feel not quite satisfied with life, or feel directionless, and not even be aware that there's a serious underlying issue. With spiritual awareness you realize you are never truly alone and that we are all connected. If you lose touch with that part of your being, it's easy to fall into these human behaviors.

What is the issue for you? What hole are you trying to fill?

Whatever the source of the void and whatever the substance or negative activity you're trying to fill it with, doing so will not work long term, my friend. Eating too much, drinking too much, using drugs, working too much, going into debt because of purchases you can't afford, having dangerous or unfulfilling sexual relationships … these are all too common and

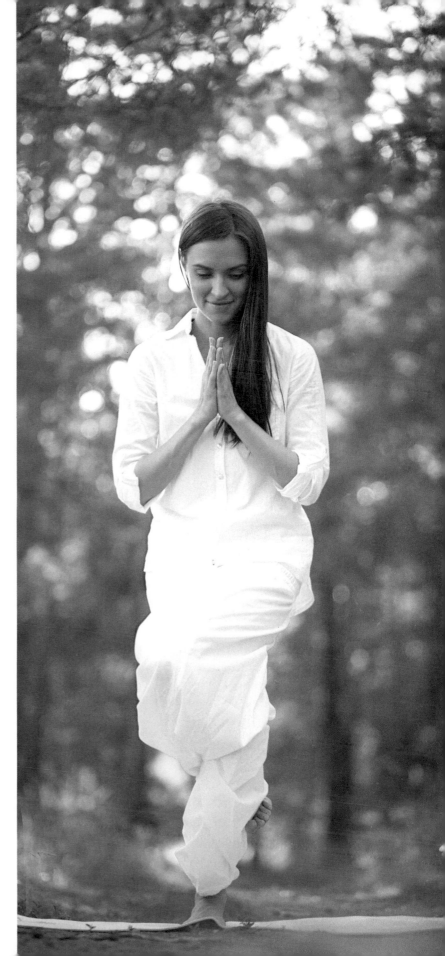

the most obvious ways we try incorrectly to fill our emotional voids. But this is like pouring water into a sieve. No matter how much you pour, it is never filled.

Worse, these negative patterns end up exacerbating and inflaming the problems you're having, causing you even more pain and emptiness in the long run. Believe me, any problems you're having with your relationship are not going to be solved by drinking, using drugs or going further into debt. And you're definitely not going to relieve your loneliness by having sex with strangers, not even if they look like Chris Hemsworth or Megan Fox.

What Does God Want You to Do?

I'm sure you can see that these void-filling behaviors are not healthy or effective ways to go about looking after the things in your life that need looking after. Instead of sowing the seeds of health, happiness and prosperity, you are sowing the seeds of neglect. Come the fall, you will have nothing to harvest. This was clearly the case with my mother. She unknowingly neglected herself for years while looking after me and later my brother and sister. Over time she tried to fill her own unfulfilled needs

"With spiritual awareness you realize you are never truly alone and that we are all connected. If you lose touch with that part of your being, it's easy to fall into these human behaviors."

with things she had seen her own family using while she was growing up, namely alcohol and prescription drugs. She eventually paid a hefty price through a destroyed marriage, what she felt was a horrible, dysfunctional relationship with her children, financial instability and, if it

weren't for God's grace, extreme poverty. Ultimately, those same seeds of neglect resulted in her untimely death at the age of 51.

So the question is, how do you resolve this and keep such disaster out of your and your family's lives? If you have bad habits that are caused by your trying to fill a sieve with water over and over again, then how do you stop this behavior and fill the void with what you truly need?

First, you must recognize that your behavior, which may not even make sense to you, stems from the need to fill something you feel is missing inside you. Once you recognize that, you can try to figure out what that might be. If you clearly understand that your problems with drugs and alcohol stem from the feeling that you aren't good enough, that you don't deserve love or to be treated well, or even that you don't belong in the world at all, in really bad cases, then you can work toward finding an environment that's more nurturing and supporting of the magnificent creation God made: you. Find the people who love you, fulfill you and add to your life, who see the best in you when you don't see it in yourself, and who help propel you in the direction you want to go.

Second, you must decide your purpose. It can change over time, but commit to a meaningful cause today. What does God want you to do to help the world around you? If you don't know, the answer is simple; ask to be part of His work. Trust me, he will soon make it clear what he wants you to do. This was the case a short time ago when I felt I had reached most of my own goals. I had remodeled my mom's house for her after my dad's death, and was so excited by the joy it brought her that I wanted to do more. I asked God to use me to help in whatever way I could.

The next day, I listened to a podcast where an author was talking about when he met Mother Teresa. She was a guest on his radio show and he asked her after what he could do, hearing she was sleeping on the floor in a nearby hotel, refusing a bed. He wanted to help with her ministry. After several efforts at begging her to let him help, which she declined, he made headway and she caved in. She said, "Ok, if you want to help me, here's what I want you to do. Tonight, after midnight, I want you to go out deep into the city. I want you to walk for a while until you find someone homeless living on the street who believes they are alone in this world, and I want you to convince them they're not." Wow. There I was on the Step-Mill at the gym, moved to tears hearing this loving tale.

That next night, one of the most miraculous synchronies occurred. I was heading home from a movie with a friend, and he wanted to get something from the store. We went to the nearest store but it was closed, (divinely intended, as God would have it) so we had to go to a 24-hour Walmart. It was two days before Christmas. The snow was falling and

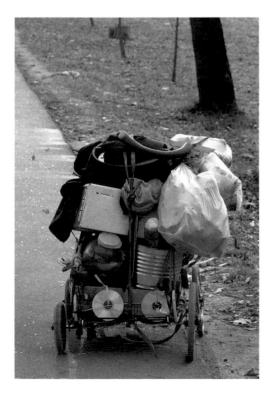

in St. Louis the wind chill was below 0. We pulled into the Walmart lot, which was all but empty aside from a snowdrift. Then I saw what appeared to be a huge heap of metal, with lit Christmas lights attached to a wheel of some sort, making its way through the lot. My friend and I were perplexed and drove closer, but couldn't make out what it was. We parked and I jogged ahead, curious to see what this could be. As I got closer I realized it wasn't just a heap of metal; it was a woman in a wheelchair, hunched over with a blanket overtop of her, one arm trying to move herself across the lot and the other pushing a pole attached to a cart in front of the wheelchair, which housed all of her belongings. I asked if I could help, noticing her bare arms. She had only a short-sleeve shirt on. I asked what she was doing and she said she was waiting. I tried not to be rude but asked who she was waiting for, since it was nearly midnight. She said not to worry, that she was fine. This didn't feel right and so I probed further. She asked that I just wheel her up against the side of the building and she would stay there. I asked if I could do or get her anything but she said no, she had all she needed.

I walked off, not feeling right and not quite understanding. My buddy said, "Hey man—she's homeless, that's what's up." Suddenly, God flashed Mother Teresa's story I heard the day before into my mind. Without a second thought I told my friend I'd be right back as I dashed back to her, knowing this was all meant to be. "Excuse me, but can I ask, would you give me the gift of letting me get you a room at the Holiday Inn?" There was one across the lot. She looked perplexed and assured me again she was fine. I knew what God wanted, so I insisted. I walked her over and paid for a week in the hotel, breakfasts included, so she would spend Christmas in warmth along with good food. God answered my prayer to be used in His work—and He will answer yours too—just ask, and listen.

We do not all have the same calling. Some are called to work with the homeless while for others it's to create a neighborhood garden, or to volunteer at a youth or senior's center. You will know what you are meant to do for the greater community by listening to your heart. Once you've heard the call, *follow it!*

Consistent Positive Choices

When you discover the cause of your empty feeling, you can fix it. Sure, you can find any excuse not to, but you can. If you hate your job, then find another. Can't find the job you want because you lack schooling or experience? Then get the schooling or experience! Sure it might take you some extra time, but the time is going to pass no matter what. Better to find yourself closer to your goal in one, two or even five years instead of farther away from it or, at best, stuck in the same place you are right now.

> Even if you can't figure out what you are lacking and therefore trying to fill, you can still resolve it. You can do this by taking positive steps in the direction you want to go, and filling your time with positive action. You may very well find that with these steps the void will fill itself, just as mine did.

Remember, consistently making the small choices that move you toward your goal will eventually bring you there. Some of those choices will be how you react when some part of you is telling you to behave in ways that are

not beneficial to your end goal. These choices will be different depending on your goal and your problem behavior, but the correct ones will help bring you to fulfilling your destiny as a successful, happy and valuable member of your community.

Instead of drinking alcohol or flirting with a stranger when you and your spouse have been arguing, how about going for a walk? This will help calm you down, it will help clear your head and it will not create the negative effect that alcohol or an affair will. Then the next time you can ask your spouse to go for a walk with you. Really?? Yes! Walking together helps create a feeling of warmth, togetherness and intimacy, and it can give an opportunity to discuss things in a non-confrontational way. So not only are you making choices that don't weaken your relationship, you're making choices that actually strengthen it! It will start to bring you both back to the place the relationship started, true presence in being with one another.

If you're trying to gain control of your finances, then going shopping when you're stressed out is the last thing you want to do! How about taking the time instead to get your paperwork in order, or negotiate a lower interest rate with your credit card companies, or arrange a consolidation loan, or see a credit counselor? Think in terms of becoming wealthy, not debt free. The wealthiest people are often the most frugal, not because they are worried about money, quite the contrary, because they respect it and are not frivolous with it. Choosing positive, constructive behavior not only helps fill your perceived void, you have also helped move yourself in the right direction.

Some issues are not so easy to resolve. If you feel unloved and unwanted then it's hard to find something to fill that void. But a very good first step is to work toward loving yourself and taking good care of yourself. If you do not love yourself then taking part in behavior you will

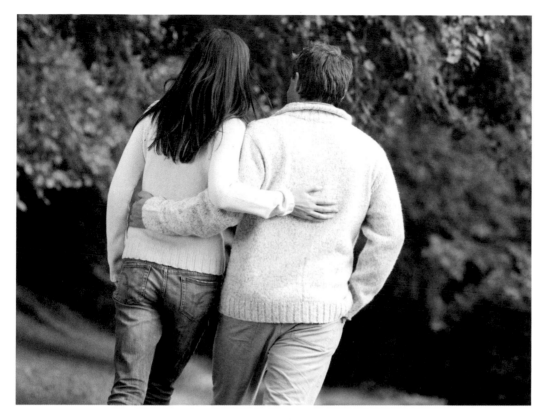

come to regret, whether that's binge eating or picking someone up at a bar, will only make you hate yourself more. Get out and do some positive things with friends, or meet people who have the same positive outlook as you do now. Taking positive steps by making these little daily choices will help you feel good about yourself, and that in turn will make you less likely to engage in those behaviors down the road.

Get some exercise. Learn how to cook a healthy meal. This does not need to be about weight loss; these are healthy habits that help keep you in a positive space. Invest in your own education, even if it's informal. Read books or articles about people who have overcome terrible odds to succeed. Read books about other things you want to learn about. Learn how to do something new, like play guitar or create stained glass.

"Remember, consistently making the small choices that move you toward your goal will eventually bring you there."

You may have heard of what I call the "defeat whirlpool," where bad thoughts or behaviors compound, bringing you further and further down to depression and negativity. There is also what I call a "success vortex!" Learn how to do new things that support your goals. Make positive choices each day. Be choosy about who you spend your time with and make sure they are worthy of you. Learn new things. Before you know it, your void will be filled with all kinds of new experiences and love for yourself. Once that happens, you will have so much love abounding within, you won't be able to do anything else but share it with others. You won't have to act loving, you will be love.

Focus on the Little, Achieve the Big!

Often we shy away from taking on major challenges because they seem overwhelming. What we fail to realize is that things that truly matter are rarely accomplished quickly or momentously. It is our small daily choices and habits that ultimately lead us to where we want to be in life. Just like drops of water make an ocean, it is the accumulation of these small everyday decisions that dictate whether our life is grand.

Here are two scenarios that illustrate how seemingly meaningless choices are incredibly important in guiding the direction of our lives, and how a little strategy and forethought can make a huge difference not only for yourself but also for everyone around you. In both you start work at 9:00AM and have a 30-minute commute:

Scenario #1

You stay up late the night before. You have a beer and eat some potato chips in front of the TV and end up staying up too late not because you're watching anything special, but just because you're feeling too lazy to move. You set your alarm for 7:30AM but when it goes off you're still tired. You push snooze. You push snooze again. By the time you get up, it's 7:50. Now you have to rush. You don't have time for a shower or breakfast because you have to get the kids up and to the school bus.

You finally leave at 8:30 on the nose, thinking

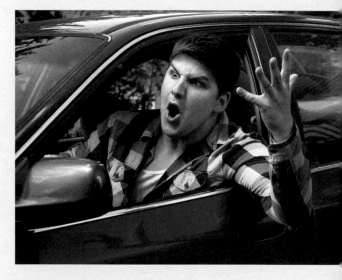

you'll make it but traffic is a little slow. You get into an irritated rage on the highway because you're not moving fast enough. You honk angrily at a driver you believe is slowing you down even more, even though you're all in the same boat. By the time you get to work it's 9:07, meaning you are late. You're also grumpy. You complain to your coworker about the traffic and snap at your assistant for no real reason. Your assistant was smiling, but not anymore. You are spreading your bad mood around the office. You're hungry but you have no time to eat, and that's putting you in a worse mood and giving you a headache. You drink your umpteenth coffee but now you're getting jittery.

Your coworkers are steering clear, so you miss it when they start talking about the new position coming available that you'd be perfect for. By the time lunch comes around you are so hungry you devour far more calories than you should, contributing to your weight problem and making you feel lethargic. Through the afternoon you're not snapping at people anymore but you're sleepy and ineffective. Your boss is not terribly pleased with your performance these days. It's not bad enough to get a warning but it's not good enough for you to move up the ladder. The afternoon passes finally and you can't wait to get home, but you just have no energy. Instead of spending the evening with your family you just want to veg in front of the TV again, and so it goes.

Scenario #2

After an evening of riding bikes in the park with your spouse and kids, you're ready for an early night. You set the alarm for 7:00AM so you have time for a healthy breakfast with your kids before getting them on the bus. You always make sure to leave yourself a few extra minutes to get to work because traffic can slow things down, so you're on the road by 8:20. Good thing. Traffic is a bit slow but you're in a good mood and unhurried so it doesn't bother you. You signal to the merging car to go ahead in front of you, figuring the driver might pay it forward later on.

You arrive at work a few minutes before 9:00, giving yourself enough time to head to the kitchen for a coffee, where you exchange pleasantries with your colleague and assistant before you begin your productive day. People enjoy your company so you're the first to know about the new position opening up. After your work is done for the morning you spend part of your lunch hour planning your approach to your boss. As you deliver your morning's accomplishments, you pitch yourself for the new job. Satisfied after a great day, you look forward to heading home to spend quality time with your family.

See how these little choices each day make such a huge difference not only in your own life, but also on the world around you? Every day, you influence your spouse and kids foremost, but also other drivers on the road, co-workers, people in line at the coffee shop and anyone else you might encounter. Most of all, those choices affect you!

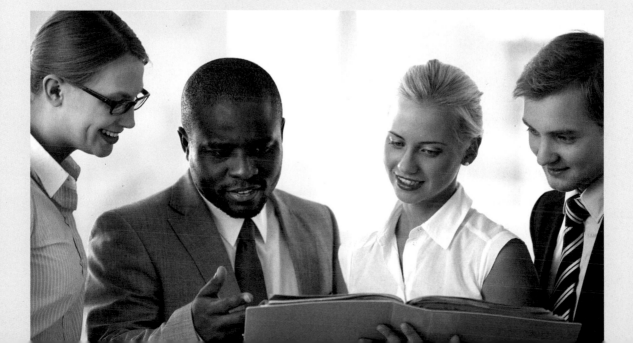

CHAPTER FIVE

You're Not Alone: Accepting God's Purpose for Your Life

"Man surprises me most ... He sacrifices his health in order to make money. Then he sacrifices money to recuperate his health. And then he is so anxious about the future that he does not enjoy the present; the result being that he does not live in the present or the future; he lives as if he is never going to die, and then dies having never really lived."—**Dalai Lama**

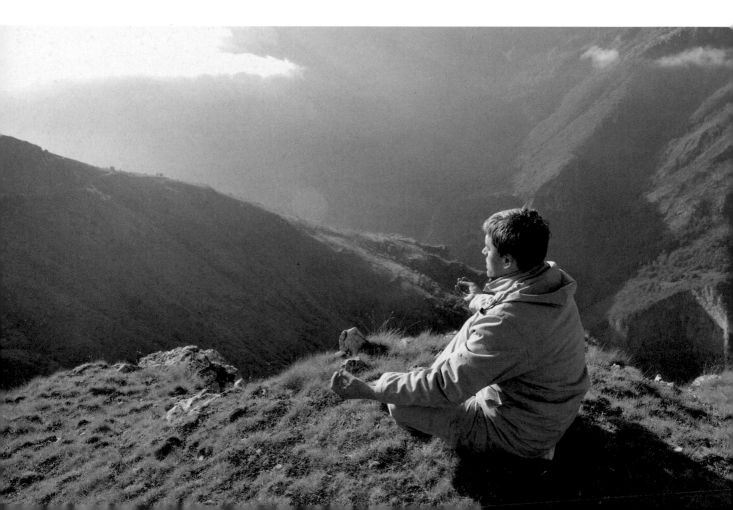

Purpose is powerful. You think something will make you happy, but once you get it and the aura of newness wears off you find you feel just as empty as before. You might also find this after you begin making changes toward a goal in your life. You know what needs to be done, you've thought about all the compelling, magnetic reasons that have you ready to follow through, you've even created a bona-fide action plan that you're willing to be flexible with, and then the unexpected happens. After a month in you find yourself stalled out, falling backward into your old habits. You've hit a slump. It's not that you lack the information you need; it's that you're finding it difficult to continue forward in the application of your plan. You've taken a little time to look around, and during this pause doubt starts to creep in insidiously, like smoke filling a closed room through the air vent, slowly enveloping your positivity in a cloud of uncertainty. This is happening because you've lost touch with your purpose.

Purpose is what keeps you moving when your circumstances don't look promising. Periods of consolidation—adaptation to and integration of all the progress you've made to this point in your life—is part of the process of ultimately fulfilling that purpose. Whenever I feel stagnant, I remind myself that I'm just getting prepared for another big leap forward. Remember, before you jump you have to crouch down to generate the power and lift to make the big leap. Sometimes the greatest energy we get can come from the lowest places in our lives!

Those who give up when they sense they're in this phase are those who die with their music still in them. When the negative voice is growing loud and the forecast looks bleak, it's that much more important to remind yourself of your mission. A purpose requires you to do a lot less of what you've been doing so far, that is, looking introspectively at what you're after, and do a lot more thinking about how getting what you want most will impact everything outside of you for the better.

Life Outside of You

What impact are you going to make your life have on the world? Why must you continue to persevere in creating health, wealth and abundance? Maybe you should start a new business or get that new job? The answers to these questions often become the fuel and the main determinant of whether or not you will actually get to where you feel you are meant to be.

Everything that's been created has a purpose—including you.

"No longer are you doing things only to better yourself, you're doing them because of what accomplishing them means to life outside of just you."

When you reach the higher levels of awareness, thinking about how your life is a piece of all that is, that you are extremely important and God has a reason for putting you on this planet at this time, flaws and all, your life takes on a different meaning. No longer are you doing things only to better yourself; you're doing them because of what accomplishing them means to life outside of just you.

Think of Rosa Parks, who took a stand to change the way society treated African Americans. She could have easily continued to go along with what those in control had set out, but would we have ever had an African-American president if she hadn't stayed adamant in her position, totally aligned with her purpose? We are all capable of such courageous and transcendent acts when we are freed from focusing on our own immediate needs. When instead we begin to focus on how our acts and choices fit into a much grander scheme is when we are capable of achieving the most.

When we escape the need we have to meet others' expectations or garner their approval our life flourishes with creativity and boundless provision. The less you need something, the more you'll find it shows up in your life. It's stepping into the flow of divine abundance available to us all. Sounds deep, philosophical and somewhat mystical, but in truth, it's very practical and just how life works.

> With the awareness that you are a seeker on a never-ending path of self discovery and growth, realizing that each life event has only brought you a chance to enrich your experience, you can start to see beyond your current circumstances into who you're becoming through the acceptance of yourself and your divine purpose.

Begin this chapter by celebrating and congratulating yourself on the effort you're making to be the best you at this very moment, knowing that everything you've done has brought you here today. All the things you are proud of and also those you're not, they all have a value and purpose in them. Don't judge yourself more harshly than you do others. Sometimes we are loving and forgiving to those around us but treat ourselves terribly. The commandment "Love thy neighbor as thyself" starts with the presupposition that you love who you are! You can't give out what you don't have. This chapter will help you begin to draw out more of who you are at the core of your being so you can radiate out into the world, bringing countless blessings to yourself and to so many others as you reclaim your

mission! So let's get on to understanding what purpose really is and where to find it.

First Step: Leave Your EGO At The Door

You may have heard that the word "EGO" can be considered an acronym for "Edging God Out." The first key to discovering your purpose is to ask God what He wants to do through you. What is the greater good you were brought to this world to accomplish? Is it creating a brand new industry that employs thousands? Is it raising a family of loved and loving children? Is it a combination of these things? Is it becoming a teacher and giving hope to a young lady who may go on decades later to run for president, citing your name as the person she felt encouraged by? Get out of your own way and stop the habit you have of judging what you feel drawn to doing. If God put it in your heart, you need to pay attention to it.

Most people think that their purpose is something that will make them rich, famous and problem-free. They think with enough prayer they can get God to go along with their plan for their life. They pray for something they want, never pausing to ask if this goal makes the best use of their innate talents and skills, things that GOD gave them in the first place! You don't create something without reason. Why would you ever think that God doesn't work the same way? It's been my experience that life works when we go with God's plans, not when we expect Him to go along with ours. The work comes in discovering what it is He wants for us. The short answer? Love.

Often people come to me and say they feel lost. They feel really depressed, despondent and totally hopeless. Several have even made attempts at taking their own lives before

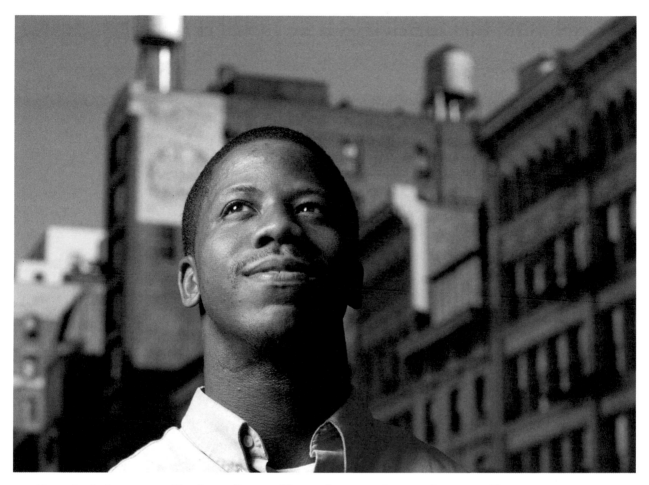

providence leads them to my office for a talk that they think will be about their body but ends up about their soul.

Sometimes our experiences can make it seem right that we lose hope. Death, abuse, trauma, sadness, loss—all inwardly focused—make us feel like we are pawns in a terrible game where we haven't been told the rules. This type of story is what many of my clients are initially focused on when we meet. They don't know where to go or who to talk to and so they come to me, someone who's been there and who they believe will be objective and nonjudgmental. Often, all you need to begin living the life of your dreams is the opportunity of having such a nonjudgmental soundboard, giving you a chance to work through the conflict safely in the presence

of love and support. Once you hear yourself put words to your amorphous thoughts and feelings, you can see you might be letting the opinions of others confuse or distract you from following your call, doing what your heart, mind and experience all tell you that God is leading you to.

Purpose Isn't Comfortable

Purpose doesn't mean feeling approved of or valued by others. Quite the contrary. It often requires you to step out of the status quo and away from comfort zones. You might be ostracized. When God has called you to be

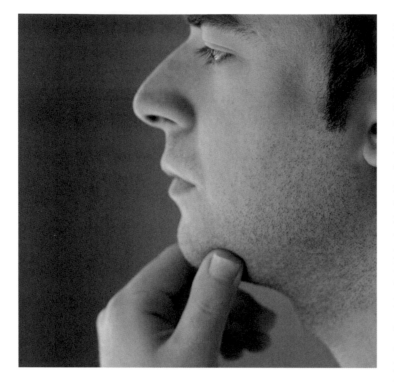

"Sometimes our experiences can make it seem right that we lose hope. Death, abuse, trauma, sadness, loss—all inwardly focused—make us feel like we are pawns in a terrible game where we haven't been told the rules."

a leader, you feel like you don't belong, and in a way that's the case. You were meant to stand out, not to blend in with the masses. Accepting this takes time. You are meant to lean upon God and work to earn His approval, the commendation of the Creator who put you here. Purpose, plainly stated, means bringing value to others' lives in the way you were designed to. It may evolve and grow over time, but its essence will always have connection to service. Understand that those who've encouraged you to play it safe in order to protect you may not understand the value in your purpose. It's often only in retrospect that the brilliance of following your dreams

is recognized. Most geniuses aren't given the label until long after they're dead.

Remember, God measures each of us in proportion to what he put into us. You have a set of talents that can become real skill but only if you commit yourself to training. You should not seek out your purpose by looking toward what society is valuing at the moment. The most popular fad of today will be a distant memory tomorrow. One thing that never goes out of style is being loving and supportive, making others feel significant and working to make today better than yesterday, for both yourself and others. The thing that controls how effective you are in doing that, the only thing, is the way you think about yourself and your life.

We all have the same hardware to work with. Our bodies can be improved and operate at peak, but ultimately our thoughts will drive our choices and future. Your mind is uniquely yours and in your full control. Talent is raw, but true skill requires practice, constant effort, refining, and a plan for putting it to use. Know that what you were born to do might come naturally, but it will still require you to grow. To uncover your purpose, look to where you are already experiencing success, already making a difference, and would do it without pay (maybe you already are)! That is a major clue as to what you were born for.

If you positively impact even one person's life, you will have an impact on the world in time, as that person's impact ripples outward. You get to choose the depth and breadth of your success. Sometimes people like to go in deep in a one-on-one way, others like to stay at the surface but inspire millions. The choice of which type of impact you will make is yours. In a society where popularity on social networks and in social media is more highly thought of than finding meaning and joy at the end of a day, changing your thinking to look for purpose and how you can serve others might take a little time.

Step Two: Purpose Requires Practice

When you discover your purpose you very well may find it is not what you thought it was going to be. You must also know that finding your purpose doesn't mean you will instantly feel powerful. It may cause you to feel incredibly vulnerable, because it's different from what others expected of us. This may be the first time you've heard the still and calming voice of God for yourself, independent of others' voices or the doubts in your own head.

No one in the family's even graduated from college, and you think you can become a doctor? You'll never make a living from being an author! What makes you think you could become President? When you're inches away from purpose, a blizzard of self-doubt and despair will make its final effort to prevent you from fulfilling God's will in your own life. If you feel you're in uncharted territory, know that's normal. Stretching beyond the little boundaries you've been living in will make you feel that way. Your purpose is about fulfilling a bigger role in life, and that means you're beginning to see that the road ahead is limitless. It's no longer about just getting what you want. The discovery of your life's purpose leads to the abandonment of immaturity, selfishness and impatience. It also requires discernment—quieting your mind enough to recognize the direction you are being called in. Like I said above, our ego will make every effort to make it about you and not about others.

"If you positively impact even one person's life, you will have an impact on the world in time, as that person's impact ripples outward."

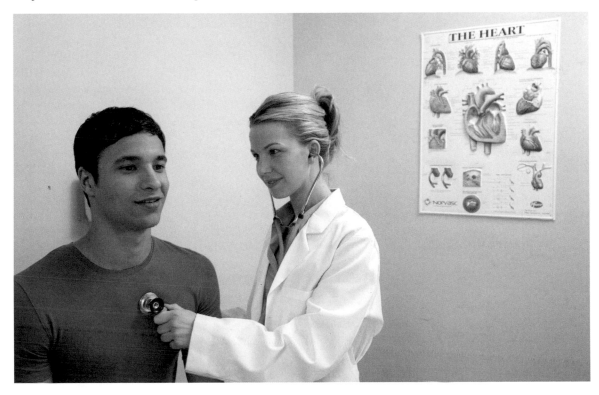

> *"If you want to look to where you're headed or supposed to move toward, look to what you've been blessed in doing and achieving so far."*

A young man I coached comes to mind. He was in a relationship that simply wasn't fulfilling. It was typical push-pull. He would get close to the girl and she'd withdraw. As soon as he backed off she'd come running after him, but once she felt she had him, she'd withdraw again, waiting for him to chase her. He had reached a point in his development where he was no longer willing to settle for this game and explained that to her. She ignored his needs and acted as if all was fine, not considering his feelings and efforts at all. Being a sensitive and loving young man, he felt leaving her was wrong. Believe it or not, this was not him being selfless. This was his EGO raising its head. "If you're a good person, you'd never walk out on someone and intentionally hurt her!" it told him. When I asked that he reflect on what God's will was as it pertained to this girl's life, considering life is about growth, he got the point. He realized he was hindering his own progress by staying with her, contrary to what God wants for us. Moreover, he was hindering hers too. He was getting in God's way. By allowing this pattern to continue, what was she learning? Nothing. When he removed himself and held himself to a higher standard, no longer settling for immaturity but continuing to send love, she would have to face her issues and either grow beyond them to attract a worthy partner or find one who was still at her level, but not my client! He came to realize he was also using the relationship, one he'd grown comfortable in, as a way of preventing himself from finding a relationship that would challenge him to become more of who he was capable of being. When you choose to live a life of purpose, progress will be constant!

In this case, the good of that relationship had long passed and both my client and the young lady were using it as a familiar crutch, delaying their own development. One thing to rest assured of is that your life's purpose will not contradict all the good that's already in your life. If you're happily married, loving your job as a music teacher and finding meaning with your charity work, God is not going to call you to leave your family and become a monk. He doesn't do that. God is an architect. He has a plan for each of us and all of us at the same time. It's hard to understand, since our Creator isn't limited by time or space. Trying to think about your life without the concepts of a history or future is difficult. Understanding life outside of cause and effect is difficult. But synchronies— the low-probability "coincidences" we discussed earlier—are beginning to point science in the direction that there is an interconnectedness— something outside traditional physics.

Pay attention to the small coincidences that are hinting to you the direction you need to head toward. I think God knows we are limited in our awareness to some degree but are also capable of significant growth, so He builds direction into your life, giving you guidance and validation through the successes you already have in certain areas. If you want to look to where you're headed or supposed to move toward, look to what you've been blessed in doing and achieving so far. Your future will always include some facet of these achievements in some way. That said, what you might think of as your greatest success so far in life is only the beginning of what God plans to do for and through you!

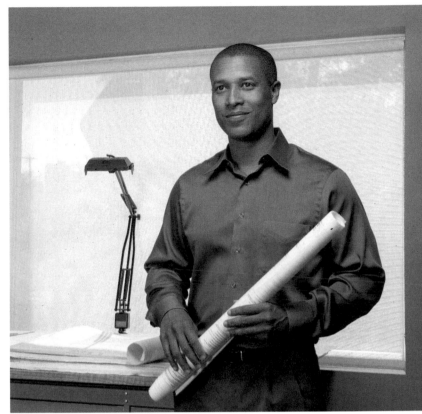

"He builds direction into your life, giving you guidance and validation through the successes you already have in certain areas. "

midst of a real tragedy. Would you be thinking about your expensive wardrobe or watch if you just lost your job? If your house burned down while you were out of town, would the first thing you worry about be whether or not your flat screen TV made it? Material possessions are irrelevant in the scheme of your purpose.

God often uses people that no one believes in to do amazing things. Look at David in the Bible. All he had was a cloth and rock, yet he took down a giant that everyone feared. When you step into God's purpose for your life, nothing can stop you. Everything that tries to divert you will be used for your greater good.

Your Task: Work Hard at Recognizing and Refining Your Gifts and Talents.

When you work hard to develop yourself and commit to being of service to others by becoming the best you, you'll always have what you need in your own life to make a difference. The money, the cars, the clothes none of those matter. How do I know? Ask yourself what you would think about in the

Once I helped a very successful gentleman who, after achieving his goals and referring clients to me, wanted to go into business with me. The human part of me was definitely interested. Because of my poor background, the security and paternal role this man could play in my life felt good and seemed attractive. Something just didn't feel right though. He was saying all the right things and doing all the right things, but my soul was not at rest. Have you ever had that happen? Where things seem like they are fine and dandy but something is telling you it "just ain't right?" Fortunately, I listened to my spirit, because it was correct. After a little homework, I found he was spread very thin in a lot of different businesses, and entangled in several legal issues. When I shared I didn't feel that direction was right for me, he acted dissapointed, but as if all was well. Soon, I noticed several of my clients he'd referred weren't showing up to see me anymore. Then a completely unrelated client of mine shared an e-mail that said this man had reverse engineered my program and was offering to waive my clients' fees!

I was devastated. I was terrified I'd lose my business. I had shared my visions and goals with this man. Still young and wet behind the ears, I didn't know what to do. This man was financially successful and I had barely begun to fulfill what I knew God put in my heart to do. But in reality I hadn't taken into account my greatest asset: God's partnership with me. God is always watching. It turns out the business the man had got involved in would close several months later as people discovered it was different from working with me. Many of those who were going to that facility came to work with me. This ended up being one of the greatest gifts God could have given me. I realized that the impact I was having had little to do with the mechanics of what I was doing, which anyone could copy, but had a lot to do with who I was.

For me, this occurrence was proof positive of my anointing, my gift, and life purpose in serving others. It wasn't just what I was doing that made the difference in people's lives, it was who I was and the love, sincerity, passion, and commitment that really made the difference. When you're friends with God, you needn't worry about anyone stopping you from reaching your destiny.

Look at all those through history who have come into the United States with nothing but the clothes on their back and a desire to work hard to make a good life for those they love, often thinking of themselves last, and who have stepped into amazing opportunities, success, and fulfillment! They weren't focused on themselves, they were focused on serving a greater good. So too must you be to get to where you are capable of going.

I once had a client who was very successful in business in Louisville. Not only was she living a blessed life, she did a lot of great work

"What has God used for a good purpose in your life that was originally meant to undermine you? Who has God allowed to witness your success, who was once one of your greatest critics? When you're friends with God, you can leave revenge to Him."

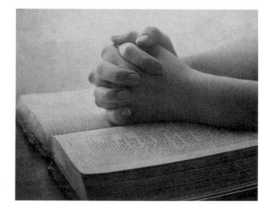

for the community, helping with numerous charities. Despite all the good she was doing for others, her husband fell ill and needed to be closer to his family in Florida. They moved down and were able to make ends meet, and then God called her husband home. Almost immediately, the support, the scaffolding that

I brought it to her attention that God's plan for our life purpose is rational and sensible. She now felt she had enough evidence that her purpose was right where she had started. When she realigned to her calling, got back in touch with what God wanted and moved back home, things began to work well for her again.

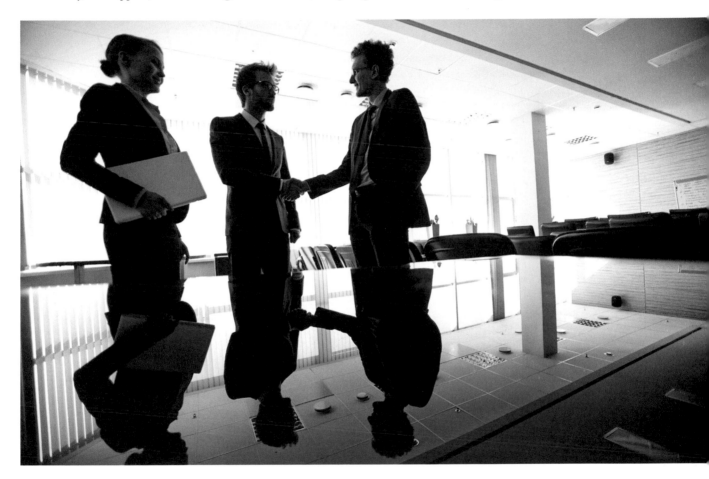

God had provided for her while she was there, came down. She loved the warm weather but her life had been in Kentucky. She felt conflicted. But though the weather in Florida appealed to her, the business success she'd experienced in Louisville came to a crashing halt. It almost felt like she'd been cursed! Every door she knocked on was met with silence. The doors that did crack open didn't offer nearly what she deserved for her talent and the value she would bring to the company.

The process of aligning with your purpose is not always an easy task. Sometimes we think we know what God's calling us to do, but find challenge in the face of its pursuit. And sometimes the challenge is the purpose as we discover more of who we are and how much we truly can handle. Prayer and reading spiritual texts can help you develop discernment in staying true to what God truly wants to use your life for.

Step Three: The Cornerstone of Purpose is Gratitude

Sometimes people tell me they feel angry at others, angry at themselves, and when they're being really honest, are often infuriated with God. Have you ever felt any of these feelings?

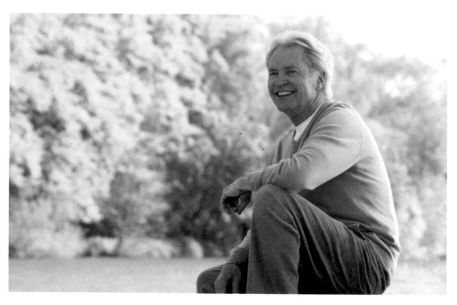

"What we see as a tragedy may be a blessing in a way we simply can't understand yet."

Mad at yourself, the world, or God? It's totally fine if this is true for you. You may find your life is not what society says it should be, or what you think your friend's lives are like by watching their Facebook pages.

The first thing you need to recognize is that every blessing comes at a cost. Rich, famous people have at least as many problems as poor people do. Always remember famous doesn't mean rich, and neither rich nor famous mean happy or fulfilled. I often help celebrities, musicians and politicians that others admire and dream of being like, but the admirers don't consider the cost, both monetary and otherwise, of my clients' success. For one thing, almost all of them need to have incredibly costly protection in place because of death and kidnap threats. They feel a constant push from the public into their private lives, and never feel like they can be "off" and just human. They have to project the image they've cultivated and people see in them. Many in the public eye listen to people around them they shouldn't listen to, falling to hubris and pride, where life changes them for the worse far more than they change others' lives for the better.

More of anything means more of everything. If you have more success, you will also have more challenges. I know a couple who tried hard for years to conceive. After months of fertility efforts, they got their wish and the woman became pregnant. The first child came into the world and over the next few years they had two more children without any conception issues. Sadly, I got news recently that their oldest was diagnosed with a terminal illness, one with a very low survival rate. With that type of news, it's easy to see how someone can get angry with a Creator who's known to be all-powerful and loving—especially considering how much they went through to bring the child into the world in the first place. We all have a vision of how things "should" be, and when they end up being totally different, we are disappointed or even devastated. What lesson could such a tragedy offer? The first that comes to mind is the reminder of just how precious and unique each life and relationship we have is. I know these parents have learned to love more deeply and value every moment that much more because of this situation.

Know that God's plan works without the limits of time. A loss to us is not a loss to Him. What we see as a tragedy may be a blessing in a way we simply can't understand yet. One thing is for sure: God will never take away something you absolutely need. You have to remember, you must be more grateful to the giver, God, than to the gift. The thing you love is only an expression of the giver's love for you. Would you give up on life or the marriage covenant you have with your partner if you lost your expensive ring he or she gave you? Of course not! Work to stay in love with God first, and everything else second. Consider that when you look into the eyes of your beloved or your child. They were given to you in love by a much greater giver, God, who works on a different plane than we do, without the same

restrictions of time and space. How can you be upset if He decides it's for the best that it is removed for their good or yours, or both? Sometimes the greatest breakthroughs in my life have come from the greatest disruptions and sadness.

When my dad died, my mom's health had been declining for some time. When he had his heart attack in June 2013, she was unconscious in the hospital, having been admitted a week prior for congestive heart failure, renal failure, lung failure, and ITP (a blood disease). To say the least, the diagnosis the doctors gave wasn't promising, but I'd been there before. For some reason, it hit me much harder though, seeing how sick she was. Come that Friday morning, I would get a second punch when my brother called me, begging me to convince my dad, who feared doctors and the news they might give, to go to the hospital. Usually upbeat and positive at their early-morning cleaning jobs, Dad had resigned himself to a folding chair and was

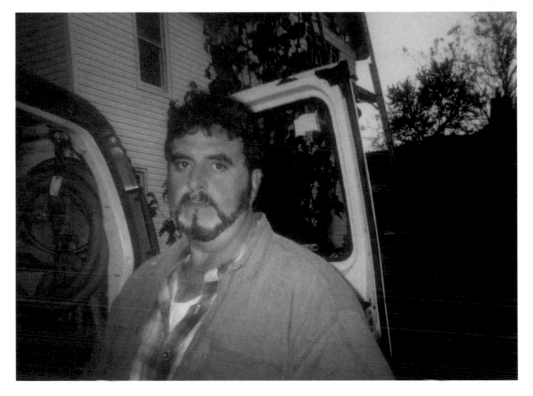

MY DAD OUTSIDE OF HIS WORK VAN. HIS RESOLVE AND CONSISTENCY TO KEEP GOING IN THE FACE OF SO MUCH UNCERTAINTY INSPIRES ME TO THIS DAY.

short of breath. Despite my brother's urging, he refused to go to the hospital. I told my brother to put him on the phone and I used every word I knew he'd understand, profanity and all others, telling him we needed him and he had to go.

For the first time, I heard my dad as a man and not as my father. I heard fear in his voice as he agreed to go to the hospital. It was providence that he did, as the ER doctors tore his clothes off immediately upon exam, saying they didn't understand how he was even walking or breathing! He had almost total blockage in his heart. One hour and one stent later, he was asking for his cell phone to make calls apologizing to his customers. He'd had this heart episode while cleaning a church, of all places! I felt relieved he made it through and had no idea that six months later, despite my grandma's warning to me that if he didn't heed his doctor's advice about rest, which he didn't, a second heart attack would kill him, which it did.

I had to tell my mom the terrible news that Friday morning, nearly six months to the day after his first heart attack. Destroyed doesn't

> "I literally felt like darkness was coming, for her. By intermission, the feelings grew too much for me, and then I noticed she wasn't talking sensibly."

begin to capture the energy that came from her. Despite the strain of their separation, a piece of her had always held on to hope that their marriage could be repaired. This news was the fatal blow that took away her hope of reconciliation and reunion.

That said, I worked hard to help create a vision beyond the circumstances. The house she lived in, the one I grew up in, looked like one of the houses you see in those reality shows about hoarding. I had it gutted, all the

dark dirty furniture hauled out and replaced with plush luxurious furniture, a big screen TV, bright artwork and colors. Despite her initial resistance, she loved the changes and began improving herself. I can't explain to you what compelled me to do this but I had a sense it had to be done then—that it couldn't be put off. My relationship with her grew deeper and deeper and we would have dinner together at least two or three times a week—all things I couldn't possibly have done if my grandma had still been living, as I spent almost every evening with her, as well as all my discretionary money.

God's timing is always perfect. I had a chance to arrange an opportunity for my mom to meet her favourite actor, Al Pacino, and planned to surprise her the week after my 30th birthday that fall, taking her to NYC for her first trip ever. I thought it would be a wonderful start to this new chapter in my life, and hers. When summer came and the house renovations were complete, God put another message into my heart: "Take your mom to NYC now!" I didn't logically see any reason for this. Why would I take her just four months before the trip? But I listened to Him and told her I wanted to take her for a dry run to New York, since she'd

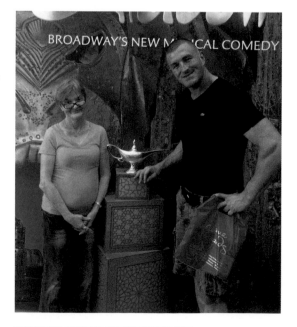

MY MOM AND ME IN NYC, ON HER FIRST AND ONLY TRIP OUT OF MISSOURI, ONLY A COUPLE MONTHS BEFORE SHE PASSED.

never been on a plane or even out of the state, for that matter! She had broken her ankle earlier that spring so walking was a challenge, but I was determined, and listened to God.

I took her and she had an amazing time. We visited all over Times Square. She ate whatever she wanted and we even saw *Aladdin* on Broadway. All the while, I had the deepest sense of sadness on my spirit. Her health issues were all the usual—not being able to manage her diabetes mellitus, trouble with walking–nothing new, but I had the worst sense of doom I've ever felt in my lifetime. I literally felt like darkness was coming, for her. By intermission, the feelings grew too much for me, and then I noticed she wasn't talking sensibly. She couldn't stand well. I tested her blood sugar, and it was over 500. I rushed her back to the hotel but she was out of blood glucose strips and insulin needles! I was scared she was going to die. She told me to just let her go to bed and I had no choice—I did. I ran down to the lobby and asked the concierge where a pharmacy was. For 45 minutes I went from pharmacy to pharmacy, wading through throngs of people under the bright lights of Times Square, dodging taxis and groups, stepping from sidewalk to street, trying to get to the pharmacies as fast as I could, but every one was closed. I was surrounded by people yet felt totally alone. Have you ever had that experience? I begged and pleaded with the store managers but there was nothing they could do—the strips and needles were controlled so I couldn't get them without a pharmacist on hand. I was sweating profusely, worried my mom would die in my arms without the medication she needed.

I went back to the hotel and to the concierge in the lobby, figuring I would have to call 911. I told him of my plight and yet again, God was right there for me. A bellhop happened to overhear me despite the noise in the bustling hotel lobby and came over quickly with a look of care and concern, sensing my fear. He told me he too was a diabetic, asked what type of

sugar reader she had, told me he happened to have the same one (what are the chances?) along with strips and syringes! He came to the room, tested her sugar and gave her the necessary amount of medicine. I was so grateful. He assured me she'd be fine and that if needed, we could call an ambulance in the morning, but her sugar was already coming down so there didn't seem to be a need. I went to my room overlooking Times Square, dropped to my knees by the window, the New Years' ball even with my line of sight, and sobbed like I never have before or since.

COMPLETING THE CIRCLE OF LIFE WITH MY MOM...SHE WAS THERE AT THE START OF MINE, AND I WAS THERE FOR THE FINISH OF HERS.

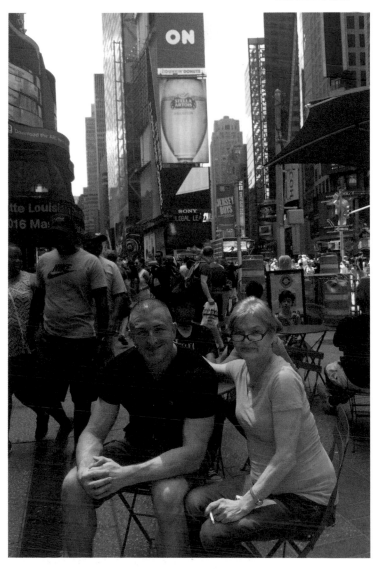

I knew I didn't have long with my mom. Despite no hard evidence, God was making it clear to me. I pleaded, begged, and bargained. I talked to Him, like I did at 17, this time pleading with Him not to let her suffer like this. I could feel her suffering and it was horrible. It was 1:00 am. I moved our flight up to depart at 6:00 am so I could get her home where her doctors were if we needed them. I could barely sleep and awoke at 3:00 am, worried what I might find when I went to her room, which was adjoined to mine. I'll never forget what I did find. It was like she was reborn. She was showered, dressed and

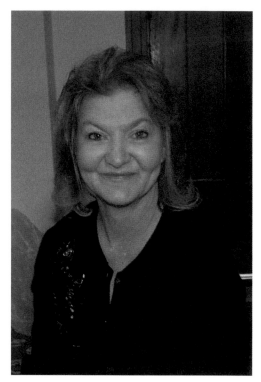

> *"God never takes anything away without giving us something that much greater. The things he takes are things we are no longer in need of, despite how we may feel at the time."*

packed. She was happy, thanking me for the trip, and excited to go home. I looked at her, stupefied, asking how her condition changed so fast. She told me that it happened to her all the time at home, that no matter what she tried, the diabetes was something she could never master. Her blood sugar would skyrocket and drop, in her mind without cause, but I would later discover it was influenced by drug interactions that no one had considered.

Nonetheless, I took the warning I'd felt to heart. I told my mom how much she meant to me, that she had always been my best friend, my biggest supporter and that I didn't hold her responsible for anything she'd ever done. I told her that I couldn't imagine life without her, and she told me I wouldn't have to, she would always be there. As I'm writing, tears are streaming down my face as I remember the look of serenity she had on her face in telling me, and the emptiness I felt, knowing that all I could have done was complete. Now, I had to give her back to God. Four months later, she

passed away on my 30th birthday, October 24, 2015. It was the hardest day of my life.

It's only now that I've realized that when I was born my mom gave me my life, and when she passed, she was giving me my life back. God never takes anything away without giving us something that much greater. The things He takes are things we are no longer in need of, despite how we may feel at the time. The woman I'd go on to marry had been put into my life by then. God wanted my entire focus to be on her and the next chapter of my life to begin, knowing that didn't negate the human sadness I felt. You too may have spiritual insight into some painful experience, but know it doesn't mean you won't need to grieve. That's the human part you need to tend to, and doing so is healthy.

The next night, I had tickets to Stevie Wonder. His show, as is usual with God's role in my life, was aptly called "Songs in the Key of Life," named after the record he had produced years before I was born. I had bought the tickets on a whim a few months earlier and at this point didn't feel like going. The week before the show, God had put in my mind to donate to Stevie's charity, so I listened and sent an e-mail asking his manager how to go about doing so. I didn't hear back until the day my mom passed. That morning, Stevie's manager called me about my e-mail. I could barely talk, as I had just left my mom's house after seeing her lifeless. I told his manager that there was really no way I could even think about it since this had happened. She said she totally understood but to let her know if I changed my mind. She told me they'd be praying for my family and me.

Hours later, I got an e-mail saying that Stevie would love to meet us if we came to the show. After a long talk with my siblings and fiancé, we thought my brother and I would honor my mom and celebrate her life by attending the show. We hired a car to take us, as I wasn't in any condition to drive. As it turned out, the driver of the car happened to be a minister, literally. He preached about God and life after death the entire way. Then things really got strange. We got to the stadium and the lights went out for the show to begin. A woman brought Stevie out, and he looked solemn.

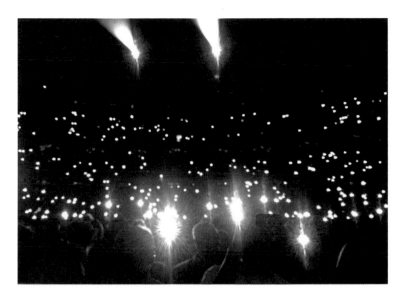

I WAS IN TEARS LOOKING OUT FROM THE STAGE AT 20,000 PEOPLE HOLDING LIGHTS UP IN TRIBUTE TO MY MOM, A PERSON WHO HAD NEVER FELT VALUED.

He said that he wanted to dedicate the show that night to the two brothers who had lost their mother, Laura D'Angelo! He went on to say that she was there in spirit and we're celebrating her life together. He concluded, calling my brother and me up on stage in front of 20,000 people who were holding lights up in solidarity as he sang and played the song "As" in her honor.

To think that God would bestow such peace and validation that He was as present as ever at such a devastating time still leaves

LITTLE DID WE KNOW THAT GOD WOULD MAKE HIMSELF SO PRESENT AT A STEVIE WONDER CONCERT!

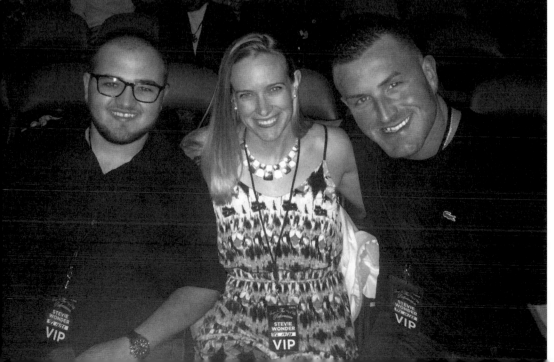

me speechless. It's one reason I'm sharing all this with you. I don't think He's done these works in my life just for me, but through me for you. He's looking to be as active in your life as He is in mine. You've just got to listen.

After the show, Stevie's team ushered us backstage and Stevie talked to me about his own mom's passing, saying she had come to him in a dream shortly after he'd decided to stop playing music—he felt he had lost his spark when he lost her, his biggest supporter. When he was a child she had told the neighbors in their poor neighborhood that he was special, and he believed it, much like in my situation. People would tell this single mother that all her blind boy would go on to do was "sell pencils." Obviously, you can see the miracle God worked through his life. He went on to become one of the most prolific and respected songwriters and performers in history.

"You can let tragedy destroy you, or you can let it touch and transform you into a more loving soul."

Stevie talked to us about how much God hates suffering and my mom had definitely been suffering, considering all I told him about her. He said God allowed her to finally come home on my 30th birthday as I was officially a man; her work was done in my life and He needed her now more than I did. Wow. After, I would realize that the passage in the Bible: "For we live by faith, not by sight" was brought to life in this experience for me. A blind man with a different kind of vision taught me more about God and my relationship with Him than almost anyone with eyesight ever could. His insight changed everything and pushed me over the threshold in deciding to write this book.

Purpose May Not Seem Practical

The more rigid you are with your vision and expectations of how things should be, the more pain you will find you have in your life, which if not brought to the light of consciousness can turn to suffering for an entire lifetime. When we shift our thinking and become conscious enough to force ourselves to find opportunity in tragedy, however, we can get a brief glimpse of the divine order of things.

We all have to guard ourselves against forgetting how blessed we each are with what we have already. If you will focus on the things you're grateful for, that you have in your life, more and more will appear. You begin to train yourself to count the small things, and sooner than you know it, they aren't so small anymore! Truly live each day and treat each person as if it may be the last time you will be able to see them. It will change your entire life.

I've softened much in light of seeing my mom as the human she was and the injustice she suffered. I don't use labels when I work with people. I see them as the unique creation God has made. I realize that much of my work is in helping people un-become what their environment and negative influences have shaped them into believing they are or have to be. Early on, as a young brazen man not yet touched by life and its booby traps, I could be impatient and too strong with those who came into my office. I now meet the people with a ferocious optimism and understanding of just how valuable is the chance they have before them, to totally change their direction and save themselves, and others, pain. I don't try nearly as hard as I used to, and yet get exponential results. You can let tragedy destroy you, or you can let it touch and transform you into a more loving soul. I chose the latter and I hope you do as well.

Step Four: Purpose Requires Patience

I know that I could have fallen into a life of ingratitude, rage and anger with my mom's issues. Easily. At the end of the day in grade school my dad would pick us up in his van. I'd look out the school window to see if mom was passed out in the passenger seat or had a beer in her lap. If Dad was alone, he'd insist we be as quiet as possible when we got home, hoping not to wake her from her alcohol and over-the-counter sleep-med cocktail that would put her into a comatose state for who knew how long. We all knew that if she awoke, all hell would break loose. Screaming, yelling, attempts to drive while under the influence—chaos. We did all we could to be sure that didn't happen.

I remember getting so mad at her and telling her "I wish she was dead," a child venting his frustration at a situation he hated, mistakenly attributing the rage at the person instead of the experience. I felt powerless. Have you ever been in a circumstance where you felt totally powerless? Even worse than powerless, I was ashamed. I thought that if people knew how dysfunctional my family was I would be judged and valued less because of it. I felt totally alone with the weight of the world on my shoulders.

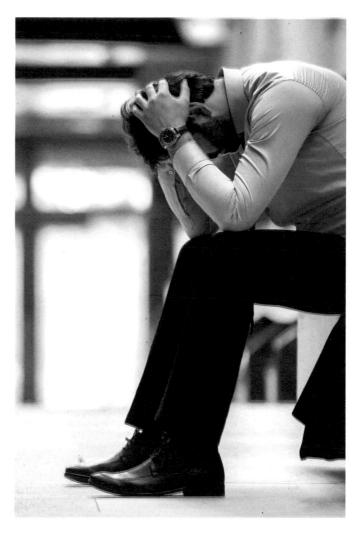

"If pain is preventing you from moving forward into your purpose, the time has come now to let it go."

The situation got worse and worse with my mom. Police were called and I'll never forget when my dad told me in tears that a male officer had punched my frail 130-pound addicted mother as hard as he could in the stomach, dropping her to the ground so he could handcuff her in our kitchen. Or my father dragging my half-naked mother into the house after she'd passed out in the yard. Atrocities. Terror. Sadness. Helplessness. It would be easy to give up if you thought

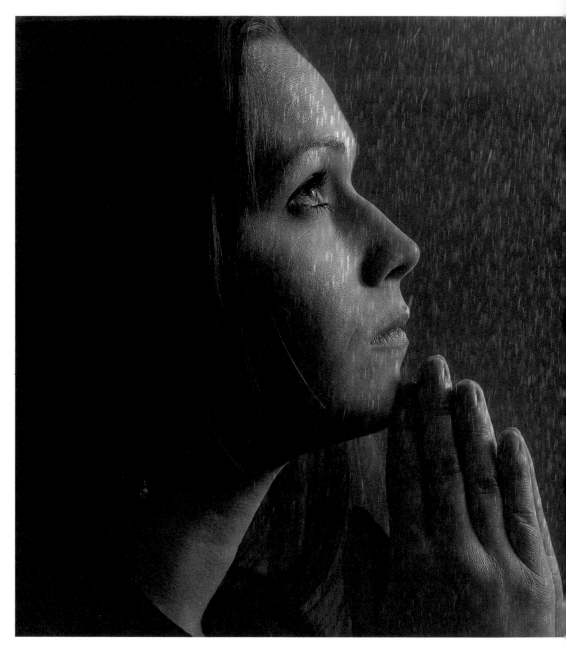

you were alone. Grace would have it that I never felt I was. I was blessed in that I never questioned what was. I accepted it. I only asked how I could use it and work with it to make it better. God was with me the entire time in my heart, mind, and soul. While certainly distraught at times, in a way I also had a tremendous sense of peace through it all, partly because of that line of thought, knowing that things would ultimately work out. Even me wrestling her to the ground, her spit and foam spraying into my face as she cursed and called me names she wouldn't call her worst enemy—these were all things I would come to feel were gifts.

That's not to say I didn't find them incredibly painful at the time. I just stayed conscious

my "real mom" was absent. Some dark force had overtaken her once she opened herself up with drugs and that force was now attacking me since I worked fiercely to free her from its grasp.

To my point, I once found her on the side of the road with a pint of alcohol protruding from her purse, staggering from the sidewalk into the street and back onto the sidewalk again. I pulled over and after a good 20 minutes, persuaded her to get in the backseat of my little Honda Civic. I told her I was taking her to the hospital and that she had to get better.

"No matter what's going on right now, do not give up on yourself or those you love. Always tell yourself, 'This too shall pass,' and know that even the darkest of storms, which wreak incredible damage, do come to an end."

She said there was no point, enraged that I was trying to help, telling me to live my own life and stop trying to control her. She told me she didn't think there was any point to living anymore, since she'd lost everything that mattered. No one seemed to need her anymore. That's how she felt in the clouded state she was in, partly due to the influence of so many substances circulating her veins. As she got angrier and angrier I drove faster and faster, hurrying to get her to a hospital, naively thinking they could stop the craziness, forgetting the dozens of times she'd signed herself out even before she sobered up.

Once she realized we were headed to the hospital things really got bad. "Let me out of this car now!" she screamed. "You better pull this fucking car over right now," yelling at the top of her lungs, the heat of her breath tinged with the scent of gin palpable in the air. Without any warning, she suddenly began pulling my hair and choking me from the

that my mother was not the person who was speaking. You must do the same. If pain is preventing you from moving forward into your purpose, the time has come now to let it go. Accept the human sadness you have, and it will weaken its grip on you. Sadness and pain are signs asking you to turn your awareness to your spiritual center. Something needs your attention. For me, I made it my belief that

backseat, all while I was driving 60 mph on a freeway. My female cousin, who had been with me, somehow managed to get her to stop. But that was only the beginning. Literally kicking and screaming, she started to open the rear passenger door, threatening to jump out if we didn't stop. I couldn't imagine her jumping from a moving car but the next thing I knew the door was flung open and in the rearview mirror I saw her body rolling on the highway, something like you'd see a stunt double do in a movie, only it was real. Fortunately there was no traffic behind us. I pulled over, wondering if she was dead. Watching through my rearview mirror, I could see she lay on her back, face up, motionless. Suddenly, like something from a horror movie, she sat straight up from her waist, looked at my car, got up and began running in the other direction. I didn't know whether to laugh or cry at how ridiculous what just happened was.

"It took God's grace, through me being unendingly loving, for her to learn she could allow her sensitivity, love and pain to come out without being afraid. When she did, little by little, she was freed. So too can you be."

We called the police and they were able to find her and get an ambulance to take her to the hospital where she detoxed, only to come back home and get wasted again.

Why do I tell you such a personal story? Because sometimes our life, if not examined, can seem futile. We think life is just happening instead of working for our greater good. But there is always magnificent opportunity for you, in even the darkest periods in your life. What did I learn about this traumatic period? I learned that I have always been who I am: a force for goodness and healing. Through what I witnessed with my mom, God chose to deepen my patience, compassion and understanding of just how deeply a person can suffer. I care so much about you because I was with my mom after she finally became clean, telling me how much hate she had for her former self, despite my pleas for her to forgive herself as we had forgiven her long before.

Through God's grace, she began to forgive. Little by little, loving herself, she started to be able to tolerate others more. She wasn't nearly as judgmental and paranoid, because she acknowledged and began loving parts of herself she had divorced herself from much earlier in her life, as numbing had been key to her own survival as a child. Unfortunately, as her unquestionably loving babies began

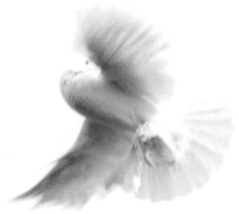

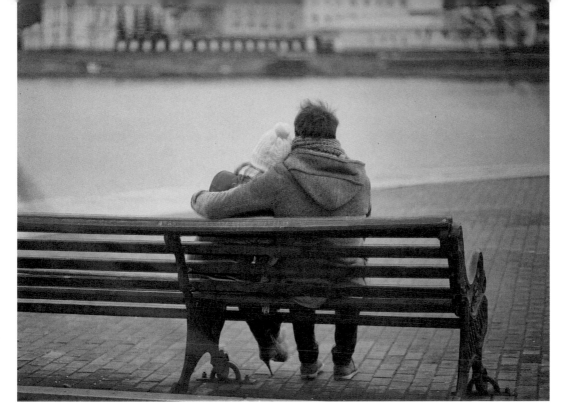

growing into independent-minded older children, she was back to her default—not feeling at all, too scared of what it might be like if she did. She had learned to deny herself the vulnerability of feelings when she was young, where she was abused and hurt when she allowed herself to feel, so she developed a skill for turning that capacity off at the first hint of pain.

I credit God's grace for my unconditional love of my mom, giving her space to learn she could allow her sensitivity, love and pain to come out without being afraid. When she did, little by little, she was freed. So too can you be.

No matter what's going on right now, do not give up on yourself or those you love. Always tell yourself, "This too shall pass," and know that even the darkest of storms, which wreak incredible damage, do come to an end. While our expectations or a particular outcome we want most may not come to pass, know that God will use the experience to better you and your life. There is peace after the storm, if you will only withstand it. Your purpose will help navigate you through the darkest storms.

"Just knowing someone else has been where you are and cares about you is often enough to give you the push you need to move onward."

Like the controls in an airplane help a pilot get through dense clouds, purpose keeps you balanced and moving onward through the inevitabilities of life.

Step Five: Step Into Relationships

To discover your purpose, you must let your guard down and let love in. Let your truth be known. Be you, flaws, scars, bruises, pimples and all. Embrace what you've been through, where you are today, and the unique vision you have for your future (or your desire to start building it!). The saying: "Those who matter don't mind and those who mind don't matter" is particularly true when it comes to living a life of purpose. You want and need to have only evolved, loving, non-judgmental, honest people in your life.

No one becomes healthy or achieves success alone, ever. And if they did, they would feel empty anyway. What do you want to do right after you receive wonderful news? You want to call all your friends and family to share it! Relationships magnify all we are and the meaning we find in our lives. They also can help diffuse much of the pain. Just knowing someone else has been where you are and cares about you is often enough to give you the push you need to move onward. Physical intimacy pales in comparison to emotional depth. When we feel like we are walking the path of life with just a flickering candle in hand, awkwardly bumping into things unintentionally, growing more anxious as we feel less and less certain and suddenly someone comes along with a lantern that illuminates everything around us in our lives, we feel less fearful, more empowered, aware of our environment and the path ahead and not nearly as concerned about our future since we can see it much more clearly. Let guides come in to be of service.

"We all must work to get to the place where we too can see the difference between what people do and who they are."

Interdependence is a critical element to success in life. Those who say you should be able to get fit, wealthy, or happy on your own just don't understand life yet. They are on their path and there is no need for you to make any effort to change them and their belief at this stage. Change yours. Being in a relationship means getting grace not just from above, but also from the people around

you. You need a steady flow of love around you and from within you. When I say "relationship" and "love" I don't mean only a romantically loving relationship; I mean relationships with all the people in your life. Other people can bring gifts of grace and love into your life as much as prayer and your relationship with God can. The more generously you pour out the love and support you have, the more space you create for it to be filled from those in your life. Give selflessly without expectation.

We need each other. Relationships of all kinds are one of the best and healthiest vehicles to grow from. If you want to stagnate, stay single and alone and you will never need to change yourself or your perception. In order to stay in any union, whether it be as a friend, co-worker or spouse, you must be mature enough to understand the world through another's eyes. That's how relationships last. When you love another for all they are even when you disagree or if you feel they are not of use to you, you know you're getting there. When you allow yourself to be known in the most vulnerable of ways and you find you are still accepted and loved, even with all your perceived faults on the table, self-hatred is replaced by self-love. By trying to avoid pain in relationships you are actually guaranteeing yourself pain. If you want to discover your purpose, you must get out of yourself and into healthy relationships.

Why would a loving, caring, good, all knowing, and all-powerful God let a child go through such an experience as I did? Life itself is the gift. This taught me that experience isn't the determinant of your future; the meaning and choices you take and make from it are. Because of the experiences I had with my mom I learned to hate the sin or wrongdoing, but love the person. Others might have used the experience as reason to reject God and live a life of hate. You too must make that distinction in your life. I remember when my grandma had a visit from a man she had known for years, but was in a really serious conflict with. It was a situation anyone would have been furious over. Rather than become enraged, she serenely said, "I love you but I don't like you. I do not wish for you to ever visit me again, please." Wow. Talk about spiritual maturity.

We all must work to get to the place where we too can see the difference between what people do and who they are. A good, smart person can do a terrible thing. It's my belief that God is with you in everything you experience, the things we label as both "good" and "bad." There are valuable lessons in each. Whether in ecstasy of a success or the suffering of a disappointment, God is there. Sometimes it's in the heart of the people working to try to bring peace back after a disruption caused by others' choices. What I did to get through all my turmoil was to remain grateful. God put the most loving woman in my life, Ms. White, my grandma, at the most critical time in my life. I think we all are given guides, mentors and friends at times we need them most. It's important to keep your ego out of the way so you don't block the blessing.

Are You Hearing God's Call?

When I was the obese teenager, any time I had a chance at a new friendship I would reach out to the person, so excited at the chance get to know someone new. All too often, I would find my e-mails would go long unanswered. The same with texts and calls. It was as if I'd never reached out in the first place. Maybe you've had this happen when you were interviewing for a new job, for example. After the interview you feel like it went great and send a thank-you note and never hear back. Or after what

"Shooting stars happen all day long, but until darkness or stillness settles in, we miss them."

you thought was a wonderful first date. You feel like it went great and so you push, trying to get a second one, and it seems there's no chance. You just can't figure out why.

In our spiritual lives, sometimes we pray and pray for something and we don't seem to get an answer, or at least not the answer we want. Since it's not the answer we wanted, we think God didn't get our note. I've reflected on this a lot. Could it be that it's not God who is ignoring us, but we who are ignoring God? Are you checking your "God" e-mails and texts by allowing enough silence and space in your life for the messages to get through? When we feel purposeless, usually it's because we are caught up in ourselves. The miracles and messages God wants us to hear are all around us, but we need to create the environment where they are getting through. Shooting stars happen all day long, but until darkness or stillness settles in, we miss them.

"You've got to be the visionary of your own life, and trust the picture God has given you for yourself."

Purpose Follows Passion, and Passion Leads to Provision

The key to discovering your purpose is to find out what you're truly passionate about. Don't chase money—instead attract it by loving every moment of what you're doing and who you're with. When you are being the greatest force for good that you are capable of being, all the material wealth you need will be available to you, either directly or indirectly through people who want to partner with you in the expression of your purpose.

Your passion is the signpost to your ultimate vocation, your calling, your purpose. The idea that you were created for a very specific and important mission that you alone can fulfill will become a truth for you that you believe when you find your purpose. Sometimes, we are moving at breakneck speed through life, not noticing much, and it can be difficult to remember that there is more to life than just doing. To find your purpose the first thing you must do is stop and listen to the inner voice tell you where you feel the happiest and most at peace.

If you were to ask a hundred people what their life's purpose is, I bet the majority will openly admit they don't have a clue, so don't feel bad if you are feeling the same way as you're reading this. Those who do have some idea are often looking for validation from others or the right conditions to give them permission to go for what they feel they were born to do, to really live their mission. No one in your circle can give you that. Often, the people closest to you are the most afraid of losing you and their connection with you, so they can't see or understand the vision God has given you. These people will grow to accept your purpose in time, but don't change your vision in your attempts to make this easier for them. Stay true.

I had a mentor who was convinced I should keep my head down, stay under the radar, be happy by helping people lose weight, and not reach out to give hope to the spiritually challenged. But God continued to put people in my life who needed hope. He put it in my

> *"To find our purpose the first thing you must do is stop and listen to the inner voice tell you where you feel the happiest and most at peace."*

heart to help these special cases despite the fears of my mentor, and there was nothing that would stop me from listening to God's direction. I did, and those people's lives improved exponentially, which made it clear that it was time to move on from that mentor. He was operating from a place of fear, and I from a place of faith. I was grateful for his care and concern and remained friends, but realized the season of his mentorship in my life had passed at that point.

You've got to be the visionary of your own life, and trust the picture God has given you for yourself. No one else has the authority to tell you what you were born to do or accomplish—not even your parents or your closest and most trusted advisors. Sometimes, the people who care the most are the most limited in their capacity to see who you really are and what you are truly capable of becoming, as their emotion and personal fear of seeing you disappointed or hurt often keeps them from encouraging you in the direction God's calling you to go. Your past connections can't feed your future because they aren't going to be there when God brings you into the next season of your life! This doesn't mean you have to remove them from your life, it just means you have to reconsider the place they have in your life going forward.

Put yourself in the presence of those who are like you want to be, making the type of difference you want to make. If you spend your time around people who can't see your vision of the future, usually the problems of the past will pull on you, keeping you from discovering and fulfilling your real purpose. The people who need to see it will, and those that don't, don't matter. You will never get unanimous approval from those around you to go for your dreams and live your purpose. You'll know you have discovered your purpose when you feel you are able to be yourself and love doing what you are doing every moment, effortlessly. A magnificent purpose can be simple—it's doesn't mean you must be extremely rich and famous. For some, purpose comes from being a good parent. For others,

"Ask yourself where, when and what led you to feel the most happiness in your life, even when you were younger."

it's helping or inspiring or teaching others at a school or hospital. A purpose is simply being part of something bigger than you or your own life. It's not without its challenges, but at the end of the day, you wouldn't trade it for anything else.

I decided long ago that I was one of God's stewards on this planet, someone He could do great things through, and it was my job to use every gift, resource, skill, connection, and talent He's given me to let more of Him be apparent to the world. At one time in my life, I didn't like sharing how different my life was (which I now call blessed), but as I matured, I realized the sharing is a gift to others. When you let your light shine, you give them permission to do the same. It shows that such wonder is possible for them too. That's why I'm so candid in sharing my life with you. I want you to know that if Charles can do it, so can you—and much more, I'm sure!

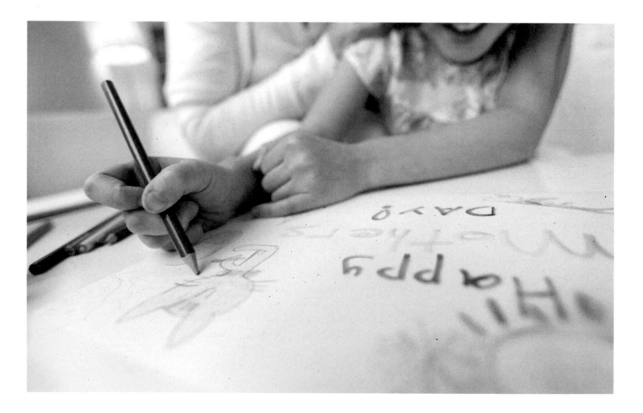

Look to Your Earliest Passions

If you are simply going through the motions each day in your job, relationship, career path, college major or whatever you're doing, frustration will eventually mount, and then anger will flood in. To create the breakthrough you deserve, you've got to align with what you were created for. What brings you joy and fulfillment? You don't have to quit your job, but at least begin to work part-time on your purpose until it becomes so strong it can take the place of what you're not feeling great about. Ask yourself where, when and what led you to feel the most happiness in your life, even when you were younger.

As a young boy, before I started turning to food for comfort, I loved metal detecting for hidden treasure in my old neighborhood and digging for fossils. I could do it for hours and hours and never get bored. I also loved playing the piano. Another favorite hobby of mine was doing magic tricks for anyone who would watch. I would even go to nursing homes as a middle-schooler to perform piano or magic tricks, sometimes walking my block looking for neighbors coming out to their cars, asking if they had a moment to see a new trick! I would sit out in my front yard waiting for the mailman so he could sit for a few minutes to hear a new song I'd taught myself by ear on the piano. At first look, you wouldn't think a young boy's interest in any of those things might amount to much. However, I would go on to love being in front of people (performing piano), helping them dig through their history to find meaning (metal detecting and fossil hunting), and eventually reach out to millions in sharing unbelievable transformations that many can't believe (doing magic). The interests of your youth are often clues of your life mission when you dig a little deeper and discover what they really are leading you to. We don't inhibit or judge our inclinations too

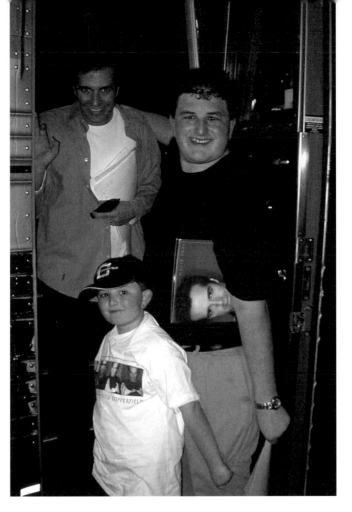

MEETING MY IDOL, DAVID COPPERFIELD, AS AN OBESE TEEN. HE WAS UNBELIEVABLY KIND WELCOMING TWO POOR KIDS UP INTO HIS BUS AFTER WE WAITED HOURS IN THE RAIN WITH MS. WHITE IN HOPES OF MEETING HIM!

harshly when we're children. If you are in love with what you're doing right now and feel tremendous passion, trace back your interests as a child and you'll likely find a connection.

To really get into alignment with your purpose requires courage. It means you have to be willing to trust God and the path ahead knowing that everything, even the painful experiences you'll encounter on your journey, are going to be part of the process and an investment in your future. Every struggle, challenge, adversity and weight in your life is an opportunity to build the spiritual muscle God needs you to have so that as you go on, things get easier and easier for you. You are on route to a cruising altitude even if you are experiencing turbulence in the ascent! For you to give birth to the new you, you have to let go of and bury who you once were. Let faith replace your fear, and you will soon be where you're meant to be.

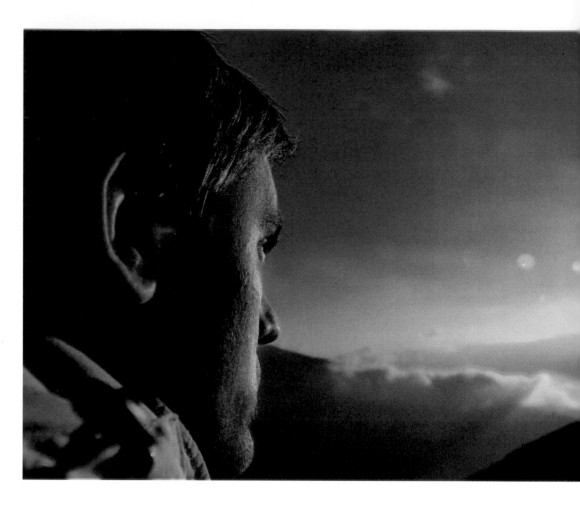

Purpose Requires Precision

You have to constantly check in with yourself and evaluate your results and progress in staying in alignment with your life's purpose. We can only improve things that we manage consistently. You can only increase the value and impact of things if you take a look at them often. If you were to check in on how you're doing with your purpose only once per year, for example, then you'd have just that one time to correct yourself if you're off course. Time will take all of us well off course if we get distracted. If the captain of a ship falls asleep at the wheel, letting even a few hours pass without checking his direction, it can cost him dearly. Don't let your life go unchecked. Be

"I finally accepted myself as I was, realized I was OK, and I decided to realize everyone else was OK too."

aware and have safeguards in place to be sure you remain steadfast and precise leading your life to the purpose you were created for.

You know about my transformation from a sad, lonely, obese teen to a lean, attractive, successful young adult with a fantastic relationship with a wonderful woman. At one time I would never have been able to imagine a life where I was looked at with anything but derision from the opposite sex, a life where I stood onstage talking to hundreds

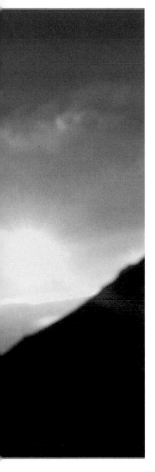

or thousands of people about how to improve their lives, or even a life where I could go for a short walk without feeling like I was going to die. And yet I've achieved all those things and many, many more. Sure, some things were difficult at the time, like saving up my money from my minimum-wage job just to buy the food I needed to lose weight while still trying to finish high school, but the process itself wasn't difficult, eating the foods I needed to eat and getting the exercise I needed each day. And that's because I finally accepted myself as I was, realized I was OK, and I decided to realize everyone else was OK too. I began to accept and understand God's purpose for me, learning to be present and joyful in the moment regardless of my circumstances, realizing that all the pain, all the challenges, all the suffering I'd gone through was going to be used in my life for the good of others. It would become heart fuel, giving me everything I needed to care at the deepest level in order to help them. I had great models in this matter in my grandparents, my dad's parents, who lived simple lives and had little fear for the future, taking joy in walking to the park with the dog, collecting and crushing cans to recycle aluminum for extra money, and taking in a movie on a Saturday night. Purpose can be simple and happiness is not the absence of problems.

As soon as I prayed to God and asked for His help in becoming a "normal" size, and when I promised Him that if He helped me I would spend the rest of my life helping others, I had the answer. I committed myself to something much bigger than myself, no pun intended. That was my purpose: become as great a servant as I could. Everything that I'd been through leading up to that point would only affect me in one way from that point on: in helping me with my new mission.

You may have said the words: "Everything happens for a reason." Or "It was meant to be." I'm going to have to agree with you. Everything does happen for a reason, and we are all part of a divine plan. I thought of calling this book "No Coincidence," because that is what I believe to be true. When you open yourself up, accept God's plan and stop trying to fight it, you will find that in every direction you look will be support for that decision. You'll see "coincidences" around every corner.

I know without a shadow of a doubt that God wants you to be happy. He wants you to make the most of your life, to find and live your passion, to be with someone who enriches and fulfills you, and to maintain your healthy relationships. He wants you to be healthy. How do I know all these things? Because He gave you everything you need to make it happen. With the hardware, He also gave you the mental software to have free will to make choices and think independently. It's your job to master your thinking so you can fulfill the purpose of your life.

Undeniable Grace: Synchronies and their Message

God has often given me clear evidence that I am living my purpose. Much like my Stevie Wonder experience, I think these "coincidences" cannot truly be coincidence. These occurrences are so incredible, the way everything fits together in an unexplainable way to us mere mortals. While they have such a low probability of happening, they do happen for each of us when we are in alignment with our own unique life's purpose, the plan God had for us when we were created. I'm going to tell you about one of the most dramatic and obvious examples of God's presence in my own life.

I met Crystal totally randomly at the airport in St. Louis. She is from California, and I was headed there to be on a national show to promote *Think and Grow Thin*. She only happened to be in St. Louis this one time as she had been visiting a cousin in Illinois, so was using the St. Louis airport to fly back home. There was a special connection we both felt that fateful day, and a long distance friendship would turn into serious dating years after.

As my relationship with Crystal progressed, I had a sense that she was the one. I felt the time had come to commit to marriage and wanted to ask her to take my hand, but like you have probably felt at critical times in your own life, the rational part of me, the doubtful critical little voice, got activated by these thoughts. "How do you know she is the ONE?"

"What if she isn't ready?" "For better or for worse, this is a big commitment; are you sure you want to do this?"

As great as our relationship had been and as much love as we had for one another, Crystal also had doubts about moving to St. Louis. She didn't have any family or friends here, and since I am such a mission-driven person, I understood her concern that she might fall in the shadow of my work. I could appreciate her apprehension and doubt about uprooting from a stable job in a wonderful city and relocating to a place where she didn't feel any historic roots. We all like the familiar.

Despite this, she said she felt God wanted us to move forward in our relationship, as I did, but we both wanted a bit more affirmation and reassurance that it was the right thing for us. Boy, did we get it! What I am about to share with you is the most clear example I've yet had of God's presence in my life.

As we were struggling with her move from Boston to St. Louis, I came home one afternoon after a long day of work. As I turned down my street, I saw my neighbor was standing in my driveway, looking a bit shaken. She had her arms crossed and was just gazing at the outside of my house. I pulled in the driveway, got out of the car, and asked if everything was ok. As if I interrupted her from her trance she asked softly, "Can I talk to you Charles?"

"Of course, what's up?" I responded hastily, as

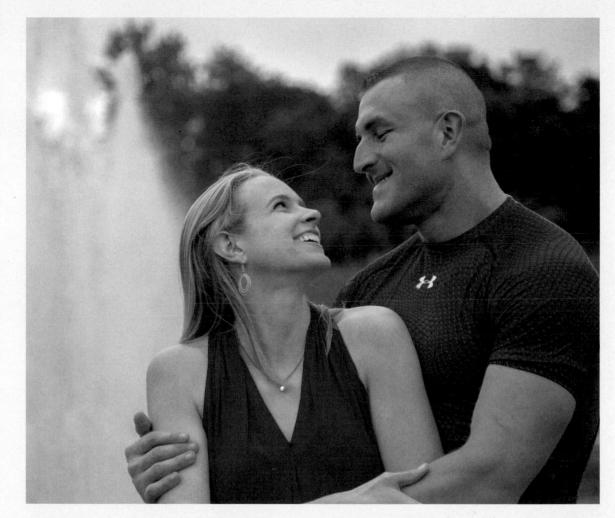

I wanted to get in the house to shower and head out to eat. "Well, I was in my kitchen washing dishes and happened to look out my window. There was an old woman looking in all of your windows! She must have been nearly 80. I watched her make her way around the entire house and even into your back yard. She was even trying to get in your back door!"

Before my mom died, as an effort to raise her spirits following my dad's death, I completely renovated and restored the old Victorian home she lived in, where I had grown up. After she died on my 30th birthday, I felt

strangely pulled to move back to the place I started, one that was riddled with many horrific memories, but also one where I felt I could lay down a new and positive history in as the man I had become, so I returned to living in our old house.

She continued, "She didn't look like she was going to do any harm, but it was weird, so I came out to try to get some information from her, but by the time I got outside, she had driven down the street in her Lexus." I found it odd someone well dressed and driving such an expensive vehicle would be trying to break into my house! Intrigued, I asked if she

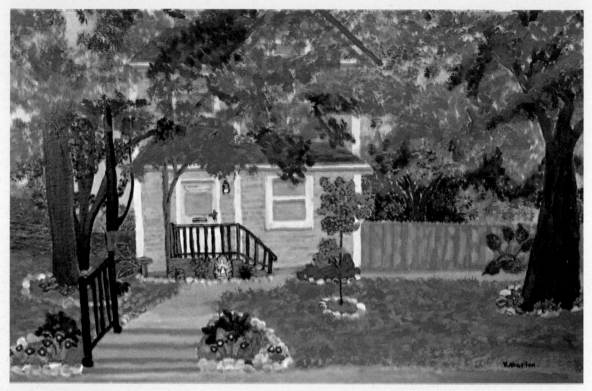

got anything, a license plate, anything at all. "Well, that's why I wanted to talk to you. I was able to wave her down and she pulled over. I told her I'm your neighbor and I couldn't help but notice she was in your yard, and I asked if I could help her. The old woman said she grew up in the house in the 1940s. It had been decades since she'd been in the neighborhood but said something just inspired her to stop by in hopes of meeting the owner for a walk down nostalgia lane. She missed her parents and many of the other people who'd long since passed who spent time with her and her family in the home and hoped to share many memories with the new owner. I told her being the historian you are, you would love to hear about it all and asked for her to write down her name and number," she finished, telling me she'd put the paper in the mail slot so I wouldn't miss it when I got home.

I went into the house and picked up the paper along with my mail, tossing it on to the kitchen table to look at later, but curiosity nudged at me. "Who was this old woman?" I wondered. Before taking a shower I unfolded the scrap and nearly fell to my knees. There were only three lines written:

Vera Lederle

Her Phone number

George and Lorraine Lederle

(Names changed for privacy reasons.)

It couldn't be, I said to myself, shocked. Why the shock, you ask? Because the last name written on that paper is also Crystal's last name, and it is a very uncommon name. The inner critic we all have inside of us barraged me at this divine moment, yelling: "You're reading it wrong." "It's just a coincidence."

But I wasn't reading it wrong. Was this God's direct answer to Crystal's and my prayer for affirmation? I delayed my plan to shower and immediately called the number. The woman's last name was Lederle, pronounced the same as Crystal's! Astounded, I felt like my heart beating out of my chest. It was one of those moments when so many words are flying through your mind that you can't speak.

I called Crystal, almost unintelligible. Was this some divine conspiracy?! Crystal was as stunned as I was. She called her brother, who had completed their family tree years before, and sure enough, this woman's father had been one of Crystal's father's relatives! Of all the houses and all the families, how could a girl I met in an airport have family that lived in the home my parents would go on to buy decades and decades later, the one I was raised in and lived in once again?!?

We agreed there was no way this could be a coincidence! It's not just the connection, though that was strange enough. It's for this to have happened at such a critical time, when we were both debating whether or not to move forward in our relationship, when she was debating whether to move here and I was debating whether she was for sure The One, the message was abundantly clear. I prayed about the matter and in short order was reassured that God's hand was guiding me. When have you had an experience like this, some call it fate or kismet or serendipity, where you feel something much greater and loving operating in your life for your greater good?

Knowing my tendency toward skepticism, God made sure he continued to affirm what I was to do in my relationship. I had fleeting fantasies of picking out an engagement ring

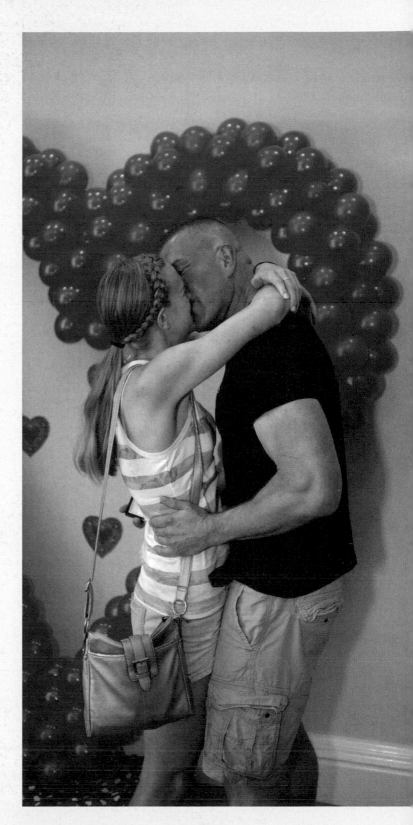

and asking Crystal to marry me. For some reason I felt a sense of urgency to do it, but again, the practical human side listed all the reasons it could be too soon, but another part of me felt I wasn't to question this pressing feeling, but to simply do it. To step out in faith.

I tried to ignore it, but God wouldn't have that! With all this swirling in my mind, I went to a play at the Muny, a well-known outdoor theater in St. Louis. Now, I'm not a flashy guy who wears jewelry. I had bought only one piece for myself in my life, from a jeweler when I was 19. It was a gold crucifix necklace that I still wear today. I had to pay it off in installments but at that time I wanted to have something to symbolize my faith. As I sat there waiting for the play to begin, thousands of people filled the seats. Moments before the show was to start, I heard a man shouting my name, "Charles, hey Charles!" I turned around and there smiling so wide he could eat a banana sideways was the jeweler I had purchased my necklace from a decade or more earlier! I had never run into him in all the years since purchasing the necklace. Was this a coincidence or a message that it was time to get another significant piece of jewelry? I was soon to find out. I went to greet him and we caught up on how life had been for both of us. Before I went back to my seat he closed by saying, "When you're ready for your big day and need a ring, let me know!" I took that as a strong sign that my heart was in alignment with God's calling on my life and set out to go the next day.

Despite this conversation I didn't want to get the ring at his shop so instead chose one randomly, a small family-owned diamond store. I waited outside the shop early Saturday morning and was the first one in the door when it opened. I spent an hour with the owner picking out what I felt would be perfect. As she asked about my special lady, I shared the story about Crystal's long-lost relative coming to my home unexpectedly, citing it as the major push behind my decision to ask for her hand at this time. Just as I was about to get to the climax of the story, revealing that Vera was Crystal's relative, a woman came out from the back of the store and said, "Hi Charles!" Figuring it might be someone who knew me from television or radio, I smiled warmly, though inwardly a bit peeved at being interrupted, and tried to go on with the story.

Instead of allowing me to continue, she interrupted again saying, "How have you been doing since you moved?" I was a little concerned at this point. Who was this woman? I did not recognize her face or name on the name tag adorning her blouse. "I'm sorry," I said, "but how is it exactly we know one another?" She seemed a little offended. "I'm your neighbor, Charles. I live right across the street from you! I was good friends with your dad and mom!" Oh my God. Out of all the stores I could have chosen, I choose one that a woman who knew both of my parents, unbeknownst to me, would be working at, even more eerily, at the exact time I was to go in and pick the ring that my fiancé would say YES to! I shared the story and the significance her being there meant to me, purchased the ring, and the rest is history!

Look for the things that appear to be simply a coincidence at first glance—there is a deeper meaning and message for you if you will only open your mind to see!

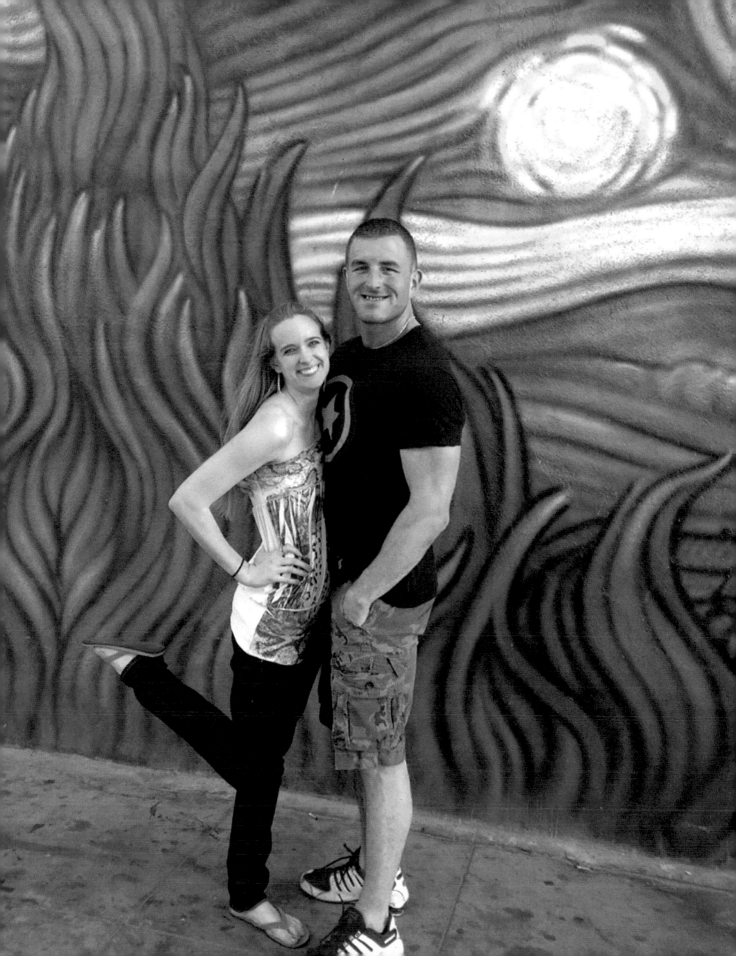

CHAPTER SIX

Labels, Expectations and Learning from Experience

So far, we've spoken a lot about how we develop ideas about ourselves based partly on our families. If you were born into a family where everyone is poor, addicted and overweight, then you might expect to be poor, on drugs and overweight, all the while using your family history as an excuse. If you were born into a family that did not strive to be its best, or maybe didn't even think better was a possibility, then you might not see that you have a way to break out of poverty in all of its facets. In this chapter, we're going to work together to liberate you from what's holding you back.

Happiness or Misery: Your Choice

Sometimes it takes a lot of pain before you will make the choice to change your life. When speaking about addiction, we refer to this as "hitting rock bottom." It's when you reach the end and can no longer live with yourself as you've become, or the results of your choices. You feel like you've tried everything to no avail, and often the people you love most have walked out. It's when you realize *you* are the issue. Not your past, not the drugs or alcohol or food, but you or, more specifically, your choices.

I like to think of moments like these as spiritual awakening opportunities. In my opinion, people who hit this point aren't at the bottom. Instead, they are on the threshold. They are at the door that will take them into an entirely new positive dimension. I don't think of it negatively at all, in fact. When you get to this threshold you take a step back and

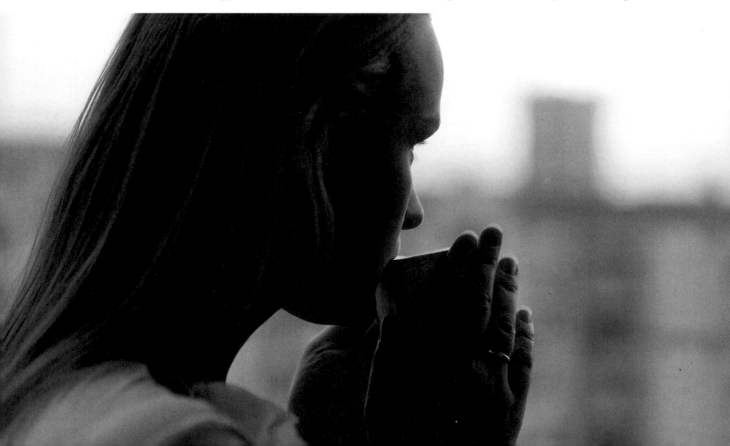

realize that all you have is this second, right now. Your past is over. It's all but an illusion. And your future is certainly not guaranteed.

Most people I've worked with who call themselves addicts are always mentally time traveling. They live in the past, when things were better or, conversely, when they did things they regret. They live in some arbitrary future, when things will be better. Some of them hold on tightly to the label of addict, because, in my opinion, facing the person they've never had the chance to know—themselves—is a scary idea. It's much safer to hold on to a label than to the idea they would have to embrace and build this new empowering identity, free of the label and the safety that comes from that construct.

While much of what you expected in your life may not have happened for one reason or another, you're still on this planet even if you've made choices that might make that seem unlikely. There is a purpose to why God has allowed you to survive it all. One thing is for sure: how your future turns out will be influenced most by your consciousness at this very moment, how you are thinking, feeling and acting, right this second.

To change permanently, you have to leave your ego behind. I think you also have to let go of expectations, the way you think things should be or how they should happen. You have to trust. You must be patient and rely on a source greater than yourself to work things out, knowing He always has.

When clients come to me, they're often shocked at how direct I am. The first realization a person must make, whether working with me or alone, is that what they're doing is not working, period. The clock on your life is ticking very quickly. Today is all that we have. If I can't offer them a new way of seeing themselves and their lives, they will be no better for it. This does not mean I think I'm better than my clients; quite the contrary,

much of my wisdom comes from making mistakes earlier in life. I don't want others to suffer a similar sadness and frustration.

Often, I will be extremely strict, just to help lay the framework that surrendering over to the process is key to growth. If a person is already doing five hours of exercise a day, I will recommend they don't do any. If a person is eating excessively and expects they will be on a limited food program, I might ask they continue to just keep eating the way they have for now. Often it's our own internal resistance to authority we must overcome. When another person helps take the pressure off you, doing something unexpected in this way can be enough to free you. When you give yourself permission to trust your own instincts and authority, you find that you will often know exactly what you should be doing to be the best you. This may seem contradictory, that I tell you I disregard what my clients tell me and in the next breath I say you need to trust your own instincts, but bear with me for a minute.

"One thing is for sure: how your future turns out will be influenced most by your consciousness at this very moment, how you are thinking, feeling, and acting, right this second."

When I challenge people in extreme and unorthodox ways, it's clear that I believe that they are capable of what I'm asking, whether or not they think so at that stage. I have faith in them, as I do YOU! However odd it may seem, this approach is far more spiritual and enlightening than it may appear. Once I've helped give them space from, and awareness of, the limiting beliefs they've long held, they can break out of a well-practiced, disempowering pattern. Without that story helping to hold them back, they can focus on making things the way they deserve.

"To change permanently, you have to leave your ego behind."

When I tell someone who says they have a problem with junk food to eat *more* of it, it totally fries their brains! I have Fortune 500 CEOs who fly in for a consultation and local kids who come to me on public transit. My approach is the same. I hold no more reverence for a person with a larger bank account. Ego has no place in personal and spiritual development. Only when you deny your negative ego, who you think you are, what others have always wanted you to be, how you think you should be treated or your expectations about how things should be going, only then can the real guide, your own inner voice—God—emerge and begin to direct your life to fulfill your purpose each day.

With weight-loss coaching, my clients choose to eat and exercise the same way every day for a period of time to truly disengage emotionally from food and develop discipline in the fundamentals. Just like legendary UCLA coach John Wooden taught, success comes from being exceptional at the fundamentals. When you're bored with the process, you can trust you're on the right track! Changing your emotional state using substances of any kind has no place in lasting success.

I quickly become less and less of a director to my clients. This is so they reclaim their personal power, as I don't believe in fostering dependency. I want you to be able to totally trust yourself once you've developed momentum. Once you've practiced basketball under the leadership of a good coach, you no longer need him to tell you how to dunk the ball. It's instinctive. So too does a good coaching relationship lead to this kind of personal autonomy and power.

When I was faced with difficulty, whether at home or school, Ms. White, my adopted grandma, was always a guide to me. I could open up completely to her, share my innermost fears, desires and concerns, and she would listen serenely and intently, making me feel

like I was the only person on the planet. It was the greatest gift God had given me up to that point in my life. Often, just hearing my thought vocalized was enough to bring peace back to my spirit. Early on she would offer clear directives, but as I grew older and neared my 20s she would most often turn the question back on me, asking what I felt was right. She didn't ask what I "thought" nearly as much as she asked what I "felt." It was as if she was telling me that the knowing, the

"Often, just hearing my thought vocalized was enough to bring peace back to my spirit."

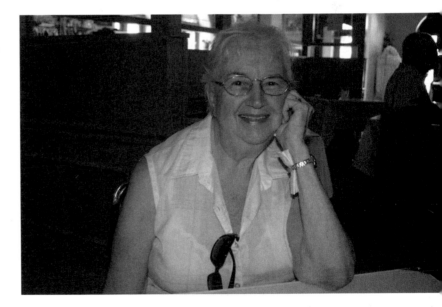

spiritual inclination to do what is meant to be, is within us. Her nearly nine decades of life experience brought great wisdom to my young mind. It's only our conditioning, which results from focusing more on our senses than our spirit, that negates that inner sense.

Do you listen to your feelings? Have you ever had a gut feeling about someone or something but disregarded it, and ended up getting burned as a result? Don't deny your intuition. It's a gift we've all been given. Be wary of any

MY ADOPTED GRANDMA AND THE GREATEST TEACHER OF MY LIFETIME, MS. WHITE. SHE TAUGHT ME HOW TO TRULY BE SELFLESS IN LOVE teacher or teaching that tries to convince you to doubt your intuitive sense. Where there is smoke there is often fire.

A spiritual life is not led through practicality. It cannot be understood through worldly measures. Your awareness, your consciousness, where you spend most of your time mentally, emotionally and spiritually will determine where you are physically. This was made ever so obvious to me when I was recently visiting New York City. My significant other and I went to see a show on Broadway. We were to meet several friends there one Saturday evening and spend time with the actors backstage after the show. That day, we

"When you enter a spiritual knowing, paradox and duality disappear. Everything just is. There is no longer judgment."

walked the streets of Manhattan. We made our way past some of the most expensive stores in the city, and in the doorways slept several disabled and ill homeless beggars. Stepping over them were men and women dressed to the nines, their arms filled with purchases. The beggars seemed invisible to them. This affected me. How could there be such disparity? Just outside the doorstep of one of the most expensive stores, beggars slept half starved and without medical care. It seemed paradoxical.

When you enter a spiritual knowing, paradox and duality disappear. Everything just is. There is no longer judgment. You get to choose which group you will be part of, but being part of one doesn't mean to the exclusion of the other. Many of those shopping could be just like those who were homeless and vice versa. This bothered me greatly. During the intermission of the play, I talked to a concession usher who had moved to New York from Texas. I told her how heavy the city felt with so many people

who were obviously in need. She said her faith led her to transcend this, and that she had trained herself to be aware when God asks her to help someone she sees.

Once I took a step back, I realized it had been my ego talking to me. I was feeling bad thinking I could have or should have done something, but being present, listening to your spirit rather than your ego, will always lead you to do what God asks. It isn't easy, but it is possible for you. When you realize that everything is connected, the beggar as well as the rich person, and that God is present in and through both, you find you don't have to suffer because of it. There was perfection in the witnessing of this truth, as it led me to open further, connect even more deeply with myself and share it with you to think about your own life experience. That experience now opens up the possibility that you will become more from it. There is no separation, even in the things we observe in an egotistical way as bad. Again, this doesn't stop the pain we feel as we witness suffering, it just reminds us that it's all part of something far bigger than our thinking. Everything is perfect the way it is right now for where we are right now. As we change individually, so will the world. War is a result of our individual consciousness that collectively compounds, leading to devastation and tragedy. When we each shift our thinking the way I'm presenting to you here, the world begins to change.

"Everything is perfect the way it is right now for where we are right now. When we change, so will the world."

The more spiritual I've become the more intensely I feel for others. Keeping yourself empathetically available and open to all those around you, even those you know are not doing themselves service by their choices, is the most selfless and loving act you can

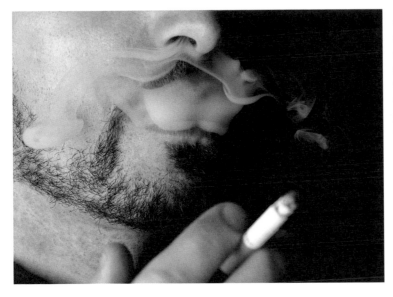

alerts us to—that something within us must change! You don't need to change the feeling of being uncomfortable; you need to address the message it's sending.

"Addict" can serve as an identity label. So can "priest," "CEO," "mom," "dad," "wife," "husband," "actor," "actress," "author," "lawyer," "judge" or "doctor," to name a few. These labels come with safety, and they obscure the notion that we are more than what we do or what others think of us. Our labels become shields we can hide our true selves behind. Whether your label reflects your position, your title, your past or a quality about yourself, even if it's negative, holding on to it meets your needs in feeling safe, important and secure. To let go of even the worst parts of ourselves means we have to embrace humility and become childlike again, exploring who we really are now and who we are in process of becoming, taking a cold hard look at the person staring back in the mirror.

commit yourself to—being a representative of God in their world which they may believe is God-less.

Addiction: Fact or Fantasy?

The reality is, we all have the capacity to get addicted to something. Some of us have empowering, positive addictions, like being of service to others, working out, keeping a disciplined routine or eating clean all of the time, others have negative addictions, like the over-consumption of alcohol, food, drugs or sex—again, often to feel some degree of control over the way we feel about our lives. Rather than spend time anticipating, planning, designing and working toward our magnificent life, being farsighted, we delude ourselves with actions that may short-circuit our life altogether. When the addiction is negative, the focus is typically uni-faceted—that is, changing the feeling of the moment without much regard for the cost against the future. We grow myopic and lose perspective when we feel pain, and we try to numb it immediately. We have lost appreciation for what pain

"To free yourself from suffering, you have to embrace that you are more than your job, your history, your accomplishments or your family roles."

To free yourself from suffering, you have to embrace that you are more than your job, your history, your accomplishments or your family roles. You are a divine spirit in a body meant to serve and enjoy all life has to offer you, and growing through all of it. Ironically, sometimes people even use religion as a way

Instant Gratification Does Not Equal Happiness

People often make the mistake of believing they want things to come easy. They dream of a life where they don't have to work so hard. They wish they could win the lottery. They want to wake up one morning and find they lost 50 pounds. They want a genie to come and grant them three wishes. But the truth is, instant gratification does not make a person happy.

Think of a person who has everything, who got whatever they wanted whenever they wanted it. Not only do we find that they can become some of the least appreciative people, they are often some of the least successful and definitely some of the unhappiest, as well. Having to work to achieve something really does serve to make you appreciate it more, and not having to work for something often makes you take it for granted. You work harder to keep what you value. If it's given to you just because you want it, then how much can you really appreciate it?

Studies of people who've created wealth shows that wealth usually disappears in subsequent generations; one individual creates a business empire, working 20-hour days, offering a world of privilege for his/ her children, wanting more for them. The children take this privilege for granted and squander their riches instead of caring for them and us- ing them to make the world a better place. By two or three generations down, the family has reverted to average, or sometimes even below-average, income.

You gain character, an appreciation of life and ultimately happiness from accomplish-ment. Little steps build esteem, which leads to confidence. You get excited when you start to make progress and you know you are the one making it happen, with God's help, of course! Anything worth having is worth working for.

You can even see this in your love life. You're crazy about someone and that person doesn't like you. Or someone likes you but you're not interested. It piques your interest when a person doesn't chase you around like a puppy dog. That's why for eons women have been advised to "play hard to get." It stimulates a man's interest when you are not too "easy" (and that's not just sexual). If you are inter-ested in a person and call or text multiple times and are always available, begging them to go out, they will lose interest in you in no time. In fact you'll probably find them run-ning away. Is this fair? Maybe, maybe not, but it's the truth. It's the same thing with every aspect of your life. Scarcity breeds desire. You take for granted anything that comes without effort, and you quickly lose interest in it.

Think of a very poor child in a part of the world where people barely subsist. Think if you gave that child the most miserable-looking ball or doll, and how incredibly happy that child would be. Here in America, kids might have a collection of video games, brand-name shoes, basketballs, sports equipment, and a toy box full of dolls or toy cars and trucks. Some of these toys may lie untouched within days or even hours after they've been opened. We take much for granted in this life, and for many of us, it's because it comes too easily.

Do you truly appreciate every day that you have a roof over your head? If you lived in a cave or on the street for a time you sure would. Maybe instead of appreciating it, you just moan about your housing situation not being adequate. God knows I don't think there's anything wrong with wanting more and wanting to achieve, but you can work for more while being grateful for where you are and without taking for granted what you already have. Do you appreciate the working body God gave you? If you are overeating junk food and not exercising, then you're not valuing that incredible gift. Maybe it's time you became honest with yourself.

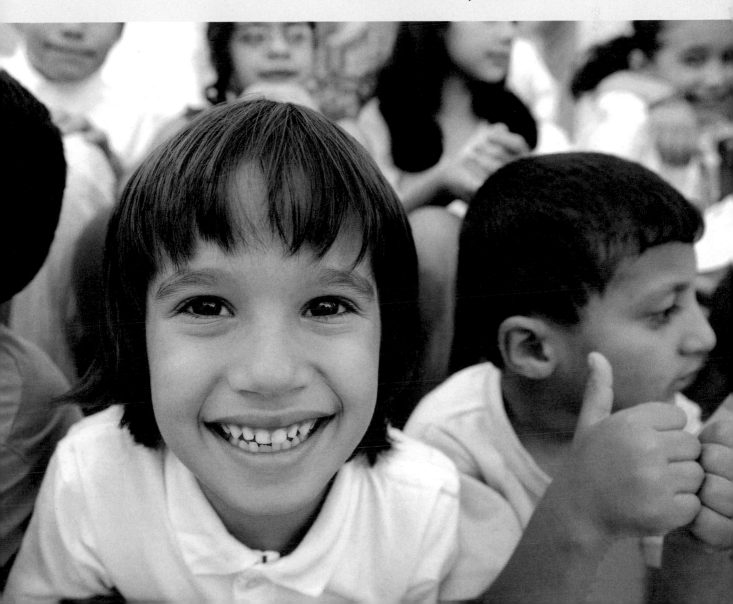

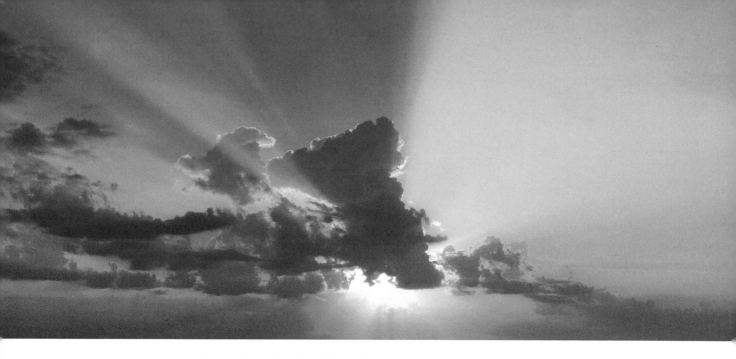

to *distract* themselves from God and separate themselves from others! They use religion as a tool against having meaningful or vulnerable human relationships.

When we look at the life of Jesus, a man who was both God and human, we see He didn't hide from the human part of himself. He wasn't living high above the city in a castle. He lived on the streets. He didn't consult with kings, telling them how to rule their kingdom. He helped people who were average, uneducated and suffering to find meaning in their everyday lives. Jesus brought divinity to places we wouldn't expect to find it. So must we. I think it's the responsibility we each have, regardless of our faith, to do the same. The streets Jesus walked barefoot on were not paved in gold; they were dusty, rough, and dirty. He was always moving, not worried about the future, just focused on being truly present with each person He encountered, being a force of love in the lives of those He called and who were called to follow Him. It's not to say He didn't have human qualities— He just stayed more centered on His spiritual nature than His human.

When you embrace spirituality and not only religion, you will find it's not that you know *about* God, you actually begin to *know God personally,* the force that connects all of

us. Being responsible and successful isn't a way to separate yourself from everyone else, with the air of superiority, it's a way for you to realize the connection between all of us, because when you become the best you, then you can be the best for all those around you. When you become financially independent because of your success, you realize, like all truly successful wealthy people do, that you're anything but independent. You choose to become involved in doing more for others, considering the blessings you've experienced and your gratitude for what you have.

The same is true for being free of illness. Most people who have struggled with and overcome some disease, or a challenge like addiction, can serve as a source of inspiration and power for others. The more they pour out into the lives of others, the larger the space within them for God to refill. As they help others grow, they become even larger and more capable in their own right.

Be present. Don't concern yourself with fame, fortune or the opinion of others. Look only to whether or not you are seeing love and goodness blossom in your life and in the lives of those you're interacting with when you want to think about whether or not you are on track. With this as your focus, joy is inevitable. Misery is attachment to expectations of how you believe people and things should be rather than to gratitude for just how blessed you are.

Feeling Your Way to God

Religions of antiquity have always said we can never really see God. I think this means God exists outside of our human experience and beyond our five physical senses. It's not that God doesn't use our senses to point us in His direction, but that the knowing of God, the intimate awareness of God being with you, and I do mean literally with you, transcends the visceral. To have awareness of God's presence with you in every moment of your life means complete absence of fear and suffering.

"We all have seasons of pain and despair, but we needn't stay there."

In the darkest moments in my own life, a profound serenity quickly brought light, quite inexplicably. When my grandma was moved into a nursing home despite her wishes to remain independent and the ability to continue visiting her seemed dubious, a "knowing" came upon me that all would be well and God was working things through. I cannot explain from where this comes, but I can tell you that the more you allow God in, the closer He comes to you.

That doesn't mean you won't experience pain or disappointment. We all have seasons of pain and despair, but we needn't stay there. Spirituality teaches us that suffering comes from attachment. What are you holding on to that is hindering your growth? Can you stop and just be present? What if today was your last day on this planet? Where would you spend your time? Who would you be spending it with?

If you were using anything excessively to numb the pain or fill the emptiness, you'd find when you raise your thinking to a higher level you would stop immediately. Why? Because you would totally immerse yourself in the now. You wouldn't eat excessively or use drugs to numb yourself because your history would immediately be rendered irrelevant, as would tomorrow. When you raise your thinking to that higher level, you won't travel the city hopping from bakery to bakery for a cupcake from each or seeking out a drug dealer for a hit. When now is all there is, you will choose to spend time with those you feel closest to, and make meaningful contributions to their lives. You'll tell them how you really feel. When you take your ego out of the picture and just observe, then what do you notice about yourself? When you become the still awareness of who you are spiritually, maybe by imagining that you are watching yourself at this moment on a theater screen, are you joyful? Is it evident in your physiology there is much that's troubling you, much that you are trying to hold back? It's not unusual for psychic pain to manifest itself physically.

"God isn't found in a particular dogma or theology or religion, he's found in you and the relationship you have with yourself and others."

There is a wonderful book on the subject by Dr. John Sarno called *The Mindbody Prescription* that goes deep into this subject if you're interested.

When I have clients do this exercise they often cry, as they've long neglected the spiritual side of themselves. They recognize there are relationships that need healing, parts of their past they haven't integrated because of the fear they have of experiencing the pain they may not have been ready to deal with at the time. Start to look at crying not as a sign of weakness, but as a necessary purifying experience, ridding you of toxic feelings about things that have happened. It's kind of like a bath. If you need to give yourself that kind of bath, do it. God isn't found in a particular dogma or theology or religion, He's found in you and the relationship you have with yourself and others.

Expectations Will Determine What You Experience

We have a way of deciding what is possible based on our past experience, and that makes sense, to a point. We have spent our entire lives doing this, from the time we were born—everything from learning how not to fall when we're walking to learning how to ride a bike. But we should use our experience to figure out how to succeed, not convince ourselves that we will fail. We need to learn from all

"We should use our experience to figure out how to succeed, not convince ourselves that we will fail."

the experiences—the good and the bad. If the choices you made resulted in an outcome you didn't want, then you can use that experience in order to make different choices next time and get the outcome you want.

The vast majority of us set extremely low expectations for ourselves, mostly because we have memories of failing in the past or because we fear failing in the future. We get so tied up in the opinion of others we forget that the only way to get more from life is to speak faith over it and act on that. Your expectations will send out a message to the universe to clothe that expectation in the nearest tangible form. If you think "I'm

fat," you'll find all sorts of temptations and references to support it. If you think, "I need to lose weight," the energy associated with that thinking in itself is negative. Rather, shift to: "I want to become my absolute best." You'll begin to set your inner GPS, your mind, to recognize the opportunities to become more than you currently are, to become your best self. When becoming your best is your major focus, your energy will flow in that direction, making it easy to follow through with the right actions.

Be Flexible—Learn and Earn from Past Efforts

As we discussed earlier, if you tried to quit smoking but failed because you continued to hang out with friends who smoke, then the next time you decide to quit smoking hopefully you will learn from that experience and not hang out with people who smoke while you're trying to quit. "I've tried to quit smoking before and I didn't manage to make it through two days, therefore I am unable to quit," is not the message you should take from that previous experience, but that is the type of logic many of us carry through our lives. This is just another variation of making excuses. It's a powerful way of preventing yourself from achieving your goals, and is the opposite of what achievers practice.

I hear this kind of thing all the time in my practice as a weight-loss coach: "I've tried everything and nothing works." What you're really saying is that you have been frustrated and disappointed so often that buying into the story seems better than stepping out to take control of your life once and for all. You have decided to focus more on your pain than your possibilities.

What you need to learn from these experiences isn't that you are a failure at every weight-loss plan and by definition can't succeed, but rather take a look at which choices you have made each time that sabotaged your ultimate success. Power and strength comes from mental flexibility. Black-and-white thinking like "Since I had that one bite of cake I screwed up my entire plan so forget

life's storms, saving you decades of pain and suffering through their trial and error, if you allow yourself to learn from them.

If you're older, stay open minded and alert to the changing times and the opportunities

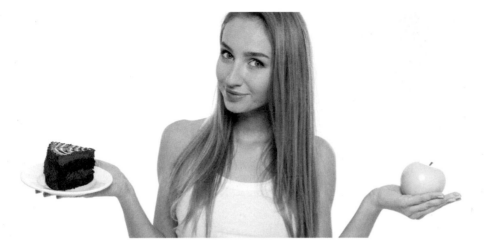

it," isn't wise. This type of rigidity leads to exhaustion—both physically and mentally. The key to lasting success is discovering the fine balance between consistency and flexibility. Despite your best efforts, you will always meet the unexpected on any journey. You will find yourself out later than you had intended, for example, and getting very hungry because you've missed the time you were supposed to eat. If you're getting control of your finances, you will have unexpected expenses such as your car needing repair. Do your best to proactively guard yourself against anything that could undermine your efforts. Expect the unexpected. Look at your past. What triggered you to break the agreement you had with yourself in your previous efforts? What can you do so you're fortified against such a threat moving forward from this point?

Important for this success preparation, especially if you're young, is to not think you know it all. The successful person is always learning and growing. Be around and learn from wise elders who've weathered many of

"The key to lasting success is discovering the fine balance between consistency and flexibility."

new research in medicine and technology can afford you. All too often age hardens one's will to the point that any unexpected change can be devastating. Maintain the hope and curiosity of a child, and you'll stay just as young spiritually!

A Contract with Yourself

To boil most of our life problems down is quite simple: we've become masters at breaking agreements with ourselves. Continually upholding your own highest standards takes work. While we all can construct wonderful stories around our circumstances to alleviate our regret over a bad decision, that story doesn't resolve the fact that you and you alone didn't stick with the program. Sometimes

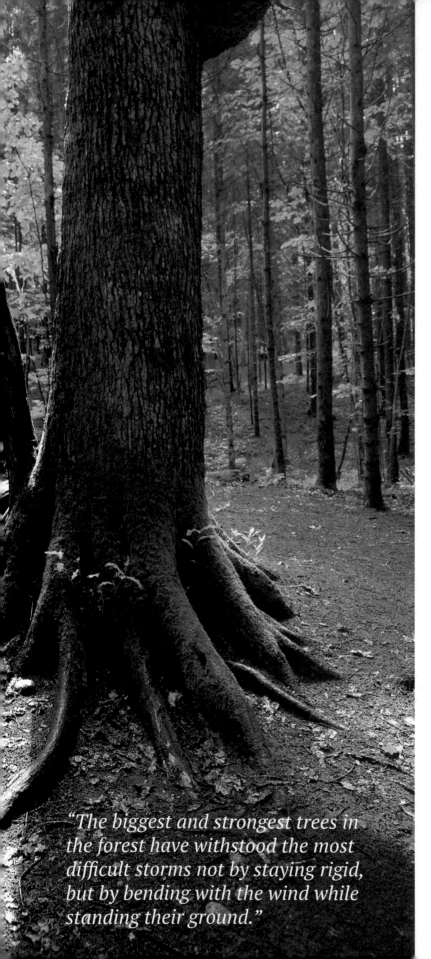

"The biggest and strongest trees in the forest have withstood the most difficult storms not by staying rigid, but by bending with the wind while standing their ground."

these seeming defeats are actually grace in action. Learn and grow from the experience, and become stronger for the next time. How many success stories have you encountered about the biggest breakthrough coming in a person's life only after their greatest letdown? What doesn't break us makes us stronger. The biggest and strongest trees in the forest have withstood the most difficult storms not by staying rigid, but by bending with the wind while standing their ground. Much like the martial art Aikido, you can learn to use the things that could break you as a force for good in your life, turning them around so they never defeat your drive! Be more concerned with winning the war than you are with success in just one battle. You need to train yourself to think long term to get what you deserve.

Replace Spontaneity with Strategy

One of the biggest problems I see with people when they are attempting to make any life change is spontaneity. I'm sure you've heard the old adage "if you fail to plan, you plan to fail," and this has become an adage because it's absolutely true. If you have started a weight-loss program but you haven't gone shopping for the foods you need, or you don't bring your lunch to work or have a plan for buying food nearby, then you are creating an environment where it's more likely that you will break away from your weight-loss plan. If you've experienced this before then that should tell you to be prepared and know exactly what and when you're going to eat each day, not that no diet will work for you. Spontaneity is the antithesis to your success, at least initially. For diet success you must have purpose and reason behind every decision of what you will eat and how you will exercise. Once you have made a clear decision and created the circumstances where it will happen, you are well on the road to success.

If you're trying to save money, then it's easiest when that savings comes directly off your paycheck and into a savings account. You've made the decision in advance and it's automated. That way you don't need to decide whether or not you're going to put money away each time you get a paycheck, and if so, how much. Whatever your goal is, you must make the associated decisions *before you begin* and *automate* them, so you are not faced with unneeded temptation that takes the energy you could expend reaching your goal!

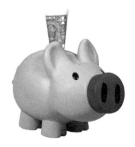

"Whatever your goal is, you must make the associated decisions before you begin and automate them, so you are not faced with unneeded temptation that takes the energy you could expend reaching your goal!"

Fortify Your System Against Threat

What you put in your body is as important as the environment you choose to have around you, and that's not just food. Another thing likely to make it difficult for you to follow through with your plans is drinking alcohol. Everyone knows alcohol lowers your inhibition, making you less likely to stay on track with any moral action. Think of what happens if you have a couple of drinks while following a weight-loss plan. Throw in a couple of friends trying to convince you to go off your diet and bam! Next thing you know you're downing your fourth slice of pizza. Pretty much everyone who's been on a weight-loss plan has had an experience like this at some point.

From this, you can learn to recognize that you are not yet at a point where you can afford a chink in your mental armor, so it's probably best if you're more secure in your positive habits before you go out with your friends under this type of circumstance, because choosing to drink alcohol with your friends makes you more likely to go off your weight-loss plan. There may be a point later on when you feel strong enough to do so, but if you feel uneasy now, listen to that inner voice and gut feeling—it knows best! Let self-direction

be your guide. Don't be faked out by ideals. Embrace the truth. Build your strength. You might love the idea of lifting a 100-pound dumbbell, but heading to the gym one day and trying it without any training would result in a serious injury. Over time and with consistent focus and determination, however, you can develop the strength that will make that dumbbell seem light. When you are willing to undertake the process of disciplining yourself to do the fundamentals now, you will enjoy the benefits.

Never Look Back with Regret

Our past can help us to learn and grow and improve, but all too often we instead use it to hold ourselves back. This can be a semi-conscious reaction when we use our experiences as an excuse for not trying, or it can be completely unconscious, when what you consider the meaning of your past may be so ingrained in your psyche that you honestly have no awareness that it cannot hold you back unless you let it.

This is often the case when people come from negative family backgrounds. If your entire extended family grew up poor, then it can be hard to place even your imaginary self into a world of wealth. Forget about the voices you hear *outside* of you. Pay attention to the voice *inside* of you, that voice from your past, working hard to convince you to stay the way you've been, despite your unhappiness. The idea of being rich in all senses of the word may seem very foreign and unusual to you. But you are no different from the people already in that land of wealth. The only thing stopping you from being there are the choices you make every day.

Thoughts → Emotions → Choices → Results

I grew up in a poor household with a poor extended family, but I managed to climb my way out of those low expectations by opening my mind up and expanding my awareness of what was possible. I did this by looking at all those in the world who had what I wanted. I wanted it, I had emotional hunger to go for it, and I chose it. The daily choices I made brought me out of the place I had felt stuck in, and you can also make those choices.

> *"The daily choices I made brought me out of the place I had felt stuck in, and you can also make those choices."*

No magic genie came out of any lamp offering to make my wishes come true, but I did begin truly listening to God. I had to act on faith—things that didn't make sense to me but made sense to God. Luckily, my conscience, the Holy Spirit, intuition, whatever you want to label that "knowing" as, was always there to guide me. I just had to trust in it, as do you. God led me to everything I needed to create the life I wanted, a life far from where anyone

would think I'd have ended up from looking at my family background. While no magic genie came to me, the story of *Aladdin*, which appears in this book multiple times, does have a lesson for you. We all loved the Disney film with the big blue genie that granted a poor beggar three wishes. When I saw the play in New York, the real meaning of the story became clear. The boy Aladdin yearns for the opulence he sees in the Kingdom of Agrabah, and fatefully meets the princess, who is sick and tired of the limitation she feels such a privileged life brings. She's moved by his generosity when she sees him, although starving himself, offer a loaf of bread he's stolen to an old beggar woman who is also hungry. The princess doesn't like the disparity between the way she lives and the way others in the kingdom live.

Love happens at first sight, but providence would have it that an evil sorcerer, Jafar, also has interest in the boy Aladdin. Jafar has been told the boy is a "diamond in the rough"—he has purity of heart and can therefore get the magic lamp that will give its owner anything he desires. The evil sorcerer seeks out Aladdin and makes him get the lamp. Unintentionally, however, the lamp becomes Aladdin's and the genie is his, offering to grant him three wishes. One of his first wishes is to be a prince, to win the heart of the princess. Instantly, he is clothed in the most expensive and impressive garments. He is given an entourage and taken to the palace, where he intends to impress her and her father. She had already fallen in love with him as a beggar, but he thinks it's because he is a prince. Conflicted, he doesn't know whether to do what's right and reveal who he really is or play into the lie, never being his true self with her. The genie reminds him that the reason she fell in love with him and the reason he was given the grace to receive the lamp was because of who he really is: honest, loving, sincere and goodhearted.

The blessings were given to him because of those qualities. So too it is with you. You don't become a good person by becoming wealthy; you attract wealth by being the good person you can be. You need only be your true self to have all that you could ever dream of and more. I can't prove it; I can only inspire you to try, promising that I have found it to be true in my life and I've seen it time and again in the lives of all those I've coached.

Success Pitfalls

Once I began listening to God, I started reading books by people who had fulfilled their destiny despite all odds. I learned from them. I began to see the trap I had been falling into, making excuses and making bad choices, and I climbed out of that trap.

"The only things that dictate future failure are not trying again and not learning from what you've done before."

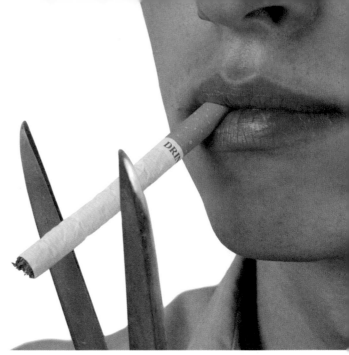

Learn from what's happened in your life so far. Grow beyond it. I began to see myself as the person God created me to be—not deficient or flawed or less than others. I began to behave the way the person I wanted to be would behave. I began surrounding myself with people I wanted to be like, and I began consistently acting in the ways that would bring me there. I acknowledged my errors and refined my approach. Lo and behold, I achieved my goals! So can you!

I decided I wanted something very different. And so I created something different. The first step was to accept God was in me, as He is in you. The second step was to admit that it was possible and even my responsibility to create the future I deserved and the reality that God wanted for me, not only for myself, but for those I love and the world at large. The third step was to make the choices that would ensure that future. Simple. My genetics, my family history or the opinions of others could not stop me any more than yours can stop you!

"We get to decide, and if we truly want the thing we say we want, then we need to create a new narrative."

Our family history, our upbringing, the neighborhood we grew up in, whether we had proper food on the table, whether we were abused or loved … all these things help to create the story we tell ourselves about why we are the way we are, and why life is as it is. Ultimately they can serve as excuses to stay limited and stuck or reasons to become more. We get to decide, and if we truly want the thing we say we want, then we need to create a new narrative. Look for what's great about your history instead of what was wrong with it. Remember the different ways of looking

"Instead of thinking your family or environment needs to change, change your perspective!"

at going off the rails when you've had a few drinks? That you can take the experience and say you're a failure and there's no point in trying or you can look at it as something you've learned from and therefore will be careful not to put yourself in that position again? What you need is a new thought process. Here's something I've heard a million times: "I've tried hundreds of diets, and none of them worked." The unwritten next thought is: "If that is the case, then trying another diet is useless because it won't work either." Maybe a diet isn't the answer, but rather, a shift in how you think about yourself is. Maybe instead of thinking of yourself as an overweight woman who needs to lose weight, you need to think of yourself as an athlete who's nourishing her body and inevitably will become fitter and leaner because of this newly embraced philosophy!

Plenty of people have had a lifetime of failure in losing weight or breaking bad habits, then suddenly they have an epiphany and turn it all around. I bet you can think of someone like this. Lots of people have tried numerous times to quit smoking, haven't managed to, and then did. I read that the average number of times a person tries to quit smoking before actually succeeding is around 12. The actual number doesn't matter, but what does matter is that the person doesn't stop trying just because he or she did not follow through on previous attempts. Once you are totally dedicated and committed you will find a way, and if there isn't a way, you'll make one!

Remember, your definition of failure is personal. The only things that dictate future failure are not trying again and not learning from what you've done before. With few exceptions, and I'm going to guess you're not reading this while serving a life sentence, your previous bad choices do not affect your possibility of having the exact future you want. They may mean you have a little further to go to reach your goal than you otherwise would, but making good choices in the future will still bring you there. You may find, in fact, that your previous bad choices can even help you to make better choices down the road.

Maybe you come from a poor background, like I did, but still can create wealth, as I have. Wealth isn't measured only in material terms. You may have poor health and obesity in your family, like I did, and still become lean and fit, as I am. You may have addiction in your family, like I did, and choose never to touch alcohol or illicit drugs, as I do not. You may have abuse in your family, as I did, and have kind, giving and loving relationships, as I do. The fact that I and so many others have done this proves that it is possible, and if it is possible for us it means it's possible for you too. That is solid logic.

When I decided to change my life as a teen, I looked for role models. I don't want you to think my family members were evil people. They were not. I am so grateful for each and every person in my family, those who've passed

on and those still here. I was loved, but in many ways their lives taught me more about what *not to do* than what *to do* for the life I wanted to create.

My father's parents were the only set of biological grandparents I really knew well. My grandparents were kind and loving, but they didn't have any formal education. My grandfather had to leave school at the age of nine, along with his brothers, to support their family. Neither of my grandparents finished school. One got to about grade three or four and the other to eighth grade. My grandpa literally couldn't read. They were hardworking, and they were able to provide a home for my dad and his four brothers, but they had very little money. They didn't know the white bread

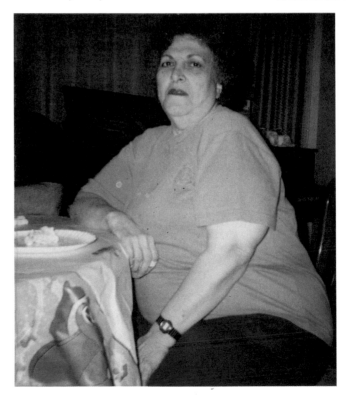

MY DAD'S MOM WAS SO JOYFUL AND LOVING, BUT DIDN'T PUT HERSELF FIRST. SHE HAD A WEIGHT PROBLEM AS LONG AS I KNEW HER.

and white pasta with butter they lived on and fed their sons would help ensure that they'd all have problems with obesity, diabetes and heart disease, but that was the case. I grew up with that same food and worse. When I was a child and felt sad and terrible about myself, which was much of the time, my mom, at that time so sweet and loving, would make me feel better by taking me to fast food place for a kid's meal, or by giving me candy. These foods did distract and give me comfort at the time, although they came at a huge cost, creating problems for my future. Instead of helping by making me healthy and providing nutrition like food is meant to, these foods deformed me into an obese and extremely unhealthy teen, to the point that I legitimately didn't think I'd be alive for my high school graduation. That all said, I am extremely grateful for all of it—my mom's love as well as the lessons I learned about bad habits. When you are touched personally by such suffering, it can motivate you fiercely.

We've talked about truth and about stories. The truth is good, and it's important to be clear on the truth in order to create a better future. It's the stories we tell ourselves, using these truths as tools in our excuse making, that are not so useful. Yes, practically everyone in my family was obese. Yes, I grew up with both their genes and their habits. Yes, I lived on junk food and used it to try to make myself feel good, like it was a drug. Yes, I too became obese like the rest of my family. Yes, my mother got caught up in a pattern of self hate—acting out in mean, violent and aggressive ways when using alcohol and prescription drugs. Yes, I was beginning to suffer from health troubles. Yes, I could barely summon the energy to walk up four stairs at my school. Yes, I weighed 360 pounds. Yes, I would come home from school and eat an

extra-large pizza and drink a two-liter bottle of soda all by myself.

All those things are true. But this did not mean that my life and future was doomed! No, no, no! Far from it. I could have continued to use all those truths to make stories that supported the excuses to stay in the place I hated, but I finally decided I didn't want to stay there! All of these things were true when I was 17 years old, but by the time I was 20 years old I was posing shirtless for *Cosmopolitan* magazine, had become extremely healthy and fit, and was already helping dozens of other people to become healthy and fit too. Soon heads of state and political dignitaries were seeking my counsel and inviting me to dinner. By the time I graduated from college, the first person in my family to do so, I had already helped many hundreds of people to lose weight and become healthy, even if they thought they'd "tried everything." By choosing my own future despite my history and my family's history, by following the path that God wanted my life to take instead of the one laid out before me, not only have I been able

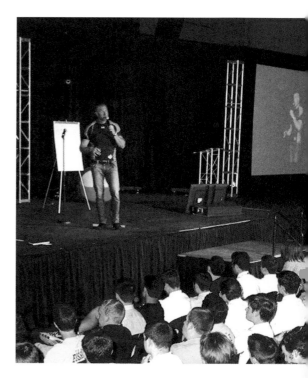

> "*I could easily have allowed the limiting beliefs of my environment to dictate my future. I had everything going against me. But I didn't want to make excuses; I wanted to make changes.*"

to provide a wonderful life for myself but also help my parents and family. I became a blessing to others because of the value I was bringing to their lives. I was able to help other people find their own way from past mistakes and improve their lives.

That has continued even more so, between my coaching, my talks and my books, to hundreds of thousands of people I've been able to positively influence. Believe me that would never have happened if I'd just said, oh, my family's all overweight. I was meant to be overweight. Of course I won't ever be fit. Or, no one in my family went to college. I won't either. Marriage, hah, all of those fail. I could easily have allowed the limiting beliefs of my environment to dictate my future. I had everything going against me.

I don't even like talking about it here, to be honest. As I said earlier, the best thing about the past is that it's over. Why relive the story? I do it for your sake. I find few people open up about what's really going on in their lives. Instead they plaster on a fake smile, pretending everything is great. The first step in making life great is admitting it may not truly be great for you right now. Start there. I didn't want to find reasons not to fulfill my dream and my God-given destiny; I wanted to fulfill that dream and find that destiny!

Three Determinates

While your past doesn't dictate your future, there are a few things that do. One is your energy. Are you excited about growing and

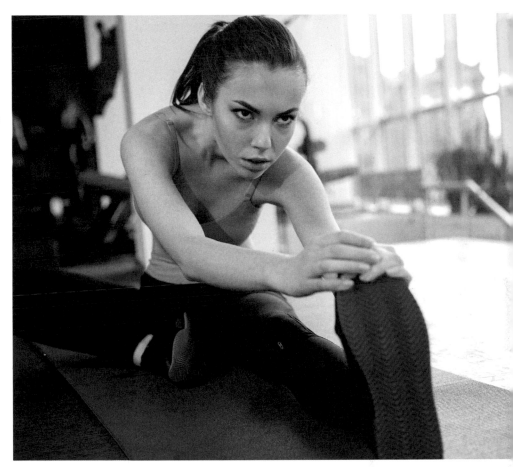

developing and achieving your destiny? If you wake up every day charged up, thinking about that goal and actually seeing yourself achieving it, you will jump out of bed, excited for the chance to get one step closer. This energy is what creates the motivation you need to see your goals through to fruition and resist temptation. When you are filled with energy, you are filled with drive and ambition. Willpower and discipline stem easily from that.

Second, your attitude. Are you positive? Do you believe that you can do this because others have proved it's possible? Or are you filled with negativity and disbelief? Are you looking for more reasons to disprove your capacity than to prove it? It takes years to paint a timeless work of art, but only a second to rip it to shreds. The cynical, pessimistic,

> *"The only real enemy of your personal success is you."*

doubtful view is fueled by fear. Recognize it for what it is. It takes no courage if you try to legitimize your despondency using data and statistics to stay the way you are. The truth is, you can find cases for both—reasons you can and those that have, and reasons you can't along with many who haven't. Which side do you want to be on? You need to believe that within yourself you deserve more than you have and are already where you are meant to be—you just have to take some small steps, one day at time, to make your current life match your vision.

The third thing that dictates your future is your worldview. How do you see the world around you? Do you see life as riddled with obstacles or with opportunities? Do you see walls and hurdles you have to jump over or do you see challenges that you'll get stronger from overcoming? If you think of the things in your life that make accomplishing your goals more difficult as a reason not to accomplish them, then you are going to create your own self-defeating prophecy. We all have things we have to work beyond. Challenges are for growth. The key is figuring out how to use and learn from them.

Your worldview is your personal perspective on life. You get to choose it. Not your parents, your friends, your teachers, your counselors, or doctors. It's how you view the world around you, and it's how you view your possibilities within that world. If you have a positive and optimistic outlook, you are more likely to be successful in your endeavors than if you have a negative outlook, even if you are at a disadvantage in other ways.

> *"Challenges are for growth. The key is figuring out how to use and learn from them."*

In one study participants were measured on intelligence level and optimism. They were then measured on their ability to make sales. Those with lower intelligence but greater optimism closed the sale 57% more often than those who had greater intelligence but a less-than-optimistic viewpoint. In other words, positivity and the idea that you can find your way around hurdles were more important than intelligence level to success rate. So attitude and worldview were the most important aspects of success. Add in the energy and you have my trifecta for a life you were meant to, and deserve to have.

That study (and many others) supported what successful people have known all along, anecdotally: Positivity breeds success, and negativity works in the exact opposite way. And that is why you need to carefully choose who you spend your time with.

Your mom was spot on when she said she didn't want you hanging around a certain crowd. No matter how good the head is that you carry on your shoulders, you will be influenced by those around you. The more we encounter something, the more we accept it, and the more you're around people the more like them you become. They say your income is the average of the five people you spend the most time with. And if you hang around with people who drink too much you will probably start drinking too much. And if your friends are overweight you are more likely to be overweight. That's the deal. If you are with people who have low expectations of their place in life, then you will lower your own.

But it also works the other way. If you hang around with people who have high expectations of themselves, then you will automatically reach for a higher place for yourself. I always say I'm not happy unless I'm the least intelligent person in the room. I love to be surrounded by people who are smarter than I am, who have knowledge bases that I don't, who achieve their goals, and most importantly, who give of themselves. Being around people like this means I'm always learning and always becoming a better person.

This is a very important step out of a past that you may not think has been optimal for achieving your goals. Very few people have had optimal lives. You usually just don't know what they've had to overcome. No one knew what I was going through as a teen. They just thought I was a very overweight, obedient

> *"Positivity breeds success, and negativity works in the exact opposite way. And that is why you need to carefully choose who you spend your time with."*

student who got good grades. The kid you grew up envying because she lived in a big house with fancy clothes and cars might have gone home to a family under constant threat of foreclosure and repossession because they had overextended themselves. You do not know what the successful people around had to overcome, but you can bet your life they had to overcome something.

The only real enemy of your personal success is you. When you see corporations fail, relationships end, people go through challenges, rarely is it something that happened overnight. It is the consequence of a long history of neglect. Not staying aware and conscious of where their daily habits and choices were leading. The process of becoming all you were intended to be is something that we are all hard wired for. You are never without the capacity to choose a different course if the one you're on isn't working for you. You can always expand your vision of the future, learn new skills, network with more people, start new meaningful relationships—the power is yours.

The time is now to make a change. Don't keep waiting for some arbitrary time in the future; you do not have forever. You know many in my family didn't take control of life until it was too late. Don't let that be you. Make this moment the time you stop making excuses and begin to create the future you want and deserve to have.

CHAPTER SEVEN

Discovering The Path to Success: Living an Unapologetic Life

Now that we've worked through the excuses and you've decided you're ready to take full responsibility for yourself and whatever shows up in your life, you need to decide what you're going to do with your power.

If you've ever watched the Oscar-winning movie *American Beauty*, you may remember the shot of the bag blowing around in the wind. To me this is a reminder of how most people choose to live their lives, being blown around in circles by the wind, as if they had no will of their own.

You are not a plastic bag subject to the whims of circumstance. You are one of God's creations. You were born to succeed and enjoy your life. You are human, yes, but more importantly, you are spiritual. Imagine! The Creator of all things, the sun, the moon, the stars, the galaxies, every butterfly and beautiful plant in nature, took the time to design and then create you for this very moment in history. Not only did He create you, He gave you power to be a co-creator in the world and impact his initial creation for the better. He made you a person with the power of choice to have an impact in the world, in a specific and important way, helping the other people He created.

How could you harbor any doubt or have any fear when you know that God is with you and on your side? You are one of His children, literally. We have flesh but we are so much more than that. We all have His spark—traits of our Creator.

Even if you were born into poverty or recently suffered an unexpected loss or life-altering accident, there is always a reason, and even when your human side tells you to be afraid, you can know that things will get better. Always. If you truly understand that you came

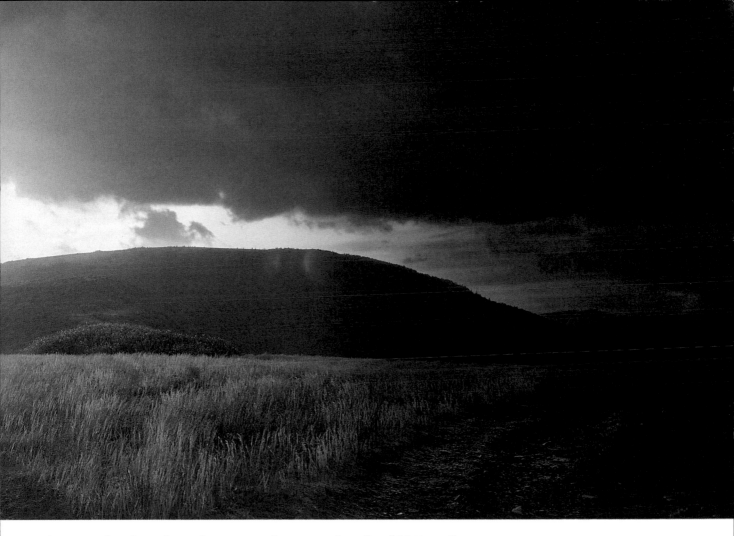

from something beyond your five senses and that grace is always operating in your life, you'll find you don't worry when the unexpected happens. It's been said that those who have attempted suicide but lived to tell the tale instantly regretted it the moment they step foot off the bridge. It's as if their lifeblood kicks in and clears out the clouds that had obscured all the good within them and in their future.

Clean Your Heart

To get better, to feel better, to be better as a person, you must begin to think better. Your thoughts, and the actions you take as a result, have far more to do with how your life is going than your situations ever do. If you start to see your life as being in divine order, including those things that don't meet your expectations,

miracles will unfold. You will start to recognize the things you call mistakes in your life as being necessary for your development into the person you're in the process of becoming.

"To get your life back in flow and find your path means not only getting your head right, but getting your heart right as well."

The major purpose of your life is to love every moment of it and be an example of love to all you encounter regardless of any blessing or difficulty—that includes loving yourself, most importantly. Many people spend time on their mental development at the expense of their own spiritual growth. To get your life back in flow and find your path means not only getting your head right, but getting your heart right as well. How you feel and how you think are interrelated. You can know exactly what you need to do, but if much of your time is spent on gossip, worry, doubt, or if you have envy or jealousy within your heart, you'll find it hard to keep your mind on the higher planes of thought and living.

or unintentional, free yourself and forgive them, wishing nothing but good to come their way. It's time to unhook your past so you can reel in your future. You'll notice some errors in life right away, like a bad haircut, but spiritual errors can take a long time before the problem becomes evident!

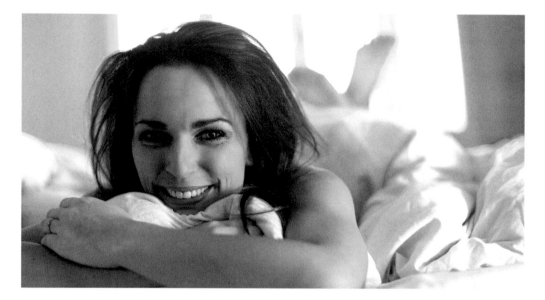

You want to be able to consistently tune into bringing about the best energy and power into your life, not just because you want it for what it gives you, but because you want to be of service for your Creator, doing what you were born to do. You want to make the formless, the invisible, become visible. To make this happen, you have to make sure you've cleaned your heart of any hostility, anger, guilt or regret—whether it is directed toward yourself or another. You need to be in a state of peace. To be a Creator you have to make sure you are operating in the image of the one who created you, God. Bringing the light of forgiveness into the shadows of your life is important. Now is time to apologize wherever appropriate and move forward. If you've felt you've let yourself down, forgive yourself. If you feel you've let those who have selflessly loved you the most down, forgive yourself. If you feel others have wronged you, whether intentional

Choose the Positive

Sometimes things that feel good in the moment aren't so good for us spiritually. The saying "sweet in the mouth but bitter in the belly" comes to mind. Are you using things and people to meet your needs without regard for the moral or ethical implications on your life and theirs? Have you misused the people that God has put into your life as gifts, seeking your own benefit but to their detriment? Have you been ungrateful for the small things in your life, or the countless chances you've been given to turn it around despite repeatedly screwing up? Now is the time to repent—and while that statement may have a religious undertone, I simply mean change your mind, and most importantly, change direction!

None of us is perfect and it goes back to the time of creation. We can see from the first book of the Bible two simple truths plainly stated. First, God created the Heaven and the Earth. Second, it says that all He created was good. You were created in his perfect image, so therefore you are good. I believe the message of the story of Adam and Eve is not that we are all imperfect, but rather that despite our innate goodness, it's through errors in our choices and actions, our human nature, that we can become estranged from God, estranged from each other, and estranged from our planet.

"Your physical self impacts your emotional, and both have an impact on all of your relationships."

To be able to channel the highest power available to you, God's energy, you must be clear minded, pure hearted, and aligned with His will. Your physical self impacts your emotional, and both have an impact on all of your relationships. This triad can help create a success vortex in your life or a death spiral, depending on how well you're managing any of the three areas. If you haven't been taking care of your body, then your brain chemistry, hormones, and ultimately how you feel will impact how well or poorly you are thinking. If you're abusing drugs or other substances, or having ineffectual or abusive relationships, then your thoughts will be clouded at best, which ultimately means you will feel lonely no matter how many people you're around. If you don't make sure you are thinking about those you love, your family, friends and community, you'll become stressed out and again, it will impact how your body is working and how you feel emotionally. We are more than just skin and bones, so you must make sure your heart, your intention, is pure if you truly desire to find your path to success. I look at it as a machine with three gears—body, mind, and

connections. If any of these are jammed, the machine called life doesn't work.

If what you want to achieve isn't loving and positive in all regards, you will be met with pain even if you succeed in achieving it. The strategies I'm going to give you can be used for good or bad. The choice of how you'll use these tools is yours, but I plead that you make sure what you set as goals are things you've spent time thinking through. There is no greater suffering than getting what you want and finding you're still unhappy. That's a clear indication that the problem is on the inside. Rather than going through all the effort to get what you want and then having to deal with that later, get it out on the table and handle it now. You don't need to spend countless years trying to figure out why you don't like yourself or what happened that gave you a negative self-image because even if you find it, nothing changes except the time lost in searching that could have been spent on growing. Instead, channel your energies into a new way of living, knowing you never "discover" who you are; instead you constantly create it.

The ultimate secret to success is becoming the kind of person who exemplifies the best qualities of what it means to be human—healthy, connected and in service to others, optimistic, unconditionally loving, understanding, compassionate, patient, committed, just, creative and honest.

If you strive to make these traits part of your character, washing away anything less out of your heart, you will make room for God to flow through you. You will ultimately enjoy what comes from His work in your life! Seeing

God's hand in your life each waking moment and in the lives of those around you is the strongest validation and reassurance you can ever experience. Even the death of those closest to you cannot shake the peace that comes from this awareness that you have the source of all things with you at every turn.

Transform Your Mind, Transform Your Life

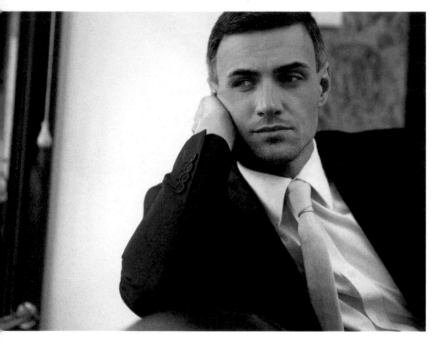

The marketplace offers us a great example of just how much our thinking impacts us in the real practical sense. Do you know of anyone who works in a similar career to you but makes multiples of what you are making? People who spend the same amount of time at work but make more money? What's the deal?

Two people can offer the same service in the marketplace at the same time, but one can earn a hundred or even a thousand times more than the other. This normally means their passion, belief and faith in what they're doing and where they're going leads to a more creative and persuasive presentation of themselves and/or their service.

As mentioned earlier, it is shown that attitude has more bearing on success than intelligence. Positivity is extremely important. But along with a positive attitude must be action. A great attitude might be helpful in recovering from a serious illness, for example, but along with the attitude must come doing everything in your power according to real research in order to beat your illness. I'm sure you've heard the saying God helps those who help themselves. That is when God knows you're really serious! You cannot ever give up, because He always has the power to help. He has the final word.

With regard to wealth, the same holds true. It's comforting to know that of the 585 billionaires in the U.S., most weren't born that way. Sixty-two percent, or 363 individuals, climbed the ladder themselves and are self-made billionaires with a capital B, (says a report by Singapore-based market research company Wealth X in collaboration with *Wall Street Journal*'s Custom Studio.) That means that most of them were just like you at one time in their life. Let that strike you. They didn't have any advantage, or elite insider connection. What they wanted was once in the invisible realm, yet they manifested it. They didn't let their senses, what they could see, hear or feel, stop them from tapping into their imagination and creativity. They went inside their own minds and created such a crystallized vision, unbridled by the present moment, thinking of the joy that it would bring them and all those they cared about, igniting it in faith.

The difference between where they are and where you are now? That very process. They had fiery belief in the probability of their dreams and much, much more. They saw their vision as only the beginning of what was possible for their future. They always knew things would work out, and with that power of belief and shift in thinking, it did.

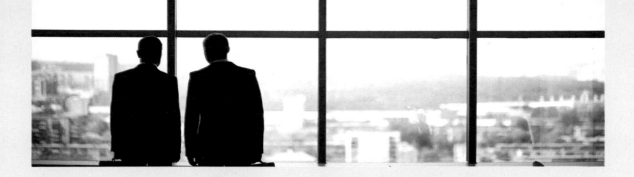

Find a Model

We are not in this alone. If you have people around you in your life who serve as great examples then that's wonderful, but you can find plenty of others. You don't have to know the person or people you model yourself after and in fact they don't have to be alive. You have tons of choices. Who do you highly respect? If you could pick any person in the world to be like, a person you respect and admire, who would you choose? Choose as many as you like. You can be like them. You just need to learn how.

Find out all about them. Read their biographies. Watch YouTube videos of their interviews or talks. Any number of people have broken free of their less-than-optimal beginnings and made incredible lives for themselves and others. Many more have come back after some very bad choices.

These people might be celebrities, like Oprah Winfrey, who grew up in a horrible circumstances yet became the not only a huge financial success but does a great deal to help others; JK Rowling, who was a broke single mother and sold so many books she brought the publishing industry back to life, or Robert Downey Jr., who succumbed to temptations after early success, losing everything, but battling back to become the highest-paid actor in Hollywood.

They might be billionaires like Warren Buffet, who came from modest beginnings, Jan Khoum, founder of Whatsapp who once lived on food stamps, or Alibaba founder Jack Ma, who began his career as a teacher. Or maybe you would rather model yourself after everyday people who manage to accomplish extraordinary things, like Rosa Parks, whose simple defiant act signaled the beginning of the end of segregation, or Candy Lightner, who founded Mothers Against Drunk Driving (MADD) and in so doing completely changed both the public's opinion and the legal ramifications of choosing to drink and drive.

I could fill a book with these stories alone – people who have triumphed over their adversity or have become much more than what their backgrounds might suggest, but let's just accept the fact that they have. And I bet you know what I'm going to say now? You are right! If they did it, you can do it!

These are all human beings. You are exactly like them. The only things that separate you from them are your choices. Whether the people you choose to model yourself after live in your neighborhood today or died in Austria 100 years ago, you can learn their habits and choose to live your life in a similar way. Act as if you are, and then you will be.

These self-made billionaires had heart, hunger, drive and determination. They married those qualities with an insatiable appetite to get what they knew was theirs; they didn't allow doubt to impact the choices they were making about their future for even one second and didn't question the calling they felt on their lives. They just acted with intention—consistently and independent of the approval or disapproval from those around them. With this kind of potential and statistic, why not decide you too will begin to live a life that will go down as legendary? One that someone else will use as a reason to pull themselves out of the impoverished circumstances they feel trapped in?

Taking Care of the Basics

One of our biggest obstacles in tapping into the higher source, achieving success and fulfillment is overcoming our own negative thinking and doubt. Without faith, we don't set a goal, and without a goal we lose direction. We have nothing to focus on, so we easily latch onto whatever feels good in the moment.

"You are the only you, that is a scientific fact. Because of it, there are things that only you can do with everything that makes you up."

To change this, you must step out in faith, accepting the probability of success and fulfillment, annihilating any shred of doubt about your dream's possibility in your life. It's looking at your life as if you are truly chosen. You are the only you, that is a scientific fact. Because of it, there are things that only you can do with everything that makes you up. Knowing that makes it easier to accept that you have a mission, one I believe God has a lot to do with. Coming to terms with this requires faith, as your environment right now may not make it seem like that's the case.

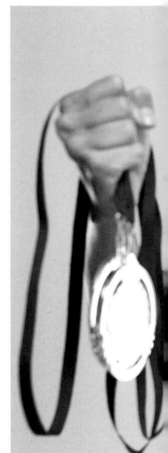

Maybe addiction has impacted your life through others, as was the case with me, or maybe you struggled with your own demons, whether drugs, food, sex, gambling or a combination of all of them and more. Realizing that none of that behavior defines who you are and neither can it stop the mission God has laid out for your life can only come to you through faith. Faith comes from hearing: hearing what you are asking, hearing God's voice in response, and hearing your Creator's message about the mission you are here to fulfill in your lifetime.

A God-Approved Goal

I always suggest to clients they take time before goal setting to ask if the things they want to go for are God approved. Be sure the things you want won't end up costing you everything you really want and can become. If the highest and best use of you is different from you becoming a supermodel, it's best you learn that before you dedicate your life to becoming one. Self-optimization, in business or life in general, is simply getting the most from what you have at the highest level possible. Is your life optimized?

How often have we heard of people who get what they want but at a huge cost, ultimately

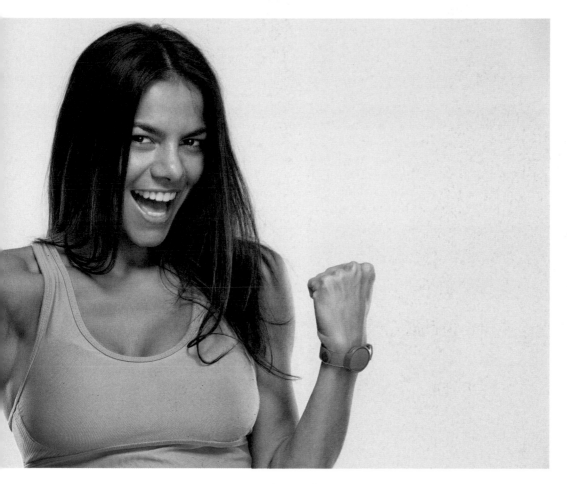

sometimes even taking their own lives? The things we think we want are not always best for us. I believe prayer and good healthy relationships infused with trust allow you to check whether or not the ideas you're putting together in goal form are from and for God or from and for your own ego. Are they meant to satisfy you or meant to satisfy He who created you? I think God wants our goals to do both.

Remember, a good goal will make your life better, your family's life better, your community's life better and our world better, all because you grow and get better as you go for it. If something you want makes you feel good but doesn't improve your character, I would question whether or not you really want to go for it. If getting what you want means forsaking your character, then take another path. It's cer-

"Remember, a good goal will make your life better, your family's life better, your community's life better and our world better, all because you grow and get better as you go for it."

tain God wouldn't ever call you to do such a thing. Also, be clear in the distinction between character and reputation. Character is who you know yourself to be—and what God sees. Reputation is what others think of you, and frankly, is irrelevant in the face of character. Reputation waxes and wanes based upon the mood of the public. Character on the other hand is unshifting. It is the bedrock of your identity. Never trade it for anything or anyone.

Shake Off Your Conditioning

Have you ever asked yourself why you're living in the city you're in? Why you eat the way you eat? Why you drive the color car you drive? Wear the kind of clothes you wear? Put make-up on? Get a particular haircut and shave? Why you look at your phone or Facebook incessantly? Take a bath every day? Shower at

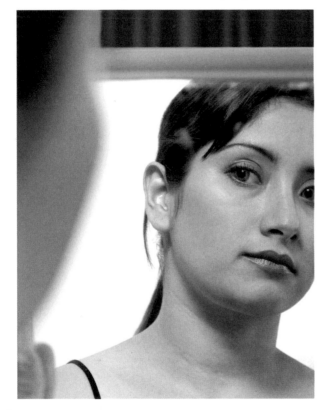

"Take a moment and ask if the things you do daily are necessary and are part of the path you're beginning to design for yourself."

the time of day you do? Many of these choices you make and habits you now have were once learned from those you were around—and as

children, we don't get to choose who those somebodies are! While we may love our family, they may not be as evolved as we hope to become.

To begin to live an extraordinary life, you have to ask where you learned to do what you're doing and behave the way you do, and if it still makes sense for the person you are in the process of becoming. This can be scary. Questioning our habits can sometimes make us feel we're losing a sense of who we are, since many of us strongly identify ourselves with what we do. What you will discover through this process is that you constantly create who you are!

Take a moment and ask if the things you do daily are necessary and are part of the path you're beginning to design for yourself. As an example, at one time it was important for me to be terribly strict with myself, hardly ever enjoying treats, but that was for the 1.0 version of me at 17 when I was learning how to be a healthy and fit person. Now, well over a decade later, the occasional indulgence is not harmful to me and quite the contrary, has become part of the definition of a healthy relationship with food. You must evolve your habits and attitudes as you grow and mature into the person you're becoming. This happens as you set new compelling goals. Sometimes we get habituated to doing things simply because we never pause to consider the reason behind our daily choices. We get caught in a rut and aren't even aware that we're in it.

When we speak of this, you might see the connection to what we've spoken of before: accepting the labels you've been given by yourself or others, and thereby acting on them almost hypnotically. To change our life we have to question the things that define that life, whether those things are the beliefs we have about ourselves, the beliefs we have about our lives or the daily habits we have and actions we take consistently. To set goals outside of your original conditioning without examining it and resetting it to allow for the person you're becoming makes it so you never can really reach these ambitious goals or maintain them. If the thermostat in your own head is set to "barely getting by" and anything above that range makes you uncomfortable, then once life heats up, what will your reaction be? Let's say you take massive action and create an avalanche of cash flow in your life, making millions of dollars in a year when your parents' combined income never came close to one million in their lifetime. Suddenly you notice you start making silly mistakes you'd never usually make. You just can't figure it out! This is your subconscious trying to bring back the former status quo—your place of comfort. People begin to do things almost unconsciously in an effort to get back to where they feel normal, in control, and in familiar territory— even if it's bad! Examine yourself and where you have the thermostat in your head set—it's time to raise it!

Once you've examined your beliefs and thought about your general goals, you must activate faith once again when fear of some outside force derailing your efforts pops up. Know that you are the only one who can create a roadblock to giving yourself permission to feel good about yourself right now. If your self-awareness wasn't reinforced when you were growing up and you never had much confidence, you will have to reprogram your thought process several times a day, indefinitely. Feeling good is key to consistent success. If you weigh 400 pounds, so what? Nothing and no one can stop you from getting lean and ripped, and you can feel good about yourself as you live through that process. Broke? So what? You can start a new path for yourself today. Divorced three times? So what? You had to go through each of those marriages to become the person deserving of your real soul mate who awaits you. Abused drugs? So what? You're alive for a reason. Now you can use your story to write a book and sponsor others in their recovery. You can always find the empowering meaning behind anything you encounter in life.

> If you're still here on this planet then God isn't done with you yet. Today can be the day that everything gets better, because you decide to get better. You can make the rest of your life a story that cancels out anything and everything you're not proud of up until now. You don't need to wait to be "successful" to feel good about yourself and your life.

Don't look back with regret; look ahead with excitement that the best is headed your way. If you'll allow yourself to experience the joy you have now in a state of endless gratitude for all of it, then your energy signature, the frequency you're on will be elevated, and more good will come. In realizing that despite it all, here you are, still standing and able to move forward, you'll reach your promised land of health, wealth, love and perpetual growth that much faster. We move towards what we focus on, and our internal feelings have much to do with the speed at which we arrive, so stay focused on what you appreciate and more will come.

Many people won't allow themselves to feel good while working toward a goal because they think it will kill their ambition and drive to strive for more and keep going. I once believed that to be true myself, tirelessly working, never looking up to really take in all the good around me, dismissing the compliments from those closest to me. This stems from a fear that if you slow down you'll stop and never start again! Whatever the reason you've come to this belief, it's erroneous. If you don't celebrate where you are right now, the small steps you're making in the direction of your ultimate goals, you miss out on taking in enjoyment through the entire process and will usually burn out as a result. The fuel for your future is found in the joy of the present. You don't want to wake up one day living the life you planned for only to ask if this is all there is.

Celebrate each step on your journey. The celebrations along the way keep you energized and charged up for the road ahead. Who wants to keep going and going like a hamster on a wheel without any sense of reward, progress or accomplishment? By shifting to a different philosophy, one where you appreciate where

> *"Don't look back with regret; look ahead with excitement that the best is headed your way."*

you're starting but know that the best is still in front of you, you embody the attitude and philosophy of the greatest of achievers, young and old.

Sir Richard Branson is a great example. He is one of wealthiest men in the world. Founder of the Virgin empire, he is involved in over 200 businesses. He doesn't try to micromanage it all; he delegates authority so he can enjoy everything he's doing. Rather than hole himself up in a castle high above his kingdom, he's a man of the people. He is one of the most well-liked entrepreneurs alive today. He believes in bottom-heavy management strategies where he empowers those working for him rather than strangling them with executives dishing out orders. Many credit this as a secret to his immense wealth.

Sir Branson defines his life not by the size of his bank account, but by the impact he makes in the lives of others. He isn't trying to control people or things as much as he's trying to enjoy and learn from them. He is infamous for taking part in incredibly fun, adventurous, and creative projects that he not only enjoys, but also lead to great publicity for his businesses. He tried to fly around the world in a hot air balloon, drove a tank down the streets of New York City and even dressed as a female flight attendant for a competitor's airline after losing a bet. He doesn't let his ego get in the way. He lives for joy, and is rich in spite of that joy, or perhaps because of it! He gets pleasure through constantly becoming a better version of himself, because he knows he is the only one who can!

He was dyslexic, and therefore had difficulties learning the way others did, but he had a spark inside just like you do. Legend has it that his mother always believed in him too, much like my own, telling others he would go on to be the "Prime Minister of England." He's certainly done well for himself. Philanthropic and joyful, he is the fifth-richest person in the UK. He didn't become bitter and stingy as he strived to become more; he fell more deeply in love with those he committed to serving. If he lost it all I bet it wouldn't take him much time to recoup it, considering all he became as a person while in process of earning and growing the wealth. My parents sacrificed a lot financially to give me a great education, and only as I got older did I realize why. The education, skill and people-talent you acquire in pursuit of whatever you're after can never be taken from you, no matter what your profit-and-loss statement looks like. With those kind of assets, you become just as priceless!

How Much Do We Really Need?

You free up your capacity for achievement when you feel good and think of yourself as a success. When you have fun enjoying the process toward where you want to go and aren't feeling anxious, worried and stressed over the outcome, doing what's necessary isn't nearly as difficult. Strive each day to be just a little better than the day before and the process will

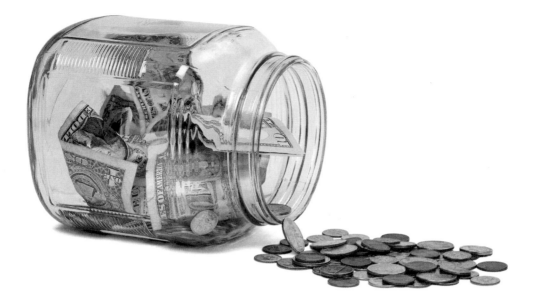

be enjoyable, filled with progress, and will not be overwhelming.

Most of us make up so many rules for ourselves that it's hard to ever be happy. We think things have to be a certain way before we can feel good, but in reality we don't need much to fulfill our basic needs. Decide today that you will make it a priority to put yourself in a position where you can focus on living in a superior way—not just making ends meet. You'll be happy with what you have and the way things are even as you are trying to make things better. You won't let little disappointments steal your joy and lead you to a life of suffering.

Making this commitment means learning to become happy from the inside out. It means getting your health in order first, then your finances, and so on. If you are struggling just to meet your basic needs, to keep clothes on your back and a roof over your head, focusing on enlightenment and self-actualization can feel like a real struggle. If that's where you are, then let's get that situation resolved first.

The cool part is that no matter where you are today, broke or rich, I bet you need much less than you've been telling yourself you do in order to be totally free from this prison you feel stuck in. If I asked you just how much

"The education, skill and people-talent you acquire in pursuit of whatever you're after can never be taken from you, no matter what your profit-and-loss statement looks like."

money it would take for you to never have to work again, I bet you don't have the exact answer, do you? You'd probably say, "A LOT!" Is it as much as you think it is? How much are your monthly expenses? Do you even know? For most people, a great part of their income is spent in ways they're not aware of. In chapter 10 I will give you an action plan for getting complete control of your finances, no matter how much money you make.

Security to Grow Into More

Focusing on your own personal growth, development, relationships and spirituality is really hard if you can't pay the bills, but no matter where you are right now, you can turn the equation around in your favor. First, by becoming healthier. You cannot be your best self if you're weighed down with a terrible diet and nonexistent exercise program, causing you to be sluggish and possibly even sick. If you've already freed yourself from that, there's now nothing keeping you from rising higher. Carrying less extra fat and freed from lifestyle-caused health issues, you can now use that newfound focus and energy on creating wealth. The key is to apply the same principles to your financial health as to your physical health. We must shape the formless into the real, just as those billionaires did. Remember most of them started in the same place you are in today! Hammer down exactly what it is you need to not only survive, but thrive.

Before moving forward with wealth creation, we need to talk about your beliefs about what it means to be rich. If you don't examine your thoughts around what it means to be rich, you could be unconsciously sabotaging your well-designed and intended efforts.

Some people cringe at the idea of being called "rich," thinking it's arrogant, pompous, and egotistic. I think it's just the opposite. If you're not striving to be all you can and make all you can so you can do all you can, you are not living your life to the fullest. I don't mind preachers who have jets, mansions and the like. I think they serve as wonderful models to their congregations of just what's possible for all of us. It's that much better that the good ones are doing God's work and living in prosperity. You too have to get comfortable knowing you deserve to be wealthy and rich, and not just in the financial sense. You will get what you ask and accept from the world.

I remember hearing a story in one of the *Tony Robbins Personal Power* ® tape programs I listened to when I was younger. He gives a wonderful illustration, telling of a late night walk he took on the streets of Boston in Co-

"You too have to get comfortable knowing you deserve to be wealthy and rich, and not just in the financial sense. You will get what you ask and accept from the world."

"Life always pays what you ask from it."

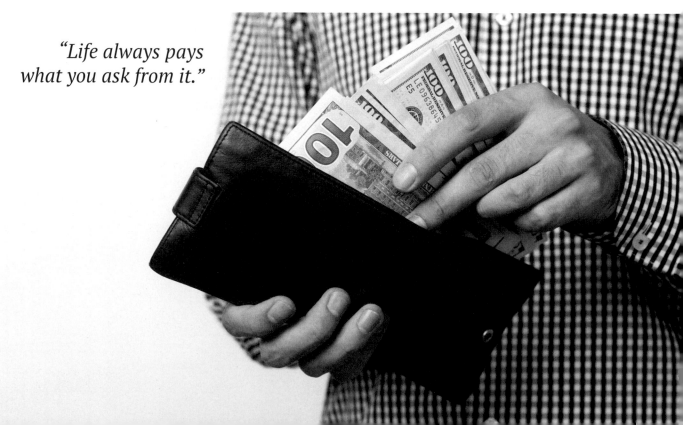

pley Square after giving a successful seminar one night. He noticed a man stumbling on and off the sidewalk, obviously intoxicated. The man approached him late this evening asking, "Excuse me sir, can you spare a poor man a quarter?" Tony, a bit taken aback by the man's meager request and rough appearance, thought this odd. He retorted, "Just a quarter? "Yes, a quarter sir, just a quarter, it will change my life!" said the man. Tony asked again, "You just want a quarter?" "Yes, just a quarter is all I need, it will change my life." Tony, seeing this as a teaching moment, pulled out his billfold, making sure the man saw the hundred dollar bills lining it, and yanked out a quarter, giving it to the man with a piece of life-changing advice, "Here you go sir. One thing I want you to know, life always pays what you ask from it!" He put his billfold back in his pocket, along with the hundreds of dollars he carried, and met eyes with the man. The man looked at the quarter, looked at Tony, looked at the quarter, and said "You're weird!" walking off. Maybe he missed the point, but I didn't.

Sometimes, at an unconscious level, people don't ask much from their life. They settle because they're afraid that they won't get it, or if they do get it, they won't fit in anymore with those they're used to spending time with. If they are making vastly more money than everyone they're around, how will they relate? In a similar way to weight-loss clients who panic during the holiday season when they think about being at a holiday party foregoing the junk food, often people with wealth goals think they will feel out of place.

Sometimes people sabotage all the good they do when they believe their success will leave them feeling lonely. Rather than deal with this incongruence within themselves, they choose to resent the people they think of as wealthy, hating the very thing they're working toward. How will you manage to follow through on the challenging journey to becoming financially free if you hate or are afraid of what you're going for at some level? Answer: You won't.

Examine yourself deeply to be sure an underlying mental conflict isn't the cause of your trouble with finances or any other aspiration you have. Sometimes mixed emotional associations are the worm that eats away the roots of your success tree. When you are at cross purposes inside like this, you can never manifest what you want, not for very long at least. You have to be congruent, thinking, feeling and acting on your outcome, consistently. Think wealth, feel wealth, and know you deserve wealth. Some I've coached talk about feeling guilty when they begin to grow wealthy but see their siblings not as well off, as if some fairy came into their life and gave them opportunity their relatives didn't have. Everyone has the same chance at success in life. While it's not easy to accept that some of those you love most will settle for far less than what you're going for, you mustn't let that hold you back. Be an example of just what's possible and who knows, maybe they'll raise their standards. Maybe they're content with where they are. At worst, you'll have so much more available to help in times of crisis if they are indeed ill prepared. Either way it can be a win/win. Let's

> "Sometimes, at an unconscious level, people don't ask much from their life. They settle because they're afraid that they won't get it, or if they do get it, they won't fit in anymore with those they're used to spending time with."

equate wealth and fitness again for a moment. Will you prevent yourself from becoming fit and healthy just because your loved ones are making poor health choices? Their decisions do not create your life; they create their own.

You will notice when you read the part in chapter 10 about financial management and wealth creation that I say to take 10% of what you make, no matter how much that is, and save it. I learned this lesson because of my grandma. She made it her first objective after we met, when I was only 13 or 14 years old, to help me become interested in the economy and in financial management. Only one week after I met her, a day that changed the direction of my entire life, this elderly lady who was all but a stranger left me a message on our family's answering machine saying God had told her that she was to help me learn how to become wealthy. Because of His instruction, she said she was giving me a sizeable amount of money (to a teenager!) saying that the only catch was I had to watch the *Nightly Business Report* on the Public Broadcasting Station to start to open my mind to how the economy works.

Honestly, how money works was the last thing I thought about at that age! The only thing that went through my head was where I would spend the money! I had never had anywhere close to that amount of money, and I didn't know what I had done to ever deserve such a thing. My mom and dad couldn't believe a stranger would act so generously. They thought there had to be a catch. There wasn't. Grandma told me that God had a special calling on my life and this was important to my future. I get emotional as I think of it now. Imagine, all of this came together just so you would be able to read this book today and hear me tell you that there is such a calling on your life, and this is your direct message from above! You must master this financial part of your life as well so you can live the life you're meant to.

When I learned I would receive the money I thought about buying my parents and siblings gifts with it, or maybe a new keyboard to play music, or maybe I could put a down payment on a car once I had my permit, or maybe a new computer with a CD burner. (Yup, back then a CD burner was a big deal!) The philosophy I lived by regarding food at that time also governed my thinking about money. I spent as fast as I earned. I was one of the many who find money seems to burn a hole in their pocket,

even with the few expenses I had back then. I had to scrounge up nickels, dimes and quarters before ordering in the drive-through to make sure I had enough for the $6.00 Super Sized meal. I had no regard for the future.

"If you act impulsively and spend recklessly, then you will find yourself broke."

This kind of thinking leads to poverty on all fronts. If you act impulsively in your relationships without regard for the long-term consequences, they suffer. If you act impulsively with your children, not thinking about their development and confidence as they grow older, you lose their respect. If you act impulsively with food, eating whatever you want when you want it without regard for how it will affect your future health, you will find yourself unhealthy. If you act impulsively and spend recklessly, then you will find yourself broke. Fortunately for me, just about the time I received this money from my grandma, a man at my high school invited me to join an investment club. It was there I began to learn the fundamentals I'm teaching you today.

If you don't have an investment account, open one today. Take this as God's direction to do so. Even if you only have the minimum amount available to open one, take action and do it. Go to a local investing bank or open an account online, and invest your money into a diversified portfolio. This means putting your money into a fund made up of a group of companies where you earn its average. The companies are in many different categories, sectors and industries, meaning you don't put all of your money into one basket such as a technology stock. Since certain areas of the market can drop out, having a diversified portfolio means you will be fortified against such risk, allowing for many pillars to support your investment and your life. If one pillar goes down, there will be many others that will continue to feed into your pool of wealth, likely

"Take 10% of what you make, no matter how much that is, and save it."

leaving it relatively unaffected or changed over the long haul. Consider something like a Vanguard or S&P index fund where it can begin to earn interest over time without your management, allowing for slow but progressive growth. Be very cautious of fees, as they can eat away at the growth of your investment. Remember, as in other areas of your life, if you want God to bless you more, you've got to show Him that you will take care of what you have right now. Think of the story of the "talents." To refresh your memory, see below:

Matthew 25:14-30
New American Standard Bible (NASB) Parable of the Talents

14 "For *it is* just like a man *about* to go on a journey, who called his own slaves and entrusted his possessions to them. **15** To one he gave five [a]talents, to another, two, and to another, one, each according to his own ability; and he went on his journey. **16** Immediately the one who had received the five talents went and traded with them, and gained five more talents. **17** In the same manner the one who *had received* the two *talents* gained two more. **18** But he who received the one *talent* went away, and dug *a hole* in the ground and hid his [b]master's money. **19** "Now after a long time the master of those slaves *came and *settled accounts with them. **20** The one who had received the five talents came up and brought five more talents, saying, 'Master, you entrusted five talents to me. See, I have gained five more talents.' **21** His master said to him, 'Well done, good and faithful slave. You were faithful with a few things, I will put you in charge of many things; enter into the joy of your [c]master.' **22** "Also the one who *had received* the two talents came up and said, 'Master, you entrusted two talents to me. See, I have gained two more talents.' **23** His master said to him, 'Well done, good and faithful slave. You were faithful with a few things, I will put you in charge of many things; enter into the joy of your master.' **24** "And the one also who had received the one talent came up and said, 'Master, I knew you to be a hard man, reaping where you did not sow and gathering where you scattered *no seed.* **25** And I was afraid, and went away and hid your talent in the ground. See, you have what is yours.' **26** "But his master answered and said to him, 'You wicked, lazy slave, you knew that I reap where I did not sow and gather where I scattered no *seed*. **27** Then you ought to have put my money [d]in the bank, and on my arrival I would have received my *money* back with interest. **28** Therefore take away the talent from him, and give it to the one who has the ten talents.' **29** "For to everyone who has, *more* shall be given, and he will have an abundance; but from the one who does not have, even what he does have shall be taken away. **30** Throw out the worthless slave into the outer darkness; in that place there will be weeping and gnashing of teeth.

This sure makes God sound scary, but there's more than appears on the story's surface. This story gives great insight into our financial lives. First, we are all always given enough from God to do what He wants us to. Be grateful for whatever you have right now, whether it be a little or a lot in your own mind. How much is your talent worth? Think of those who find a niche and become unbelievably wealthy from one skill. It's not what they have, it's how they use it to help others that matters. One talent alone can be priceless and I'm sure you have many. Each person was given a different number of "talents," and some seemed to get more than the others. But the number wasn't nearly as important as what happened once the talents were given. Two of the three servants compounded whatever they started with. That's the best you can do!

Where you begin isn't important, because it's not going to be where you'll finish. If you invest just one of your gifts and double it, you now have two. Do it again and you now have four, once more, and you have eight. All from just one. Hold on to that one and never put it out there, fearing things might not work out, and it does nothing to change your life. We are expected to make good use of all the gifts God's given us, to be stewards of the people God's put in our path, to invest ourselves fully in faith and expect our good work to flourish. When it comes time to take stock of what we've done with what we've been given, the people, the money, the gifts and possessions, we don't want to say that we simply held on to what we had out of fear that we'd lose it. Trust that when you put yourself out there with whatever you have and you follow wise advice that you've checked with prayer, good will come from it.

To make improvements on what you've been given, you need to learn an important concept called "compounding." Einstein said, "Compound interest is the eighth wonder of the world. He who understands it, earns it ... he who doesn't ... pays it."

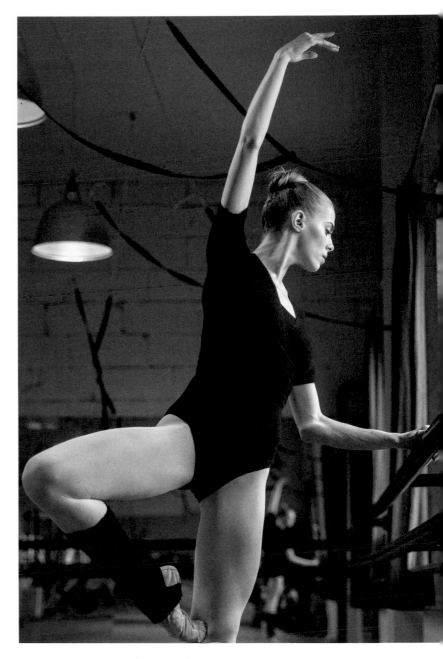

"Think of those who find a niche and become unbelievably wealthy from one skill they have. It's not what they have, it's what they put it to use doing in others' lives that matters."

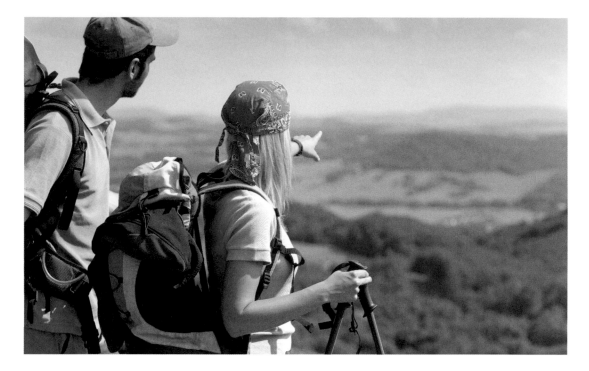

Charting the Course to Success

First Ingredient: Belief

The first and penultimate key to getting anywhere is deciding where you want to go and how you want things to be, realizing it is all possible for you. The belief is the most critical element. Once I believed, I never allowed the way I looked at 360 pounds to stop me from seeing the rippling six-pack underneath the rolls of fat. That belief and vision is what got me up early, had me working out even on the days I lost those closest to me, saying no to junk food on holidays and foregoing birthday cake on my 18th birthday. I didn't allow a shred of doubt to enter my mind. So too must you be like when deciding your future will forever be different from your present and past.

We've all heard incredible tales of survival, people using creativity and tenacity to get out of dire situations. They either figure a way out of that situation or they die. You need the same tenacity when it comes to achieving your goals. When you put yourself in a situation where your goals and dreams are things you have no choice but to follow through on, you'll make the breakthrough happen. Don't give yourself the option to stop or fail. We all do what we feel we have to. Belief is the activator of magic in our lives.

Outline Your Goals Guilt-Free

What is it you're truly after? When people seek transformation, they most often want to "look" better or "feel" better. We are all after attaining a more serene and peaceful state. We are chasing emotions. Unfortunately, many get tricked into thinking a thing or a person can give them that, when the truth is you must create those improvements. You might think you'll "look better" in a more expensive wardrobe or shoes, or you want to seem more important to those around you, thinking you'll "feel better" driving a new sports car and living in a big house. There is nothing wrong with enjoying these things, but you must harness the power of what's really driving you, a yearning for becoming more, before you decide to embark on the quest to get there. Sometimes people say they want to be a billionaire, and guess what, they are successful, achieve their dreams and get there. In the process, they get divorced three times, use cocaine to deal with the stress, have affairs, age prematurely, gain 60 pounds of extra fat, lose all their childhood friends and grow estranged from their children, all in the pursuit of this elusive goal, thinking that once they achieve it, they'll be happy. Instead they're alone with their billions. I say that's bullshit. Be happy where you are but also ambitious in going for what you want. That's the key to lasting real success.

You must have a clear vision for where you're going. That's what will determine where you put your focus and ultimately what you do. The way I help people to do this in my office is to imagine what the perfect day would be for them. Don't put any limits on yourself. Think like you're writing up a wish list as a child. Don't question if it's possible or reasonable, just write it down. The first things that pop into your mind. I would work to come up with a list of at least 100 items. For example:

What type of house will you live in? What type of cars will you be driving? Will you have a limo drive you to and from work so you can focus more of your time on creative efforts? Do you want a person to clean your house weekly? Or a live-in housekeeper? Do you want a home for every season in different parts of the world? Do you want to stay in one city, or travel as you wish with whom you wish whenever you wish? How will your body look and feel when you jump out of bed in each morning? Do you want to learn an instrument or new language? How about teach at a local school? Volunteer at a health clinic? What will

the scenery look like when you gaze out the kitchen window in your home? Do you want to have a Ph.D behind your name just for the ring it gives? Or do you want to get a medical degree and help people become healthier? Who will be at your side every night in bed? Do you want an in-home theater? Would you like to be a stay-at-home mom or dad and not have to go to work at all, but get to if you so choose? Would you like to meet or perform with your favorite actor or musician or write with your favorite author? What causes and charities do you want to support? Do you want to open a homeless shelter? Start a foundation

"You must have a clear vision for where you're going. That's what will determine where you put your focus and ultimately what you do."

for underprivileged or sick children? What will you spend most of your time doing if you didn't need any money and everything you've been told you could or couldn't do instantly became irrelevant? Where would you be investing your time? With whom? What would you be eating and drinking? When? How many hours of sleep would you prefer to be getting? Would you get daily massages? How often would you check e-mail and social media?

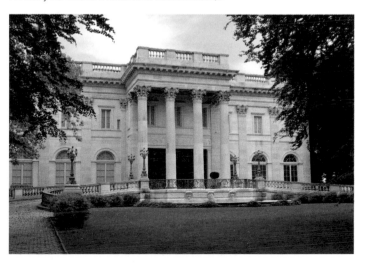

Would you even have an account on any of the platforms if you no longer were in need of money? Think of financial, physical, spiritual, emotional and mental goals.

> The key is not limiting your thoughts to what those around you and your history have conditioned you to accept as appropriate, realistic, or reasonable. Fear is the thief that's invaded the minds of the people who don't go for it. I'd rather face short-lived disappointment at a small failure than the perpetual despair of regret knowing I could have but didn't.

We all have hopes, dreams, desires, abilities, and most of all, free will. Just as our ancestors crossed oceans, climbed mountains and worked their way through thick forests to create our villages, roads and eventually cities, we as humans can certainly cross our imagined barriers, climb over perceived walls and work our way through education and other challenges to create the life we desire. It simply requires a knowing that the promise we envision awaits us.

"We have the ability to make things work, no matter the situation. Why, then, do so many people choose to be like that bag, blowing in the wind?"

Humans are the undisputed kings and queens of the world. This is definitely not because we're the biggest. Whales, bears, tigers and many other animals are larger. We are not the fastest; many different cats, dogs, deer and even rabbits are faster. We are definitely not the strongest. Ever tried to arm-wrestle a gorilla? We are at the top because we have the capacity to choose how we're going to play the game of life. We get to decide if we want to play the game setting up our own rules, or living by the rules that were laid down by others. We can decide to make our lives magnificent, operating above our most primal levels. We can elevate our consciousness and thereby elevate the standard of life we enjoy if we begin to reprogram ourselves and the way we look at ourselves and life.

As we discussed earlier, we can adjust to pretty much anything. We are able to make the best of any situation or find something to complain about during the best of times. It is for that reason that we alone can live everywhere from the coldest arctic to the hottest tropics and from the rainiest mountainsides to the driest deserts. We have the ability to make things work, no matter the situation. Why, then, do so many people choose to be like that plastic bag, blowing in the wind?

I believe the answer is two-fold. First and most importantly, they may not have yet had the chance to fully embrace the degree of power they have over their own lives and how even the tiniest aspects of their lives are based on the decisions and day-to-day choices they've made up to this point. Maybe they've never been exposed to this way of thinking. If that's the case, get them a copy of my book as a gift!

I was once in that category. While I loved my parents to death, they didn't think about "personal development," "goal-setting" or living in abundance. Frankly, I think they didn't feel they deserved much so didn't even ask. Maybe your parents were the same. Before I decided to take control of my life, losing 160 pounds of pure fat and achieving my goals of getting a good education, both formally and informally, developing a hugely successful career and having strong, loving relationships, I allowed this conditioning and my life circumstances to direct the quality of every day. At that time I never woke up and decided that I was going to make the day great, or find a benefit in everything that happened to me. I just hoped it would end up that way on its own, that the right girl, enough money and a career path would just come into my life, flashing to get my attention like a neon sign. The funny thing is, the signs were actually there but I wasn't looking in the right places. I thought I'd find the answer rather than create it. Hoping things will somehow come together the way you dream of is never the path to real success.

If a terrible person gets into power in government and you didn't vote against him, then you are partly responsible for him winnng. Hitler gained power not only because of the people who wanted him, but also because the

"Not taking action is an action. You must decide to do all you can in the best way possible to bring about your desired outcome. Only then can you sleep peacefully at night knowing your task was complete."

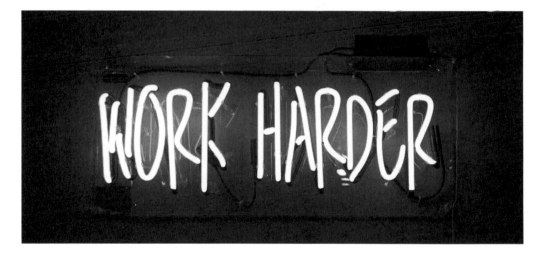

The second reason people don't open themselves up to real success is fear. If you're the one who is really calling the shots and making decisions, then you have to accept your own culpability when it comes to failure. But the decision not to decide or act is still a decision. Pretending you don't know that collection agencies are calling makes you no less responsible when your vehicle is repossessed. Not taking action is an action. You must decide to do all you can in the best way possible to bring about your desired outcome. Only then can you sleep peacefully at night knowing your task was complete.

people who didn't want him sat idly by and allowed it to happen. A brief aside: The power of a crowd is astounding. People will do little if they see others are doing little. There was a psychological study done years ago revealing something we call the "bystander effect." The studies showed that in cases of real emergency, people are less likely to offer help if others are present. The more people present, the lower the chance someone steps up to do the right thing, so people who could have been saved end up not being saved. Don't be a bystander in your own life! As you sit by and allow your life to happen, you are in fact determining your future by inaction, and it's not the future you want or deserve!

> *"To create the path leading to where you want to go, you must first determine where you want to be."*

The future you want can be created only by making decisions and choices that bring you there. And just as your ancestors created the paths that later became roads, leading them from where they were to where they wanted to be, you must do the same in your own life, no matter how dense the brush, weeds and rocks lying in front of you seem to be. To create the path leading to where you want to go, you must first determine where you want to be. Next, you need to ensure that you keep your eyes focused on that destination so you head in the right direction. Otherwise, you might end up running around in circles or in the wrong place altogether.

But how do you determine your destination? If you've lived through your life blowing in the wind and no one has ever spoken faith and promise into your life until now, how will you change that and begin acting with determination to achieve your goals? I have the answer.

It is part of the human condition to have dreams. Dreams and ideas are truly what separates us from all the animal kingdom, because it is through dreams and ideas that discovery is made. You can see how this has affected and elevated humans through history with the first basic creations of the spear, wheel and house,

"What if I use this stone to make this other stone sharp? Then I can hunt for food more efficiently."

"What if I shape that piece of wood so it's round and then put this piece of wood in the middle so it can roll?"

"What if instead of searching for a cave I take these pieces of wood and bind them with mud to make a residence?"

We were designed to innovate. God gave us the innate ability to achieve and make things better. He did not create a world in which everything is figured out for us. He gave us the ability to figure things out. To forge healthy relationships, love each other and strengthen each other because of the awareness that we're better together. He gave us curiosity and intellect, ideas and dreams. But to succeed and achieve, we have to make use of those abilities. We have the parts, but we have to educate ourselves on how they function and put them to work. A car plus a working engine plus gas do not bring you to your destination unless you put them together in unison as a vehicle and then steer, consistently directing that vehicle in the right direction knowing that you will deal with whatever is on the road to your destination.

"What makes your heart beat faster and your eyes glow when you think or talk about it, do it."

Above is a quote I've read recently, and it describes perfectly what I call God's spark. Most of us have some similar goals, like we want to be healthy, look great, and have a good relationship with our families. But we also have a great many dissimilar goals. Could you imagine how boring the world would be if we were all exactly the same? And nothing would be accomplished! Whereas I love speaking in front of thousands, lights flashing and music blaring, my brother's idea of a good time is being out on a quiet pond with a fishing pole and no one around for miles. If everyone wanted to be an actor and no one wanted to be an engineer, then the world would cease to function.

Luckily, God made each of us with a different set of talents, skills, interests, desires, and gifts. We each have a unique spark that God gave us, and that spark is the essence of us. It's our job to create the best version of ourselves with the gifts that God has given us. Our spark is found in our passion; it's what excites us and inspires us. The problem is, too often instead of fanning that spark and turning it into a roaring blaze, we douse it out, smother it and try to make it die, recalling the negative thoughts we picked up earlier in life, accepting other people's disempowering opinions as our own, as if they were the prophets of our future.

The only thing that determines your future is you, your thinking and your choices. Period. Not some talisman, doctor, shaman or voodoo curse. Even if we fall victim to the idea that we aren't as great as God created us to be, even we can't put the spark completely out. Trust me, I've seen people who've tried, cutting themselves, drinking themselves up to death's door, overdosing, all in an effort to stop the pain they are focused on and feeling. They're good people, just caught up in a bad pattern. Redemption is always possible. That spark of God is still in them, still burning, and it's people like me who have learned to listen to God that can see it, no matter how faint, reminding you of its presence. Instead of ever putting the spark out even with their most destructive efforts, what happens is people like that unhappily go about their lives with this poor spark trying its hardest to find some energy and shine as they continually smother it with inaction, indecision or fear. Goals, self love, good relationships with God and others are the oxygen needed to set the flame ablaze!

"It's our job to create the best version of ourselves with the gifts that God has given us. Our spark is found in our passion; it's what excites us and inspires us."

I want you to take a look deep inside and find your spark. Find your passion.

Did you have dreams when you were growing up that you've let go of as the years have passed? Did you have a passion for aeronautics, or fashion, or did you always picture yourself living by the ocean? Did you want to be a professor, a doctor, or veterinarian? Whatever you dream of doing and wherever you dream of being, that is what you are meant to do and where you are meant to be. And just like those past humans figuring out how to make spears or wheels, you have the ability to figure out how to make it happen.

A few lucky people have grown up with a positive and realistic message that they can do and be anything they want but have to take the necessary steps each day towards it. Most people are bombarded with negative messages practically from the day they were born that "other" people accomplish things. Success, health, fitness and financial security are meant for others.

Yes, there are families with a greater propensity for certain diseases – people who carry the BRCA1 and BRCA2 genes, for example, have a far greater chance of developing a number of cancers. Even with genetic disorders such as these you can take steps to help prevent the diseases, but certainly if your family has a history of diseases caused by lifestyle factors, like mine does, you can bring your chances down not only to normal levels, but you can even bring them down to lower than normal by a) realizing you can choose your outcome and b) understanding that it's not going to happen simply by wishing that it will.

"I knew which choices I had to make each day to reach that goal and I did whatever it took."

You can never absolutely guarantee that you will not get one of these diseases, but no matter what your family history says, unless a disease is 100% genetically determined (and few are), you can greatly reduce your chances of getting almost any disease or illness, not to mention making yourself look better and feel better, and having more energy for all areas of your life. If you do this and do end up with the illness despite your efforts, I can guarantee you will be much better off coping with it while fit and healthy versus obese and sick.

Of course this is the case for any goal, whether that goal is weight loss or a better job or an improved financial situation or anything else. Some people will have an easier go of it and some will have more to overcome. Some people are born with a silver spoon in their mouths, others are born into poverty. Is it easier to keep wealth when you have it to begin with? Yes definitely, and yet some people born into wealth end up in poverty and some people who are born in poverty end up billionaires.

When I was at my peak weight, I couldn't look to my mom and dad to show me how to work out and eat right. My parents felt they had bigger things to worry about at that time than if I had my chicken breasts and broccoli for dinner. But I had a goal. I wanted to be a normal size and feel good. Heck, at that time I wasn't looking to be as fit as I eventually became and as you can become; I just wanted to be able to walk into a normal clothing store and buy something that fit. Really what I wanted was to connect with others. I wanted to feel love and passion. I knew which choices I had to make each day to reach that goal and I did whatever it took. I wasn't ashamed to walk on the treadmill, legs chafing so much that I had to

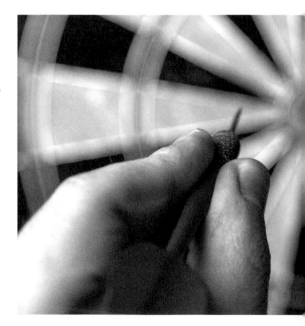

put Vaseline on them, making it look like I'd wet myself. I recognized the embarrassment would be short lived if I stayed true to my plan. So, still in high school, with help from grandma and money I saved from my part-time minimum-wage job I joined a gym and bought my own food. Would it have been easier to have lost my excess weight if I'd had a supportive family to model myself after? Yes, probably. Did the fact that I didn't have that support make a difference in the outcome? Only in the sense that it gave me jet fuel to go for my dreams to honor them!

You will achieve your dream by making the right choices each day, period. It doesn't matter where you come from, who's for you or who's against you.

The flip side to those thinking they can never have what they want is another (increasingly large) group of people who expect to have everything they want without having to go through the necessary daily effort to get it. One example of this is the type of person I mentioned before, someone born into wealth who ends up in poverty, but there are plenty of less extreme examples.

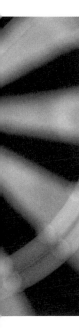

These days teachers often find that parents come to speak with them, angry that their child got a bad grade. Are these parents angry at their children for not doing the work necessary to get a good grade? No! They're angry at the teacher because somehow that teacher should have seen their child's miraculous, though invisible, work! They don't want to see that their children need to perform better. Teachers are pressured into giving higher grades than children deserve and passing kids who in reality fail, because the kids' parents are smoothing their children's passage. These parents feel like a smooth passage will help their children to a better future, but they're wrong. When

these kids hit the real world, they find they are met with major disappointment. Potential employers don't care about who they are or where they come from, they care about the impact a prospective employee will have on the bottom line—results.

"You will achieve your dream by making the right choices each day, period. It doesn't matter where you come from, who's for you or who's against you."

I feel my experience with bullying represents a similar way of thinking. While these days there are different types of bullying, such as anonymous and online, in my case it was the traditional male physical bullying. I needed to learn to become more confident, assertive, and prepared to protect myself. When I confidently took a stand against a tyrannical bully, it ended the pattern in my life.

After months of me getting soccer balls kicked in my face as a middle-schooler, my parents didn't know what to do. They had meetings with the principal, threatening to withdraw me from the school since the bullying I suffered was so intense. One teacher advised me to physically take control, and finally one recess I did. The leader of the pack that bullied me kicked a ball in my face and instead of retreating, I lunged up, threw him on the ground and began to wail on him, bloodying his nose. All the kids stood around paralyzed at seeing the timid fat kid take a stand for himself. I hated myself for it but the bullying did stop afterward.

The temptation on the part of parents is easy to understand: an easy passage makes an easier journey, which makes your child more likely to reach the distant shore. But life is not like that. While yes, there will be lovely islands to visit along the way and toward which you must navigate, there is no "distant shore" any more than there was once an end of the earth. All of life is the journey. You may have heard the saying: "A smooth sea never made a skillful sailor," and that is true of life. You have to learn to navigate through life's difficulties, keeping your eye on your next goal or destination and maneuvering as you must. Otherwise, you will succeed only when you are in a perfect environment but when you have challenges to face, you will crumble.

> *"You have to learn to navigate through life's difficulties, keeping your eye on your next goal or destination and maneuvering as you must."*

You see this with people who go to weight-loss camps or on TV weight-loss shows. When you are in an environment where everyone is focused on weight loss, when you don't go to work, when you don't have family struggles or friends inviting you for margaritas and nachos after work, where a personal trainer brings you to the gym for hours every day and every ounce of food that passes your lips is decided for you, losing weight can seem incredibly easy. When the weight-loss camp is over and you get back to real-life challenges, relationships and temptations and no longer have the number goal hanging over your head, things often don't go so well. Note: The journal *Obesity* recently reported that of 14 weight-loss contestants they looked at, 13 had gained most of the weight back.

So on the one hand we have people who never even attempt to get to their dream destination and achieve their goals because they believe themselves incapable of getting there before they even try, and you have another group of people who think they will magically end up at their destination as the seas part before them. These two perspectives are equally incorrect and equally likely to result in disappointment,

and it does not matter where you start from for this to be true.

No Limits

So now that you understand you have choice in this whole deal, what are you going to choose to do? What do you dream of doing and becoming? What will give you satisfaction and make you feel that you're fulfilling your true destiny?

The great thing is, there are many aspects to your destiny and achievements. Once you understand that you get to set the outcome and decide the course, you can navigate your way through any waters and achieve everything you

> *"There is absolutely no reason to limit yourself, and as you succeed in one area you will almost inevitably find that you succeed in more than one area. Success breeds success."*

desire. There is absolutely no reason to limit yourself, and as you succeed in one area you will almost inevitably find that you succeed in more than one area. Success breeds success.

My original goal and focus was weight loss, but once I saw I could change myself so drastically, I knew the disciplines could be applied to all other areas of success in life. Why stop at extraordinary weight loss? I could be the first person in my family to graduate from college. I could start my own successful business and become financially independent in my early 20s. I could write a best-selling book. I could become the type of man to deserve the woman of my dreams, get engaged, and ultimately marry her. I could create the exact life I wanted, down to every last detail! Does

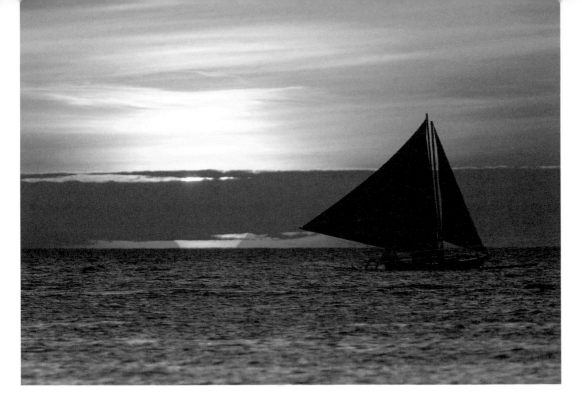

this mean everything just falls in my lap? Far from it! But I know how to set goals, discipline myself to pay the price for their attainment, and I'm still going. I will always have more goals and I will continue to achieve them. I think this is critical for all of us. It just takes a little daily discipline correction along the way to keep you on the right path.

Building the Discipline Muscle

You may have heard the term "exercise your discipline," and this term exists for a good reason. It takes a little effort to develop your discipline and willpower, both of which are necessary to accomplish your goals and achieve your dreams, but as you continue to put this effort forth it gets easier and easier, just like physical exercise.

If you're out of shape then beginning an exercise program can be overwhelming, even doing something simple like walking for a few minutes on a treadmill. Those first few times at the gym might feel like the hardest thing

"It takes a little effort to develop your discipline and willpower, both of which are necessary to accomplish your goals and achieve your dreams."

you've ever done, and you might be able to do only a small amount. But as the days turn into weeks you find it easier and easier. Soon, you end up having to challenge yourself more and more because what you used to find difficult is now so easy!

Like building stamina and muscle at the gym, the secret to achieving your goals is just a matter of consistency, making small changes but following through with them every day. When you see how just a little discipline enables you to make the right small choices each day and then how those choices have such an enormous impact, compounding just like the interest we spoke of earlier, that discipline muscle becomes stronger and stronger. Things you once felt were insurmountable now seem easy. Achievement becomes addictive.

"Things you once felt were insurmountable now seem easy. Achievement becomes addictive."

So now you understand that the navigation of your life is completely in your hands, where will you navigate to? Will you become fit and healthy and finally get the body you've desired and deserved all your life? Will you rein in your spending, get control of your debts and finally start saving some money? Will you go back to school and train for the career you've always wanted and know you'll be incredible at? Will you start your own business as you've been wanting to do for years? Will you finally buy your own house? Will you rekindle the love and passion in your ho-hum marriage?

You know you want to get there, you are now convinced you can get there, you have faith that you can exercise your discipline and make the right choices each day to navigate those waters, but now you might ask, "how?"

We are so lucky right now to live in a time when we can learn anything we want. We have literally millions of books at our disposal and we don't even have to pay for them! We can get them at the local library. You can study exactly how billionaires made their money and you can learn everything imaginable about which foods you should eat for your best health and which exercises produce the biggest benefit. If you want to learn how to do pretty much anything you can learn it by watching YouTube.

It's a great idea to find someone to model yourself after, a mentor who's achieved what you're after. You might also hire a coach or helping professional to accompany you on your journey, but if you can't afford it you can still find all the information you need. The internet has gathered the knowledge of billions of people and made it all accessible to you. Debt problems? You can learn exactly how to budget your life and how to deal with creditors in order to get control of your finances. Want to fix your relationship? There are loads of forums and relationship experts online to help you think of possible solutions. Want to switch careers? You can learn which courses to take

and exactly what employers in that field are looking for. Want to renovate your house? You can learn how to do everything from taking down a wall to moving a toilet. Of course you have to be choosy with who you lend credence to in this new information age, and just learning how to complete a task or discovering a different way of looking at things does not necessarily bring you to your goal, but it can at least help you learn what you need to do in order to get there. Once I made the decision to change my life, I began realizing that God had put everything in front of me that I needed to succeed. But here's the really exciting part: it had always been there; I just never saw it until I was ready! And you'll begin to notice this too.

You see whatever you're focused on. If you're concentrating on how much worse off you are than everyone else, you will see barriers everywhere you look. If instead you are focused on finding ways to get where you need to be, you will see that God has placed opportunities all around you! If you focus on the challenges, you will never see the opportunities. If you put roadblocks up then you will see nothing but brick walls. If you look for ways to get where you want to be, you will see doors and windows.

Mentors are hugely important to your journey. You don't need to personally know this mentor, although that can be helpful. You'll find as you move toward your goal you will naturally meet people who will be in this role for you. A

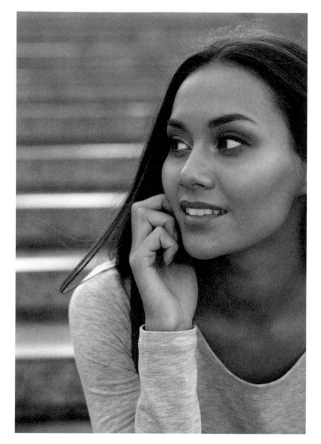

to build his body, his example pointing me in the right direction. The psychology professor was a mentor whose opinions challenged my faith, but ultimately strengthened it. Who will you choose to be your mentor?

We've spoken many times about how you will achieve what you want by acting as if you're already there. You want to be fit and have a six-pack and look like a physique model? Believe me, physique models are not sitting around every day eating junk food and moaning about how they can't lose weight. They have a planned workout routine, they continuously examine their bodies, decide on areas that they feel need improvement and then set about improving them—even when they don't feel like it! They have treats on occasion like almost anyone and they have occasional days off, but they go right back to their planned diet and exercise regimens. When I was losing extra fat, I visualized exactly how the body I wanted would look, and pored over information from the guys' who already had it. Every day I did what I'd learned they did, and over time I ended up like those I aspired to be like because I made the daily choices they made.

mentor doesn't have a big "mentor" nametag. A mentor is someone who is doing what you want to do or has accomplished what you want to accomplish, and who you can learn from, whether or not you actually know that person. I value them highly.

Walt Disney is a huge mentor of mine. He died many years before I was born and he was in a completely different field from mine, but he's still my mentor because he succeeded against all odds and I was able to learn from him. He saw what he needed to do in order to accomplish his goals and he did it. But he was far from the only mentor in my life. I've had many. In high school, the dean, a former military man was my mentor, laying the foundation for me in living a disciplined life. When I first began going to a gym, the gym owner became a mentor. He knew what to eat and do

"Find people who are doing what you want to do and who are in the place you want to be, and learn their steps and habits."

This is the case no matter what your goals are. Find people who are doing what you want to do and who are in the place you want to be, and learn their steps and habits. If you dream of being a makeup artist then you are not going to do it by stocking the cosmetic shelves at a store. Take any necessary courses in the evenings if you have to, ask everyone in the industry how they get jobs, learn from them and do as they do.

Here's something else you'll discover. As you start finding mentors and learning from them, your social circle will change, and it should change. You will begin spending more time with the people who inspire you and who are more like the "you" you're becoming, and because daily time is finite you will automatically spend less time with the people whose habits are more like the "you" you're trying to change. This does not mean you have to stop being friends with people or avoid family functions (although you may choose to do that, depending on how negative the individuals are), it just means that automatically more of your time will be spent in a positive environment and less of your time will be spent in a negative one. Successful people tend to be successful in multiple areas, because they have the habits that breed success. Surround yourself with successful people and that will assuredly increase your success rate. Do not underestimate the power of those you associate with. An unintended but wonderful result of being around successful people is that you will find it easier and easier to make daily choices that bring you to success as unconsciously you strive to be more like them, simply to be able to stay in rapport!

Here are the steps you need to take each day to bring you to where you want to be. In chapter 10 I will give you more specific instructions to take for specific goals.

1 Decide clearly where you want to be. Don't limit yourself! Get excited! Remember energy is what helps see you through to your end goal instead of just becoming motivated and then quitting. You can do and accomplish anything you want. Dream big.

2 Seek out people who are doing what you want to do and are in the place you want to be. Model them! Ask questions! Don't be afraid. Almost every successful person loves to share what they've learned and help others become better. When you've achieved your goals you will want to help others as well—and it's your obligation to do so, in my opinion.

3 Remind yourself every day that you are already the person you want to be. You just need to make a few different small choices, and make them consistently.

4 Remind yourself of the pain of the past. Before today, you made decisions that brought you to a place you didn't want to be, but you won't continue making those decisions. Remember the catastrophe you were in or headed toward, and remind yourself how you do not want to go there ever again.

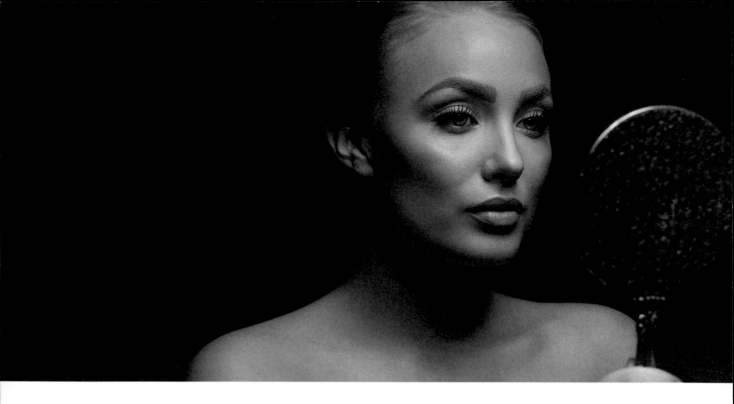

CHAPTER EIGHT

Acceptance: See the Reality and Go From There

If there's anything we humans are, it's adaptable. We can adjust to just about anything. We have adapted to living at the furthest reaches of the icy north and in the steamiest tropics. Humans live on islands and in deserts. We live in overpopulated cities and in the barren Steppes of Mongolia. We can learn to live on a very small amount of food doing high volumes of exercise, or huge amounts of food and do far too little. It is this adaptability that made us the only species to thrive in every part of the world, but it is also this adaptability that sometimes causes us to live under conditions that are not the best, when we could certainly do and expect better. Adapting to an environment or circumstance doesn't imply happiness

"I want to teach you, so you too can choose to go down that path with a no-limit mentality, achieving and contributing whatever you decide."

or joyful living, however, and the distinction between apathy and acceptance is a fine line.

Throughout history, humans have often had to accept whatever they could manage to get, and in many parts of the world that continues to be the case today. Even now, there are people who live in caves in Afghanistan, people in Somalia who have to walk miles for water and people in many countries who do not have access to rudimentary education. The basic necessities are their focus because those who live in such poverty have no concept that there might be more. Here in the developed world, however, you can't escape the fact that more is possible for you. Watch the TV, listen to the radio, login to Facebook—companies are all competing for your attention, trying to convince you that you can and should have more. I'm here to tell you that while there's nothing wrong with having more, *becoming* more is far more important. When you become more, the having is inevitable since you'll be contributing so much more to the world.

Every day you can see people who seem happier, wealthier, in better physical condition, more recognized or famous, or perhaps making a bigger difference in the world than you are at that given moment. They've tapped into the Source, God, and are living boundlessly because of it. I'm not saying by any means they are better or more capable than you. I'm simply pointing out that they've found the path that helped them get to where they wanted and decided to be, and that that path is available to you as well. They have learned and taken a different route and approach to living life—and it's the one I want to teach you, so you too can choose to go down that path with a no-limit mentality, achieving and contributing whatever you decide.

The Right Questions

People often circumvent their power by misdirecting their focus to open-ended questions that cannot be resolved and make no difference: Why does she get that and I don't? Why am I so fat? Why am I so poor? Why did my parents treat me so terribly? What's wrong with me? Why was I born with this disability? Why are things always so messed up in my life?

This pattern of thought leads to a feeling of helplessness, and in severe cases, worthlessness. The error is not you, but rather in the way you are running your mind. When you have a choice to ask why, stop and redirect your mind to ask "what do I want?" Once you've decided what you want, then you must replace the question "why" with the question: "What action must I take to get to where I desire?" Asking why is only important if it generates possible solutions.

If you find yourself broke, don't adopt a poor attitude that perpetuates the problem. Step out of that mindset by doing something generous for someone even less fortunate than you. This act of faith begins the process of getting beyond your limited way of thinking that there's only so much to go around. Behave as the person you want to be and soon your reality will shift as your actions do.

Broke is not a state of being; it is a state of feeling. Plenty of billionaires have lost it all, finding themselves broke on paper, but they don't lose touch with who they are. They don't let the situation undermine their confidence. They won't allow a "poor" attitude to overcome them. Attitude about your circumstances determines in large part the outcome you'll ultimately achieve. If you look for a lesson and opportunity and don't personalize unfortunate circumstances as having to do with you, if you keep your ego out of it, you'll find—like many of the wealthiest people, who have been broke several times over—you will recover and usually end up in a better financial situation than your former one, as long as you take the appropriate steps! Start with an attitude of gratitude and generosity, and you will set the stage

> *"Broke is not a state of being; it is a state of feeling. Plenty of billionaires have lost it all, finding themselves broke on paper, but they don't lose touch with who they are."*

for success. If you seek out the blessing in adversity a day will surely bring, you will never meet a day you are unhappy with. You have the total power to do this as you continue to learn to change your programming—your thinking.

When I was a teenager, my grandma helped me understand that how I felt about what was going on in my life was actually more important than the events transpiring. She once gave me a copy of a poem on this very point, which

I want to share with you. Here is the famous writing, called *Attitudes*, by Charles Swindoll:

Attitudes

The longer I live, the more I realize the importance of choosing the right attitude in life.

Attitude is more important than facts.

It is more important than your past;

more important than your education or your financial situation;

more important than your circumstances, your successes, or your failures;

more important than what other people think or say or do.

It is more important than your appearance, your giftedness, or your skills.

It will make or break a company. It will cause a church to soar or sink.

It will make the difference between a happy home or a miserable home.

You have a choice each day regarding the attitude you will embrace.

Life is like a violin.

You can focus on the broken strings that dangle,

or you can play your life's melody on the one that remains.

You cannot change the years that have passed,

nor can you change the daily tick of the clock.

You cannot change the pace of your march toward your death.

You cannot change the decisions or reactions of other people.

And you certainly cannot change the inevitable.

Those are strings that dangle!

What you can do is play on the one string that remains – your attitude.

I am convinced that life is 10 percent what happens to me

and 90 percent how I react to it.

The same is true for you.

---

you'd have a good job and a nice house. Most of all, you'd be happy. This life you have dreamt of is now within your reach. It comes from making the right choices, starting now. You are lucky to have been born in the right place and at the right time in history. Never before has there been such opportunity. That isn't to say this time is perfect, of course not. We're talking about reality here. The reality and what you need to accept before you can have that life you want is this: it is your choices that brought you where you are right now. And now, your choices from this very moment forward will bring you to where you want to be, along with much more than you ever dreamed of.

Do understand, the acceptance of where you are and the inevitable responsibility that stems from that doesn't mean you won't have unexpected challenges and difficulty. In fact, the more potential and promise you have in your future the more problems and pain you'll have in your history. The devil works harder to derail you when the positive impact you are capable of having is great! We all have to deal with difficult issues. You will either allow them to keep you stuck or begin to see them as training for your future, learning things from them that will empower you to be that much better for upcoming opportunities. You can have exactly what you want and need in life. Just remember you have a ladder to climb. We all do. The happiest and

Convert Pain to Action

I bet when you were young you had some exciting ideas about what your life would be as an adult. You would find the partner of your dreams, you'd have some wonderful children,

wealthiest of us have climbed it rung by rung. The most successful don't care where they start, but rather how high they want to go. The choice to change your life's direction happens in an instant, but the wonderful manifestation of the blessings that come from this one choice continue to blossom over the remainder of your lifetime. You may be afraid of change, but you will find you get far more than you ever expected on the positive side and encounter far less negative. Be more frightened about how terrible it will feel staying where you are and things getting even worse. Let that pain motivate you into action. You probably already know what not having what you want feels like, so what's to fear about experiencing what real achievement and fulfillment feels like? You can always go back to being unsuccessful if you so choose!

God rewards those who become stewards of their own life, working to become their best so He can do more through them for the good of others. Don't ask God to do for you what you can do for yourself. He has bigger things to think about. Trust that.

Most of us are somewhat optimistic. So when you look to some arbitrary time called "the future," you probably see things as being either as they are or better than they are now. Just like when you were a kid and you dreamt of the life you thought you'd have, like you saw on your favorite TV show. But things don't just get better all on their own without you making better choices. You have to take steps to get there. That, coupled with grace, guarantees you a legendary life.

"The Future" may feel somewhat scary and unknown but you can see into your future right now. You can discover where you're going to be next year. The future is not something that's waiting for you; it's something you are creating right now. Reading this page at this moment is a wonderful investment into that future.

To discover where you're going to be next year, look at where you were this time last year. Consider the direction your life has been taking. Are you happier than you were last year? Are you healthier now than you were 12 months ago? Has your blood pressure dropped? Are you in better condition? Are you pleased when you step on the scale? Is your job more rewarding? Is your relationship with your partner more satisfying? Are you getting along better with your coworkers, kids or parents? Do you have more in your savings account? Do you have less debt? Do you feel fulfilled in your work or mission?

If you answered yes to most of these questions then congratulations! You are on your way to an even better next year! But if you're like many Americans, and like me when I was a teen, you answered no. What if you are actually in worse shape this year than last year? Then I'm telling you, and I know this to be true as much as I know that God put this book in your hand for a reason, if you don't change your path, if you don't make the simple choices you need to make each day to get where you want to be, then you will continue to head in the opposite direction of your purpose and dream, and when you decide in the future to change you will have even more ground to cover, if you even get the chance!

"Progress happens when you direct change, and progress doesn't come until you become unhappy with the way things are right now."

You may feel that you don't want change but that's not true. You just have connected pain to the idea of change. Let me assure you, change is inevitable whether you want it or not. Do you look exactly the same as you did 10 years ago? I don't think so! But it is your decision whether that change will bring you to your dream. Progress and change are not the same. Progress happens when you direct change, and progress doesn't come until you become unhappy with the way things are right now. I'm all for celebrating success, as small changes and small successes over time become big successes, but don't let a small success stop you from being consistent and following through to your ultimate goal, achieving what you re-

ally want. If you allow yourself to be satisfied with relatively insignificant improvements, then you will stop taking the necessary steps to affect the change you truly want.

"Allowing yourself to be comfortable at a place you don't really want to be ensures that you will never be there."

Here's a typical example to illustrate what I'm saying. Usually you weigh 160 pounds. One day you decide to weigh yourself after a year of avoiding the scale, and you find you weigh 180 pounds. You knew you'd gained a couple of pounds but you didn't know it was that many! This upsets you and makes you start a diet. You are really upset at your weight, and therefore determined and excited to change. You throw out all the food you shouldn't be eating and you follow the diet strictly, until you get to around 165 pounds. This feels comfortable to you. Your clothes aren't really tight anymore. You're not upset with yourself. In fact, you feel pretty good. While you're not at your goal, you still have five pounds to go, you decide you've been "good" enough and lost lots of weight, so you deserve that pizza night you've been craving. You break the agreement you had with yourself to get down to 160 pounds and stay there. You cave in, reinforcing the very habits that caused you such pain. And soon the needle on the scale starts inching its way up again.

How did that happen? It happened because you did not accept the reality of where you were. Instead of saying, "I'm still five pounds heavier than I want to be," you said "Great! I'm awesome! I lost 15 pounds! Now it's party time!" You didn't work on the part that's most important, integrating the habits into your identity. If it's weight loss you were after, great, you did it. Now what? You've got to take it one step further and ask why you want to weigh 160 pounds. Who must you be to maintain that standard? With a focus on why you started and who you are becoming, you recognize using food like a drug when you're not at the place you've wanted to be doesn't make any sense. Allowing yourself to be comfortable at a place you don't really want to be ensures that you will never be there.

Most Limited Resource

Here's the thing. We always feel like we have lots of time. People in their 20s say they're too young to start saving money. They want to have fun and they're not ready to invest in anything! By the time they're ready to buy a house in their 30s, they think of all the money they could have easily saved and wish they'd started sooner. People in their 30s and 40s think they don't have to start worrying about their health yet. They'll start looking after themselves later. They're too busy looking after their families. Someday they'll get to it, they tell themselves. They still have time.

But you never have as much time as you think you have. My parents didn't start thinking about their health until they were in their 40s, but then my dad died at age 54. Fifty-four! It wasn't until he suffered a heart attack at 53 that he really got serious and came to me for weight-loss coaching. I helped him lose 50 pounds. He did the right thing, taking charge of his health, but it was too little too late. The damage had already been done and the 50 pounds wasn't enough. He suffered a second heart attack that ended his life, far too early. His focus had been so much on everything outside of himself that he never had the chance to enjoy living and being. He was always trying to hurry up to get more work done to pay bills, support my mom and send us kids through school.

I've spoken a lot about my mom so you already know that the year after my dad died, my mom died at 51. Just like you, maybe, they both thought they had time, that somehow their bad habits would magically disappear and their health would magically recover.

"You never have as much time as you think you have."

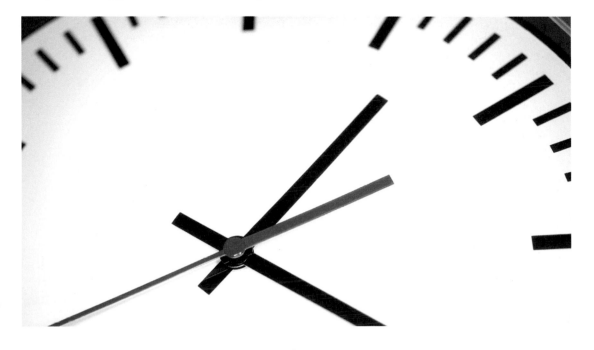

Habits do not just disappear. You have to be the magician. You have to figure out which habits are keeping you in a place you don't want to be and where they are, and you have to make the choice to replace them with better ones that meet your needs. Choose habits that invest in your life and future, not withdraw from it. Your life will not magically start taking a different course than the one you're currently on. There is no magic. You have to fully and consciously decide to change the course you're

> *"Your life will not magically start taking a different course than the one you're currently on. There is no magic. You have to fully and consciously decide to change the course you're on or you'll keep traveling in the same direction."*

on or you'll keep traveling in the same direction. It's time to bring the light of awareness to all of your choices and truly examine their impact on your present and future. Turn your car around and consciously move in a different direction if you're dissatisfied with where you find yourself today. For this to happen, you have to take a good hard and honest look at yourself, see where you want to improve things, and let yourself get very uncomfortable about it. And then you can get excited about what's possible. Now is the time you will make the change.

Accept that the world, the people, the situations are the way they are at this moment and are intended and providential in the lessons they can offer you. You don't need to change *it* or *them* for your life to change. The world operates perfectly without our interference. God is with you right now. Acceptance of that and the implication it has on the power it can release into your life is monumental for your future. You need only begin to do all you can to design the life you deserve. Whenever

you give it your best, making every effort to make your life magnificent, let go at that point and leave God to take care of the rest. I'm telling you that ever since I started doing this myself, nothing but blessings have flooded my life. They will yours as well—it only takes you making the choice that this is the way you will begin to see your life.

Use Your Privilege

If you're reading this, I'll assume you are privileged enough to be living in a developed country, where we have access to everything we need to have an incredible life full of health, happiness and success, and yet many of us act like it's not available. You have the world

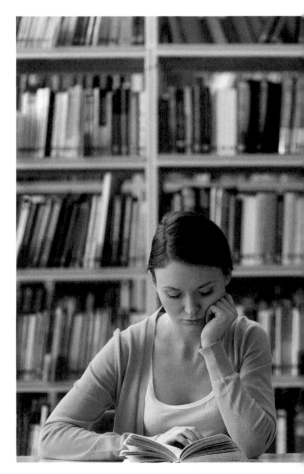

of knowledge at your fingertips, and you don't even need money for a computer and Internet for this to be the case. Libraries abound, and they are filled with volumes and volumes of information on the very things you may hope to achieve. Whatever you want to learn, whether that's piano playing, being a better communicator, parenting more effectively or anything else you can think of, the information is there.

We all also enjoy another privilege in our part of the world: literacy. Most people in developed countries can read. That is not the case everywhere, and we often forget to count the small things with which we're blessed. Even when those on food stamps in America are living better than the 71% of the world who live on less than $10 per day.

Knowledge of this is not power. Action is. Who was it that said that if knowledge were power librarians would all be billionaires? Well they'd be the world's leaders at least. Obviously, knowing what to do, like the importance of a good attitude, is only part of the equation— activating that knowledge through consistent action is the second and most critical step. It is through that application of consistent and flexible activity in pursuit of what we want, that success begins.

Those who are successful at life are not any smarter, better or more spiritual than you— they simply have begun to love themselves, tapping into the truth and feeling that they too deserve the wonders and luxuries that a rich life affords all of us. They've learned the laws of life, accepted them and learned to play by those rules, using them to their advantage to further their personal aims, to succeed and to improve the lives of others in some capacity or another, whether in their own community or across the world. They've accepted themselves for being human, know who they are authentically, realize they don't need to be more or have more to be happy, are independent of others' opinions, at least to the degree that others don't influence how they feel about themselves. They learn to love themselves as people who can always make progress at becoming more when they see areas that need refinement, while being content in this process of their own spiritual growth.

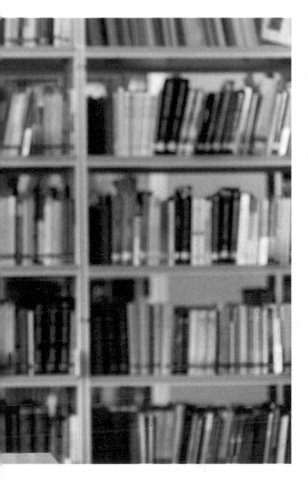

"Those who are successful at life are not any smarter, better or more spiritual than you—they simply have begun to love themselves, tapping into the truth and feeling that they too deserve the wonders and luxuries that a rich life affords all of us."

Know you are "self-employed" and the CEO of your life even if you have a job because, in truth, we all are.

Your employer can replace you at any time, markets can drop, and industries can be eliminated in less than a day with the speed of change in today's world. The idea of being taken care of when employed as an adult is an outdated illusion. The best philosophy is to make yourself as close to irreplaceable as you can be, however you create an income. Become the person who everyone comes to when they need to get a job done. Jesus had it right when he said "The greatest among you will be a servant." When your purpose and motivation aren't what you're getting or the money you're making, but rather being joyful in the service

"The best philosophy is to make yourself as close to irreplaceable as you can be."

you're rendering, you'll never have to worry about the money.

My dad, who owned a janitorial company in an extraordinarily competitive industry where he truly was the little guy, built his company into a well-known brand without any formal education in business, marketing or corporate training. He loved people. He loved helping others. He was able to make money not because of a fancy business card, van, or the most cutting-edge equipment, but by his desire to be the best servant to those who chose his company. He made himself available 24/7, and had strong relationships with and loyalty to all those he worked for. It was only at his funeral that I realized the impact he had. Many of the millionaires who owned the companies my dad had cleaned for attended. They wept uncontrollably, seeing his coffin in front of the altar, and shared meaningful and thoughtful things my dad had done for them over the years. Several said my dad's lightheartedness, sense of humor and can-do attitude inspired them to work harder, be better and care more about their own employees. My dad was the type of guy who would say yes to doing something and then learn how to do it after he committed!

Many of these leaders at my dad's funeral were C-Suite executives—not the people you'd think would know much about the janitor of their building, a man who in his entire lifetime earned a fraction of what they made in a year, and yet he touched their lives. It moved me. No matter what you think of yourself or where you are, you too can make a difference by committing to bringing hope and love into every interaction and place you go, just like my dad did.

I do advise you, however, to take a look at balancing your life so you don't burn out or suffer an early demise because of the drive you have in business. You have to be your own best advocate because no one is going to work harder for what you want and deserve in your life than you alone can.

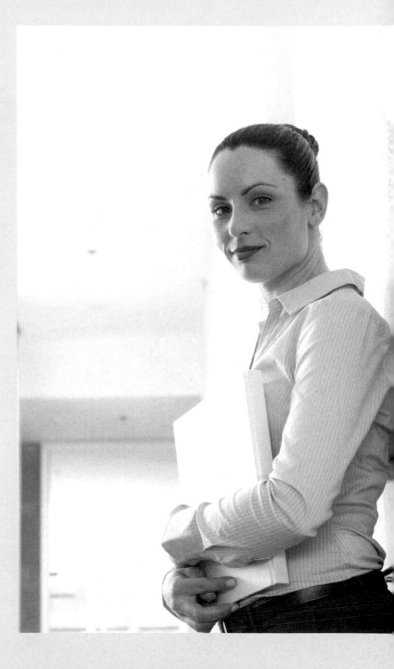

Our ability to adapt combined with a fear of what we consider an unknown future, one in which we are captain and not passenger, can cause us to adjust and lower the expectations we have for ourselves. If you just realize that the road called uncertainty is the only path to any growth, you will quickly click into gear and choose what you've long known in your heart and spirit is best. When have you ever accomplished anything of significance where you didn't feel unsure, shaky, or straight-out terrible about how you were doing, at least early on? All great achievers were once horrible at the things they've now mastered. I'm sure even such a comedic legend as Robin Williams was booed early on! Look at early tapes of great entertainers and speakers. They "fail" their way to success. They just don't have the same definition you do of failure! Their vision of their future is so strong and compelling it pulls them through the temporary disappointments we all must face. What others might consider failure, to them is trying out new material discovering what will and won't work. Many of them had to go through hours and hours of intensive coaching and training on the use of words, intonation, and vocal inflection before they earned the reverence of the public. Many even had speech impediments they overcame!

Achievers give as much to an audience of one as an audience of a thousand. They are in love with what they do but never rest on their laurels and grow complacent. They always want to be better. They never lose their desire to refine their gift and ability. They understand that a few stumbles and turbulence are inevitable in the ascent toward their ultimate calling. Since life is all about growth, we too must choose this route, ensuring that everything we're doing is progress oriented. If you don't, you have only yourself to blame, it's truly your fault. The only things in life that survive are those that continue to develop, grow, and contribute. When your life's purpose has been met, your life will end! That which doesn't grow and blossom inevitably gets weeded out. Choose not to accept a life far inferior to the one you could have, simply because you are presently ok with the status quo. Life has a funny way of shaking us up into action if we don't take it upon ourselves to shake things up on our own.

Raise your expectations of yourself and your life will change this moment. Move beyond your comfort zone. If you're out of shape, go to a gym where the other people are in great shape. Befriend people who have more, who can do more than you. Don't surround yourself with those who are settling in order to make yourself feel comfortable with your own negligence. When you raise your game, putting yourself in a room where you no longer are the smartest, best looking, healthiest, most successful or fulfilled, you will inevitably begin to raise your standards and grow. If you're not outgoing or social, make it a goal to talk to at least three or four people a day. People in sales often make it a goal to get at least 10 "no's" per day.

Find people who have achieved what you want to achieve, are in the career you always have dreamed of, who work for the company you want to work for, who earn the income you've dreamt of earning, and give them the gift of a dinner out. Is it worth the tab? You'd better believe it! Having access to someone who's at the level you hope to be is invaluable. The bible teaches: "As iron sharpens iron, so one person sharpens another." Who are you spending time with who is helping you to accept less, even though in your heart you know there is more meant for you?

Time to Check Yourself!

Do any of these statements sound familiar to you?

☐ You no longer enjoy shopping for clothes because even if you manage to find clothing you like that will fit, when you try it on you don't like how it looks.

☐ You keep your favorite clothing in the back of your closet, thinking one day maybe you'll be able to wear it again and you can't bear to get rid of it because that means admitting your size.

☐ You used to feel so close to your partner, but now you feel like you both just go through the motions.

☐ You and your partner don't share the passionate intimate life that you once did.

☐ You are in a position at work you don't like, where you don't feel respected.

☐ You dread Mondays to the degree that you get anxiety on Sunday evening.

☐ When the alarm goes off, rather than meet the day with excitement and anticipation for what's to come, you hit the snooze button and pull the covers up over your head.

☐ You would like to live in a nicer neighborhood, or you'd like to be able to send your kids to a better school, but feel you can't because you don't have the financial resources or backing.

☐ You want to start playing a sport, participating in a group activity or socializing, but you just don't feel like you're good enough, or think you won't fit in.

☐ You want to travel the world, enjoying the rich experiences life has to offer, but you feel you can't afford making the dream a reality.

I can relate to many of these things from one time or another in my life. I too was once the guy who had to think carefully about what food to buy, hoping I had enough to cover the bill! I went door-to-door in the summers asking neighbors if they needed to have their lawn mowed so I could go to the movie theater and get a ticket, a popcorn and soda. I wasn't always aware of the abundance that is available to all of us. I once heard a speaker say that what's available to us through God is as vast as the ocean. The trouble isn't the size of the ocean, but rather, that most people go to the ocean with a thimble!

You have the power and ability to change all of these things and many, many more, simply by changing your mindset, but at this point you've adapted, you've grown accustomed and you've created a belief system that this state of being you call "life" is where you are meant to be. At this very moment, there are others who are vacationing more than half the year, living life on their own terms, spending time with the people they want to spend time with and creating a legacy not only for themselves, but for anyone else they so choose. If they can do it, so can you. That said, you don't have to do what the so-called "successful" people do to earn the title. Success is moving toward what you want more steadily and consistently than you have been. You get to determine the details of your success, but in simple terms success means becoming more of what you

"Success is moving toward what you want more steadily and consistently than you have been."

can be. The military's saying, "Be all that you can be" comes to mind. Break out of the routine you've found yourself in to grow into what God planted in you. The notion that you're reading this book is proof that you are the kind of person who has it in you to do so.

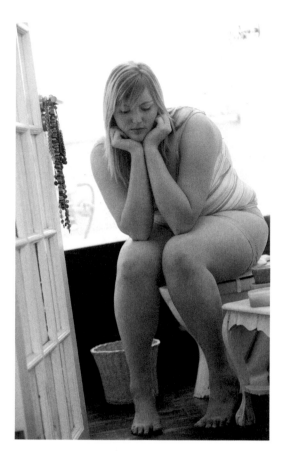

If you are not happy with your health, emotional state, relationship, career or life's purpose, your story is not over. Quite the contrary, it's just beginning this second. This is the first step in beginning to realize what indeed is possible and even probable when you embrace the daily disciplines needed to have and deserve that lifestyle. Misery is not where you were meant to be. This is where you've allowed yourself to be, probably because you have told yourself that you have no choice or power.

This belief system is often passed down from generation to generation, which at least in part explains the adage, 'The rich get richer and the poor get poorer." It's not who you are that explains why you have or don't have what you want, it's what you've chosen to believe and how you make choices based on those beliefs. You have removed yourself from the flow of abundance that life offers. Psychologically, it takes the pressure and ownership of responsibility off of you and puts it on something outside of you. If your belief system has been that the choices you've made up until now have nothing to do with the outcome of your life, then you can't possibly fail—because it's always up to someone or something else for you to have a better life.

Have you ever caught yourself saying any of these things?

- I'm overweight because my whole family is overweight and that's just the way I'm built.

- I can't possibly work out or get healthy with all the people I have to take care of.

- I have a job I hate because that's the only job I could get. If you lived where I do, you'd see what I'm talking about!

- I have relationship issues because my spouse doesn't listen to me. I'm only in this because I have to be for the kids now. I'm out as soon as they are grown.

- If you were abused like I was as a child, then in all the different dysfunctional relationships and failed marriages I got mixed up in, you'd be just as messed up too!

- I'm broke because things are way too expensive and my workplace doesn't pay me fairly, so how could I possibly get out of debt with a paycheck like mine?

You can adapt to a life that's less than you would like it to be in a number of ways. One is by seeming to relinquish control. One is to invent reasons or excuses for why things are not as you might wish. These are both demonstrated in the statements above. Another important way to adapt to an inferior life is to tell yourself it's not all that bad: "I'm better off

than my parents were." Or "I'm in better shape than I was a year ago," even though you know your progress has halted and you may even be sliding backwards.

People who have always been of a normal weight have a difficult time understanding how a person can become obese, as they don't understand that the obese person blinds him- or herself to the obesity. In general, we go into denial or think thoughts that serve only to keep us trapped in that disempowered state, feeling our condition is permanent, bad, and we're helpless to change it. Obese people make certain they don't get on a scale. I was guilty of this type of thing when I was 360 pounds. When a school nurse once saw my flushed, beet-red face and wanted to pull me from class to take my blood pressure, I refused, delusionally thinking if I didn't acknowledge the truth it wasn't actually true. People like the teenage me don't typically look in full-length mirrors or want to be in pictures. Once their weight gets to a point that they are having a hard time mentally dealing with it, they stop dealing with it because they stop facing it. At this point it's almost inevitable that their weight will continue going up further, because they are not seeing it.

This is very similar to people who have problems with debt. They are unable to meet their payments, so debt collectors start calling. Because debt collectors are calling, they stop answering the phone. Bills arrive in the mail and they don't open them. They somehow feel subconsciously like if they don't admit the problem then it's not real. Some people are so out of touch with the reality of their financial state that they will continue to go further and further into debt even while refusing to admit the problem exists—going shopping, racking up more and more debt while not paying the debts they already have.

I'm sure you can see logically how this refusal to come to terms with reality will never result in you achieving the goals you want, but it can be a little more difficult to see when it's your own problems, your own goals, your own excuses and your own avoidance. What are you distracting yourself from dealing with by not acknowledging the real situation? Has it been way too long since your last doctor's visit? What's your blood pressure? How's your cholesterol? How happy are you and your spouse with your marriage? How many times have you consumed alcohol in excess this year? How much do you and your teenaged kids talk? Have you not checked your retirement accounts since the beginning of the recession because then you can just "believe" it's better than it really is? Not taking any action is taking action—just the worst possible action you could take in these situations.

Don't leave your future to chance. You can't manage what you don't measure. The first step to change is accepting where you are. Acknowledge the truth. When you don't check in honestly on where things are in your life, it can lead to a state where you are never quite

> ## "Not taking any action is taking action—just the worst possible action you could take in these situations."

happy with your reality, but also never quite ready to create a reality that you will be happy with. When you are faced with unavoidable proof—you are unable to fit in a restaurant booth, for example, or your car gets repossessed, or you can't remember what you did last night after a few too many drinks—then out come the excuses.

The excuses might make you feel better briefly, but they do nothing for your long-term goals and happiness. To actually reach those goals and achieve that happiness, you have to accept reality for what it is. Denying it doesn't make it any less real. Currently you are here. You would like to be there. Why you are where you are is not nearly as interesting to me as your commitment and plan to get where you

deserve to be and enjoy it! What will you decide to commit to today? Now is the time to create a plan.

This is simple, but simple does not always mean easy. If your goal is to become debt free, then shift your focus from "debt," which is negative, to wealth creation or accumulation. It does take some work to earn what you deserve, but making the choices to accumulate wealth will be far easier psychologically than "putting money aside to pay off a mountain of debt" that you may not fully believe will ever happen, because you're so used to being buried under it. You have to change your thought processes from excuse making to path creating, designing a personal road map to success and following it. What you will find is that once you make the first, most important shift, choosing to accept where you are and decide where you want to go, the flow will start. It will seem as if the universe is conspiring in your favor with the right people, opportunities, and ideas popping into your awareness. Often my clients experience remarkably divine synchronies and positive affirmations that they have discovered their life's purpose shortly after accepting their current reality as well as their responsibility to direct their life from here on out.

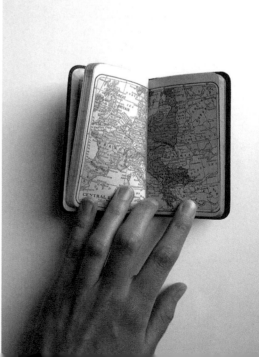

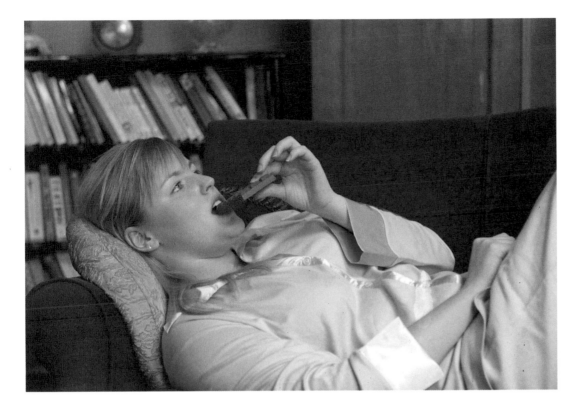

Acceptance x 2

Many people, including the former me, hold on to the following philosophy for far too long. See if it resonates with the one you've had up until now: "I'd have to be crazy to think I can change my reality. I just have to accept that the cards are stacked against me and settle for what I have. I'm going to be alone and miserable forever. It's too difficult to do things differently. I've tried, and I have no idea how to make the necessary choices in order to make my life any better. Screw it. I'll just drink, smoke, spend, sleep, eat and medicate myself more, and make myself feel better." This way of thinking makes us give up before we try, too overwhelmed by our own self-perceived barriers.

Is this you? The things you're not happy with, do you just set them aside, put them on the back burner and think "one day I'll get to it"? Do you feel sorry for yourself? Have you mis-

"If you educate your emotion, you'll soon recognize that often what feels good in the moment results in long-lasting feelings of guilt, remorse, resentment, and even lower self-esteem when clarity returns."

labeled your self-punishing behaviors like junk food, drugs, illicit sex, gambling, overspending or alcohol as a reward or pleasurable behavior when the reality is maybe at your core you simply just don't believe you're worthy of having more?

It's not uncommon for our egos to delude us into thinking that the things we do that ultimately destroy us and rob us of our futures are gratifying. If you educate your emotion, you'll soon recognize that often what feels good in the moment results in long-lasting feelings of guilt, remorse, resentment, and even lower self-esteem when clarity returns. Think about it.

So maybe you want to lose some weight. Maybe because of that weight gain or other reasons you don't feel like being intimate with your partner anymore. Maybe your relationship is ok but now the passion is gone. Or

"A successful relationship comes from a selfless desire to love and contribute not what you want to give, but what your partner wants and needs from you."

maybe your relationship is truly on the rocks and you're thinking about ending it. Maybe you drag yourself out of bed in the morning wishing you didn't have to go to work because you think it should make you happier than you are.

Or maybe you hate your job so much that your misery doesn't wait until morning—the night before you lie in bed dreading the next day. Maybe your finances are not good. You are having problems with debt, you struggle to pay the bills each month and the phone is constantly ringing with calls from collection agencies. Or maybe you're in that gray zone of life where you're not terribly upset with how things are, but you certainly aren't happy. You are sitting on the sidelines. Every aspect of life could use some improvement, but you don't make changes in that direction. 'What's the point of it all?' you ask yourself as you sleepwalk through another day feeling never quite satisfied.

Acceptance. The word can have two very different connotations. On the one hand, you can accept where you are and never really question where it's possible for you to be. You grow complacent. This is probably where most of the people in the world are, accepting what they consider to be their lot in life, never realizing that by making just a few small choices each day their world can be entirely different and a million times better. Maybe, like many who have come to me for coaching, you've even achieved all the measures of success you thought would make you happy. You have the relationship, the money, beautiful house and expensive cars and clothes and yet you still feel empty. Is this you?

The other way you can look at the word "acceptance" is to accept or admit the way things are instead of deluding yourself. This is the divine path. This can also be thought of as honesty. If you're 50 pounds overweight and it is impacting your health and quality of life then telling yourself that while you could stand to lose a few pounds you are in an acceptable weight range does not help you any, and it certainly doesn't help you to be the fit person you truly desire to be. You can rationalize any position you are in, but doing so keeps you in that position, or, more often than not, guarantees it will only get worse.

Rationalization and justification is easy. I'll do it for you: "My marriage isn't great and we don't have passion anymore, but what do you expect? We've been married for 15 years and have two kids. No one expects passion to last. Anyway, most marriages end in divorce. All of my friends hate their marriages. If you're smart, you never get married!" Wrong! While you might be in a relationship that you don't feel fulfilled by, these are gross generalizations. A successful relationship comes from a

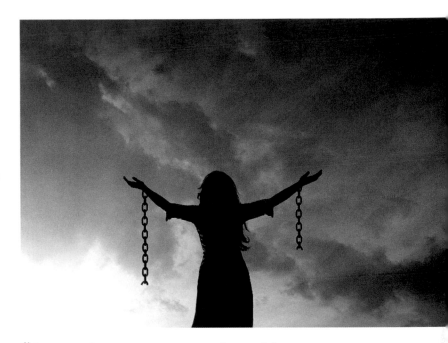

"Don't choose to stay miserable. You have endless possibilities, but limited time."

selfless desire to love and contribute not what you want to give, but what your partner wants and needs from you. It's meeting them on their terms. It's ego-less and God full. When you realize that relationships are God's gift to us to magnify all the joy we get to have on this planet, your worldview changes. Rather than going into the relationship expecting to receive, you go into it wanting to give. That giving guarantees a shift. If you are honest with yourself and truly have practiced that for several months or years and don't see your partner shifting or working at their own development in this area, then perhaps the time has come you consider leaving the relationship, but not until. With this strategy you can leave knowing you did everything you possibly could. The act of shifting to this approach guarantees you will attract into your life someone in harmony with that, a person who is a giver as well.

Again, it all comes back to you. If you're not happy, stop complaining and change it. Truly

"Get angry if needed, and transmute that anger into activity to climb the ladder to have and become all you're capable of."

give it your all and if that still honestly has no impact, leave and know you are better for it. You have given your ex-partner the greatest gift: unconditional love and support. Now you deserve and can have more than you did because you've grown beyond who you were! I believe and know that you can have a passionate loving relationship until the end of time if you choose to.

"If you don't have money to give, offer your time"

Maybe it's not your relationship that's troubling you, but rather your job. "I hate my boss and I can't stand my job but it took me a long time to find something in my field and there aren't a lot of jobs out there so I'll just have to suck it up. Besides, my family depends on this income. What am I supposed to do?" I'll tell you what to do: stop trying to find happiness outside of yourself and enjoy what you can in the position you're in, remaining grateful instead of needy. Maybe there is a lesson or person you're meant to connect with at the place you're in. Maybe this is a stepping stone. Trust that if you will work hard on yourself while you're there, doing all you can to the best of your ability and learning all you can, you will grow. When you have the attitude that you are preparing yourself for the next opportunity, expecting it to appear when that time comes, then it will, like magic.

Neediness does not precipitate getting what you desire. That's not how life works. Whenever I ask anyone for anything it is always with an offer to give much more than I'm asking. Never go with an empty hand extended. If you don't have money to give in return, offer your time. It can be more valuable than money.

Your job doesn't exist to make you happy; it exists to provide something necessary to your employer, and then in return you make a living. If you own your own business, you know that you have to provide your clients with outstanding service or you may not make a living at all. On a personal level, it's your mandate to discover happiness in everything you do, and that takes mental and spiritual discipline. If you can't change the actual thing you're dissatisfied with, like you can't change your job right at this moment, then you have to at least challenge yourself to change your perception of it. A shift in your perception of the thing changes the thing itself. When you treat someone as the person they are capable of being, despite whatever behavior they have exhibited in the past, it's fascinating how that expectation activates within them the ability to live up to your higher expectations. Make a decision and either change the thing you're unhappy with or change how you see it. Don't choose to stay miserable. You have endless possibilities, but limited time. You could work full-time at your job and part-time on a hobby that in time could grow to a career. You could take courses to grow your skill set so you have more to offer at your current place of employment or so you are better prepared when another job becomes available. You do not have to be complacent in a dismal, dead-end, life-sucking job and delude yourself into thinking that's all there is. I've known plenty of happy people in less-than-perfect situations but I've never found a rich, fulfilled, happy person with a terrible attitude. Even if your situation sucks, your attitude doesn't have to.

"A shift in your perception of the thing changes the thing itself."

Embrace Your Dissatisfaction

"This debt is crushing me. I make minimum payments each month but the principal never gets paid off. I just can't get on top of it." The truth: you can't get on top of it if you're choosing not to. If you're making only the minimum payments each month, and especially if you're accumulating more debt, you're right. You're never going to get on top of it, at least not in the near future. For things to be different, you have to make some changes. You can appreciate the fact that you have had the opportunity to enjoy the luxury of whatever you purchased on credit. That's a privilege, and you will definitely be paying for that privilege. Make the decision that you will not allow yourself anything more on credit until that is paid off. When you commit to a discipline like that, it's typical that you automatically feel better since you've made a choice to no longer worsen the situation you're in. But be grateful that first you're unhappy, because dissatisfaction is what usually provokes and accelerates rapid and massive change.

The critical ingredient to change is dissatisfaction. You need to find your current situation unacceptable before you will change it. Get disgusted with how things are. Get angry if needed, and transmute that anger into activity to climb the ladder to have and become all you're capable of. Certainly, it requires effort to make this type of progress, but the effort is worth it. Just ask anyone who stepped out of misery and into the uncertainty of something new, accepting their dissatisfaction and embracing their responsibility to change it. They will tell you it's the best thing that ever happened to them.

Take a good look at where you really are. The truth. Get out your bills. Write down the amounts. Get on that scale. Get in front of a full-length mirror. Don't rationalize or make excuses any more. Make this next year the one when you turn your entire life around. Don't talk yourself into feeling better about where you've ended up, negating God's promise on your life and future. Accept where you are and know you are the only thing that needs to shift to make it different: your perception and everyday choices. Get uncomfortable. Get angry. Get upset. Most importantly, get busy! Instead of asking yourself 'why me?', ask how you will get to where you've always wanted to be.

A Few Laws of Life

Law of Familiarity

That which we have access to all the time, even if we were once enamored or obsessed by it, becomes the norm and thereby loses its apparent value, even though we may recognize the value when we consciously think about it.

Think about when you first fell in love with your partner, how you couldn't wait to spend time with him or her. While you were at school or work, the love of your life was always on your mind, and you'd go out of your way to make him or her feel extremely wanted and special by doing really thoughtful things. Then, after years of dating or marriage, the relationship may have grown stale and boring. You started taking the relationship and/or your partner for granted. This can take place with any of us, in areas inside and outside of relationships. Far too many of us take our

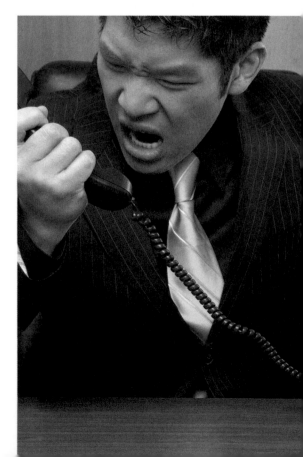

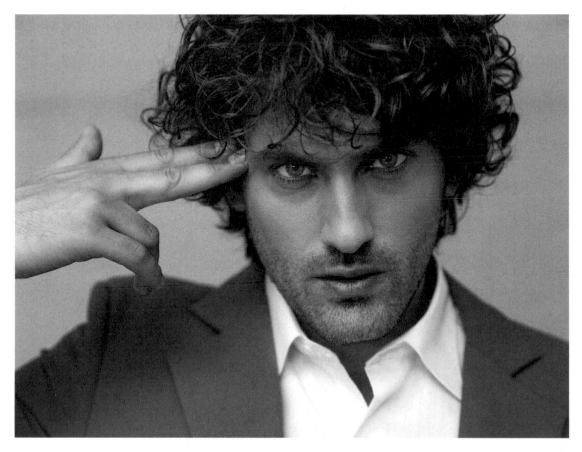

health for granted until we come down with an illness. Then we appreciate what we had after it's gone.

Guard against this by staying grateful, perhaps journaling at the end of each day. Write down several things you appreciated that were unique to the day and could see as gifts from your Creator.

Law of Proximity

The impact of a message is greatest soon after you encounter it. That's why, as we discussed earlier, you'll be excited after leaving a seminar but a few days later barely remember the message. And this is the reason achievers say they never leave the site of setting a goal without doing something immediately to move toward it. When you let the emotion fade, so too

"Be sure your thoughts harmonize and vibrate with what you have decided you want for yourself or you'll find that despite your good intentions, they'll fall on rocky soil."

does the probability that you will take any real meaningful action toward getting what you want and deserve! If you had time to think about doing it, it's clear you have the time to start doing it!

Take action while the emotion is high and you will progress. Otherwise, the negative emotions of doubt, fear, despair or simple distraction creep in, leading you away from something that is inches away from you! If you want to take action toward something you feel inspired to do, act now! Make the call, write the note, order the book. The strength to make the breakthrough is at its highest when your emotion is driving the thought!

Law of Reciprocity

If you think the "bad guys always win" or "nice guys finish last" you might have to reconsider. While it's rare to see a return from the field you sowed your seeds in—that is, if you treat someone badly you will probably not get your just desserts back from that specific person— when negative energy or vibrations are put out into the universe, it's not long after that it boomerangs back. I've seen this in my life. Be sure you are sowing seeds of harmony, love, care, authenticity and compassion. When you meet people with a smile, you'll notice they can't help but smile in return. We are wired to give back when given to. Expect kindness from others and you won't usually be disappointed.

Be the first to give and you'll never have to worry about receiving.

Law of Attraction

This law had a tremendous amount of hype when mentioned in a number of books a few years back. Simply stated, the premise is this: what you put your focus and intention on comes to you, almost magically. The words you speak have amazing power. When you speak words over your life that are negative, it seems you pull more and more of it to you. When you say "Losing weight and getting sober is so hard," the universe will find people, experiences, and references for you that reflect those words. Be careful that you are speaking only words of promise, joy, wealth, health and prosperity over your life. At the same time, my personal belief is this: While thinking thoughts of health, happiness and wealth are helpful, they are not enough in and of themselves.

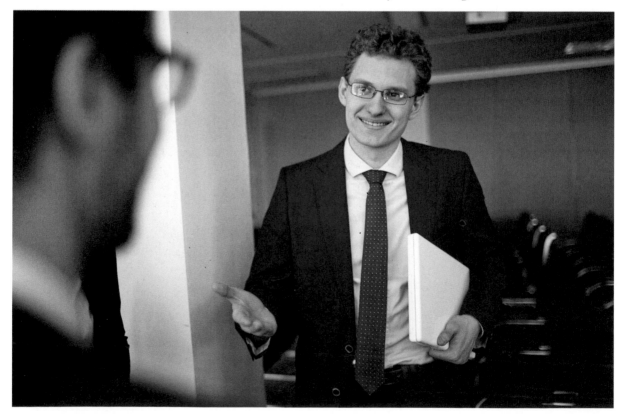

In my experience, this law is more about how you filter reality. For example, if you are thinking negative thoughts about others, it's not likely that you'll trust people. Since almost no one succeeds alone, that negativity dispels the chances that you'll connect with anyone who could open a door that you alone couldn't—perhaps with a potential business or relationship partner or investor.

Be sure your thoughts harmonize and vibrate with what you have decided you want for yourself or you'll find that despite your good intentions, they'll fall on rocky soil. The mind is the soil. When you think more positively about everyone around you, welcoming people into your life knowing that life is furthering your divine purpose independent of your efforts, that life is guided and that most people are good and sincere, you increase the probability you will experience more good from others. We come to receive what we expect. With that worldview, if you do happen to encounter one of the rare few people that aren't good and sincere, you'll take a valuable lesson and be more experienced and have more to invest in your journey because of it.

Law of Responsibility

Self-responsibility is critical to achievement. You are the only person who can make any difference in the quality of your life. Others may speak to you about how much better life can be, and might even be willing to financially support you, but only your choice about that can impact your life's trajectory. You must learn to feel in charge of your life.

This book's power is only that it can help you take action after reading it. Others may say they can change you and make a difference, but it's simply not true. You make the change. They can inspire, motivate, and empower you with strategy, but you are the only person who decides what you're going to do with whatever you take from the experience. And that's as it

should be! Do you really want your future to be left to someone else's whims?

Many people avoid thinking about their own power because they fear failure, but if you didn't know before starting this book you definitely know now that if you don't get what you want with your first efforts you have not failed; you have simply learned that you need to shift your strategy until you get it. It's that simple. What you do at this point is critical. Anyone who is successful is constantly moving closer to what they want. They see themselves as the most important determinant of their own future, and everything they encounter as an opportunity to further their personal growth and mission. They define themselves as "learners." What is it that finally allows for a child to walk, after countless falls? Believing, trying, learning, and persisting. While the baby's muscles and coordination grow and strengthen with the effort, the success comes solely from the mind—not giving up.

That same kind of change can be yours right now. You can decide right this instant that today is a totally new start. Nothing that has happened to you and no action you've taken up until now matters, because you're going on an entirely new self-oriented and inwardly directed path. Belief is the magic ingredient that gets activated when you take responsibility for where you want your life to go.

When you begin to make choices from this perspective, acting as if you are already where you want to be, you will take more risks, and the greater the risk the higher the reward. You will begin to move toward that very future you've always dreamed of! Learn to become self-reliant and count on yourself as the greatest advocate for your future!

The day I decided I was responsible for everything that happened to me—even if I got a flat tire and was late—was the day my life changed. If I was late because of a flat tire it was my fault, not the fault of the nail on the road or the tire. If I didn't have a backup plan, what could I have expected? I could have thought about having AAA, or I could have learned how to fix a flat tire. Bottom line, it was my responsibility. Have lines of defense ready when changing yourself, many plans to fortify yourself against the inevitable, so if the first doesn't go as planned you have back up.

When you take responsibility for your life in this way you don't have more stress. You anticipate challenges without unnecessary anxiety because you are focused more on problem resolution than problem description. A dead giveaway that someone isn't ready for real lasting change is when you hear them talking more about why they are where they are than about how they are going to get to where they want to go or how they will never allow such a situation to occur again. What is your inner dialogue focused on? Are you spending more time thinking about why things are the way they are, or are you constructively focusing on how you're going to make yourself better so you can influence things on your own terms?

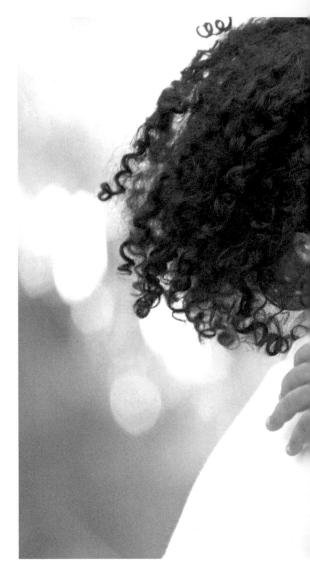

Law of Unconditional Love

This law is very important. It teaches that no matter what a person has done that may cause you offense or harm, we are to hear their message as either a "Loving Message" to us, or a "Cry for Help." The book *A Course in Miracles*, by Helen Schucman, goes much

deeper into this, but for now understand that it means you suspend all judgment, replacing it with compassion. Consider that even the most diabolical and cruel people are operating from a place of meeting their own needs. This obviously does not mean you should allow harm to come to you or those you love; you need to learn healthy boundaries so people in that state don't have free access to you—but you still send love and warm wishes their way. Having coached so many people, I can't help but have tremendous empathy for everyone, even leaders who seem cruel and heartless. If

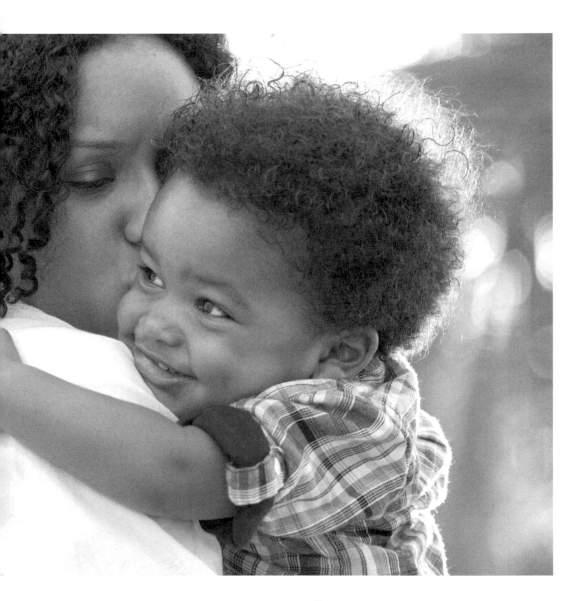

we had the privilege of watching every waking moment from their birth to the present as God does, I don't think we would be as quick to lay judgment. When you consider the person you abhor was once an innocent child, you'll find yourself responding differently. Some people, despite aging physically, are emotionally infantile—and I don't mean that in a judgmental way. Age isn't just chronological. Some children have the maturity of someone who should be decades older. When you encounter an adult whose behavior you just don't understand, then take into consideration

"This perspective can also do wonders to reduce the anxiety you may feel about others' opinions. They have just as many insecurities as you do, and often more so!"

that things you don't know about fed into their development. This can do wonders when you feel less than loving toward them. This perspective can also do wonders to reduce the anxiety you may feel about others' opinions.

They have just as many insecurities as you do, and often more!

There is an art to learning this law, as it doesn't excuse the other's responsibility in doing unjust things as an adult and it certainly does not mean that you should put yourself or your family at risk (mentally, emotionally or physically), but it does mean having the hope that they reconnect with their purpose and highest selves in time, thereby improving the quality of all of our lives. It was Abraham Lincoln who said, "(If) I don't like that man, I must get to know him better." Always remember we rarely know the whole story in even the most tragic of situations. I prefer to let God be the judge.

This law also requires that we personally find a reason to be grateful for everything in our life, that we find the lesson in every problem. As the greatest motivational speaker of the 20th century Dr. Norman Vincent Peale said, "Whenever God wants to send you a gift he wraps it up in a problem. The bigger the problem the bigger the gift." Find the gift in every adversity. Once it's gleaned, you'll find the challenge will dissipate like a puff of smoke, and you'll never have to relive the pain the lesson brought again.

Law of Abundance

This law teaches that there is no scarcity in our lives. The only thing that can block us from tapping into the overflowing abundance that surrounds us is our own thinking. What you want is already seeking you out. Like the Sun, what we need is always available. We need only have the intention, take the seed God's given us, plant it in fertile soil, nurture it, and from something as small as an acorn grows a massive tree! The same is true with the thoughts you translate into action and continually act on with the firm faith that things are moving even if they aren't apparent on the surface yet! Thinking, backed by strong

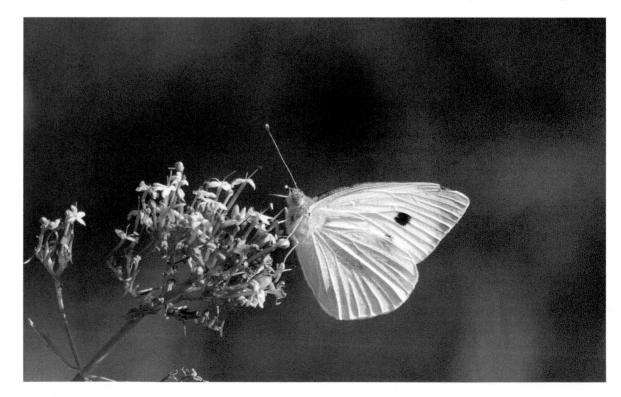

feeling, followed through on by flexible action is the recipe for success.

How valuable is an idea? It's nearly impossible to put a price tag on something that can change the course of your life or the course of humanity. The printing press, channeling and storage of electricity, the phone, the car and now the Internet and smartphones are all ideas that resided inside a person's mind and through activity became reality. There is no limit to where our thoughts and action can bring us, and the first step in tapping into the abundance available to all of us is that recognition.

What stops most people from ever tapping it? Conditioning. Fear. Worry. Looking to the wrong examples and being influenced by them. The secret to utilizing this law is recognizing how the desire within you gets activated. Once you acknowledge that, anything you want for yourself is possible. When you seek to be happy each day, authentically happy, you find that all the tangible measures of success—relationships, health and wealth—flow to you rather than you having to chase them. Like a butterfly landing on your shoulder, the state of tranquility and calm attracts that which is in harmony. Never chase what you're after; become the type of person that naturally would attract the conditions you're seeking.

Do you have to tell your heart to keep beating? Do you need to remind your lungs to expand and contract? No, there is an intelligence inherent in each of us. We simply have to relax in the knowing that what needs to happen will when we are aligned with God's purpose for our lives. When you stop to think about how your body has an intelligence all of its own how, your lungs, heart and blood all know exactly what to do without any of your interference, you relax into knowing you're part of something far greater than what your senses would have you believe.

When I was about five or six years old I had to have a hernia procedure. I don't remember experiencing any fear, worry or anxiety over it. I trusted that my parents knew what was best and went through the procedure, no problem. As adults, sometimes our mind begins to run us instead of us running it. We lose faith in ourselves and at times, doubt our Creator. President Franklin Roosevelt once said, "Men are not prisoners of fate, but prisoners of their own minds." While God has given each of us more potential than we may ever manifest, you have the free will to choose whether or not you are going to develop your talents into marketable and applicable skills for your life and family. How much better will your life be if you accept everything with joy—the ups, the downs, the unexpected wonderful surprises as well as the unanticipated tragedies—knowing that it's all working together for you and us? How would your actions toward yourself and others change if you recognized we are all connected and what you do affects every other person on this planet?

"Never chase what you're after; become the type of person that naturally would attract the conditions you're seeking."

The people I've worked with who are the wealthiest, happiest and most fulfilled understand these laws. They don't wish it wasn't the way it is or spend their lives trying to change the laws any more than someone would try to change the gravitational pull of our planet. When the Wright brothers attempted to create an airplane, their objective wasn't to change gravity, it was to build something that worked with the law of gravity to their advantage. Learn how life is, why people do what they do, how things work, and ask what you need to do and learn from that to make your dreams come true.

CHAPTER NINE

Specializing in Your Own Transformation

The D'Angelo Scary-Easy Plan to Achieve **Any Goal**

1 Define Your Dream

2 Convince Yourself It's Possible

3 Concentrate Your Power

4 Ritualize Your Routine

5 Partner With The Ultimate Venture Capitalist

My claim to fame was as "The Weight-Loss Coach" because helping people take charge of the ultimate driver of their success, their health, was my unrelenting focus. People would come to my office wanting to lose anything from an extra 10 pounds to well over 300 pounds. Many of the people who sought me out had almost completely given up and thought they'd tried everything. But the truth is, I'm not really a weight-loss coach. I never have been. I'm a transformation coach.

"But isn't it a transformation when people lose weight, Charles?" you ask. Well yes it can be. And it might not be. It really depends on how you look at it.

Changing your outward appearance is not a transformation in my opinion. If I put on a mask or a Halloween costume, am I transformed? No of course not. What if I get a new hairstyle and outfit? I may look better, but have I been transformed? Nope. To be transformed, a person or thing has to change from

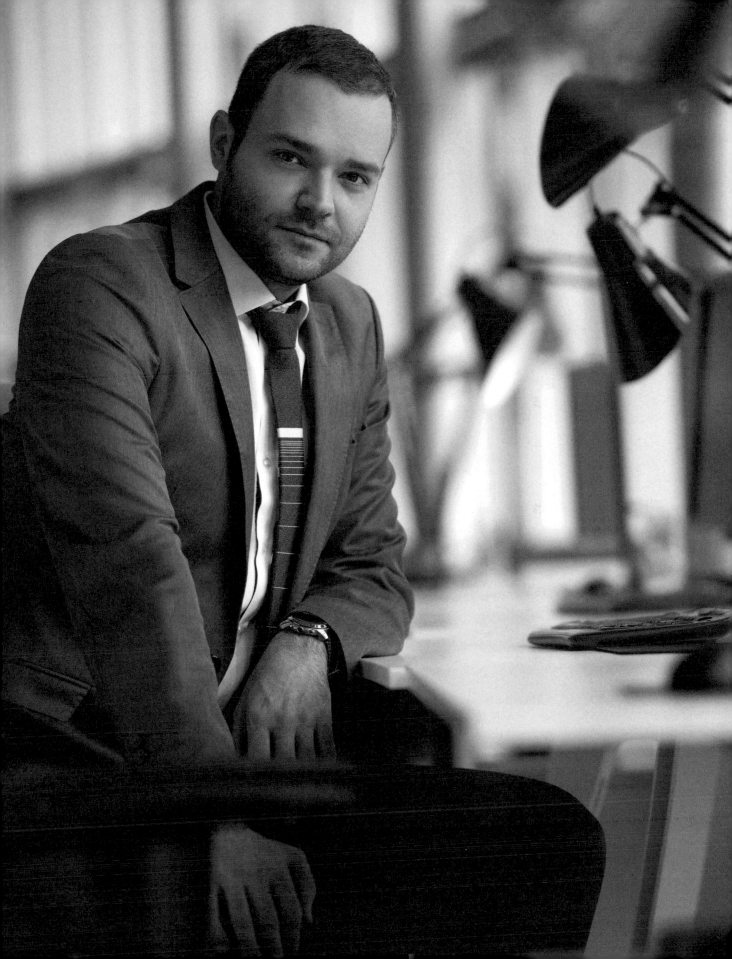

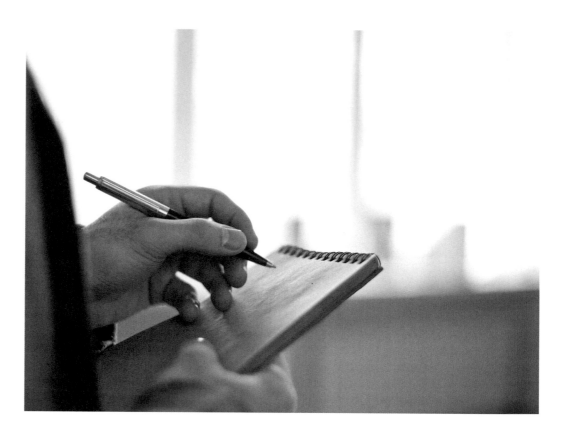

the inside, not just the outside. Until you've shifted your personal identity—who it is you believe you are—nothing changes. How many people do we know who've lost weight only to gain it all back, and more?

This has probably happened to you with one goal or another. You get so upset with yourself, you feel so much pain from your current situation, that you decide to make a change. You're excited. You're motivated. You are finally going to do what needs to be done in order to achieve your goal. And you do! You start your diet. You throw all the junk food out that you won't be eating. You buy all the healthy food you need, you buy a blender for your protein shakes, and make a dream board with pictures of people you want to look like and you are excited! You lose the first couple of pounds so easily that you feel this time it might be for real, it just may be effortless!

But this doesn't last. After a few days you find life's challenges are making it a little more difficult to stay resolved, and the struggle begins. By the next week you've slipped up a few times. By two weeks in, your life-changing diet is forgotten, and a couple of months down the road you weigh more than you did to begin with. This pattern is extremely common. People lose their motivation and their focus and don't stick with the plan until they reach their goal, because they didn't work on the unconscious beliefs and mental drivers behind their daily actions.

The reality is that you can also actually stick with the plan, achieve your goal and still not be permanently transformed! For example, some people manage to stick to their diet until they reach their goal weight. That number is magic to them. They inch closer and closer and then, finally, after all that hard work, they reach it. They celebrate! They're so happy! And at the same time, so confused. Scared, even.

That number was the goal and they've made it. So after the celebration they start sliding back into their old habits. Before long, they gain their weight back and then some.

Although they have managed to change their outer appearance they did not truly transform themselves, because they are still the same on the inside. They still deal with life and its inevitable challenges the same way. They still see their true selves as being the person they used to be, so they feel like an imposter. I am often asked how many of my clients keep the weight off. The truth is I can never give an accurate answer, at least not until all my clients are dead! Transformation is a lifelong endeavor. If you start out with the idea that there is a finish line, you are finished before you even start.

Let's unpack the steps of a transformation so you can get to work on creating lasting change in your life.

1 Define Your Dream

There is an effective and simple way to break the disempowering pattern I mentioned above. First of all, you've got to be extraordinarily clear what it is you want, and why you want these things. What are your goals? What is your purpose? We've been through this in depth already. From there, you have to concentrate all you've got on getting what you want. You must shift your focus from what others are doing and thinking to what you will think and do to make your dream happen. Every fiber of your soul has to be invested. Some people suggest this is unhealthy. I totally disagree. Anything I've achieved, whether physical, mental, emotional or spiritual, has been a result of unrelenting mental focus. I eat, dream, sleep and talk about it to anyone and everyone I can—anyone who is willing to listen and be supportive, of course. Don't share your dream with unsafe people. Dreams,

like infants, must be protected and nurtured until they can stand on their own feet! Don't let anyone or anything attack your dream. If God put it in you, it's for you to accomplish, but don't get your ego involved by trying to excite others who are more interested in feeling significant by demeaning your ambition. Sometimes when a person isn't achieving success, their only way of feeling significant and worthy is by tearing down others' dreams.

If you think back, I'm sure you can remember times when you felt like everything else had become almost irrelevant because you were

"If a goal or dream is in your mind's eye, know beyond everything else that it's available for you to get it. You've already proven this in other areas of your life."

so focused on something you wanted, or more specifically, something you felt you absolutely needed. You can train yourself in this process, making your goals become part of that category— a must instead of a want. Back it with huge reasons, how achieving this goal will truly impact your life.

But maybe your goal isn't just something you desire in life. Maybe you've been diagnosed with a serious illness. No need to accept the diagnosis. God has the final word and can flip the situation around any moment. Norman Cousins was said to have healed himself of a crippling disease via self-induced laughter by watching comedy every day. No one, I don't care what degree or experience they have, has the final say on your life outcome. If your dream is to be free of illness, the principles to aid in manifesting it are the same.

To discover more on this, look into the work by Dr. Deepak Chopra. He talks at length about a new emerging scientific field called "epigenetics." In short, science shows that there is intelligence above the genetic code that environmental and lifestyle factors play a big part in. Long story short, how you think, sleep, meditate, eat and move have a far more significant impact on the expression of your genetic predisposition than the story your DNA can tell. Even if you have bad genes, they don't need to express themselves if you have other things in check!

② Convince Yourself it's Possible

I'm sure you have things in your life now that at one time felt like an impossibility. At one time, maybe getting yourself a computer or your own car was just a dream. Then one

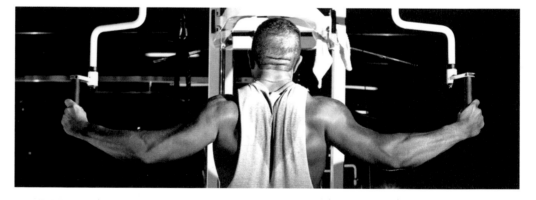

day, you had them both. Obviously, you know that what seems impossible can one day be achieved. After you've decided what you will transform in your life, you must train your mind to believe in it as completely as a child would, persistently taking action. Have complete confidence that what you want and who you want to become, while it might seem contrary to your life at the moment, is meant

for you. The reason is God has equipped you with a natural mechanism in your own mind to achieve all that you can conceive. If a goal or dream is in your mind's eye, know beyond everything else that it's available for you to get it. You've already proven this in other areas of your life.

Most people weaken that innate mental power by starting several projects serially or simultaneously rather than starting one thing and staying with it until it totally matches the picture they have of it in their mind. If a roadblock comes up, as they do in every journey, rather than interpret the stumble as a small and trivial meaningless blip on the road to their dream, they over-interpret and shift their focus to something else or another project. What you really need to do when this happens to you is ramp up the effort in order to break through. See this challenge as a test of your will and commitment. If you want more than others have, you must be willing to do what they will not. This means staying with it even when it doesn't seem that things are happening. When you make a decision to go for something in your life full-out, it means you must cut off all other options until the vision you have for that is fulfilled. Don't give yourself the option to fail.

Much of my personal power comes from my choice to fully immerse myself in whatever I have sitting in front of me. I'm totally present when tackling any challenge or goal, and you also can train yourself to be. That means you must eliminate all distractions. I had a picture in my mind of having a washboard stomach, and I would not stop until the mirror reflected the picture in my mind. People told me I looked "good enough," but the issue wasn't vanity. It was accomplishing what I had long before decided I would accomplish. Don't allow your family members, friends, your spouse, TV, radio, Facebook, Twitter or any of the many other things that clutter up our day bombarding all of us to distract you from being totally relentless in the pursuit of what you want.

As inventor and visionary Alexander Graham Bell said, "The sun's rays do not burn until brought to a focus." Channel all you've got in becoming all you can be. If anyone or anything in your life conflicts with your conviction that what you are dreaming is possible, they have no place in your life at this moment. As Psalms 1:1 says: "Blessed is the man that walketh not in the counsel of the ungodly, nor standeth in the way of sinners, nor sitteth in the seat of the scornful." Put more simply, God's will can't be stopped even if you don't believe in what God has placed in your heart and in your head, but that disbelief can raise doubt, making the road rocky at best. You've got to replace fear with faith, if not in yourself, then in God, and better yet, in both. Learn to hear and see everything in your life in connection to the attainment of your goal. If you start to ask how you can use the things most would see as challenges, you will make progress.

To manifest what you want most you have to be congruent. There needs to be total harmony between the heart and head, otherwise your consciousness will refuse the dream you have and you'll just get more of what you've always got. Whether you help yourself stay congruent by reciting an incantation emotionally such as

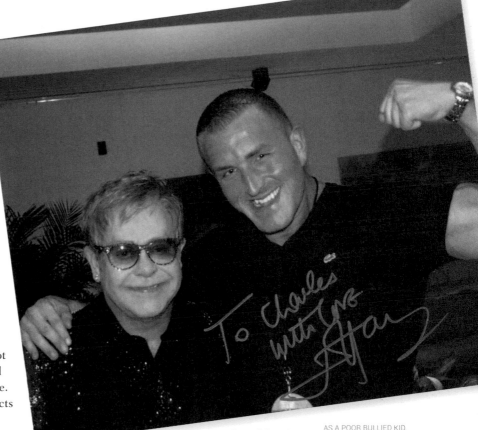

"Healthy, Wealthy, and Successful" or by putting up images that inspire you throughout your house, surround yourself with an environment that nurtures your vision. Visualization is a powerful tool in achievement. See what you want as clearly as if it's already here.

In my office, I have pictures of some of my life's most magical moments professionally framed and hung. Most of the images are the perfect match of the vision I once had only in my head, and now have become realities. I wanted to thank Elton John: done. Share my story with Paul McCartney: did it. Positive energy emanates from those photographs, so much that you can't help but feel good sitting in my office. You can do the same for yourself, creating a sacred place of success in your own home or office to reflect what you've already accomplished that once had seemed impossible.

AS A POOR BULLIED KID, I TAUGHT MYSELF PIANO BY LITERALLY WATCHING HUNDREDS OF HOURS OF ELTON JOHN PLAYING ON VHS, ONLY DREAMING OF MEETING HIM, THE MAN WHO EPITOMIZED CONFIDENCE, CREATIVITY, AND LOVE. GOD BLESSED ME WITH THE CHANCE TO DO SO AND SHARE MY STORY!

Whatever your goal, you need to know that if anyone can succeed, that means it's possible, and with your new congruent way of thinking, you will be that person. Perhaps you just found out you are dealing with a serious life-threatening illness, and you are reading the scary statistics. If 1% recover from the illness you have, then focus on being in that 1%, not on the negative statistics that feed your fear. If the 1% got better, so can you! The enemy to healing is fear. There is only love and fear. What isn't love, is fear. When you are in a fearful state, it robs your system of its power to recover. Fear's antidote is education, problem solving, and a strong connection to others. The more you know about something the less afraid you will be. Find people who've had a full recovery and learn all you can about and from them. This will empower you, and will work wonders in your life.

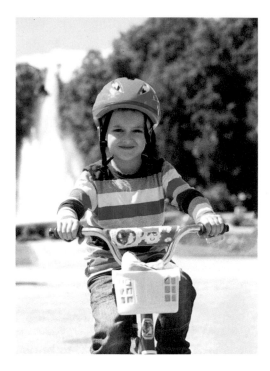

3 Concentrate Your Power

As soon as you make the decision that you want to achieve something and have cut off any other option, eliminating anything in your life that's in conflict with achieving it, the next step is gradually developing the confidence and certainty that you will really get it. Begin the journey that second, that very second.

I recommend that you create a list of things you've done that once seemed they would be only a dream. Go way back. Remember when you were a kid and those young adults were graduating from high school and you felt like you'd never get there? This is an incredible tool to help stir up your self-esteem. Read,

"Just like learning to ride a bicycle, you can have the best teachers in the world tell you how to do it, but you and you alone can achieve your dream."

listen, talk to others and watch inspirational programs until you start to see you are making progress in the direction of what you've decided. Just like learning to ride a bicycle, you can have the best teachers in the world tell you how to do it, but you and you alone can achieve your dream. Just staying upright on two wheels is not enough, however. You've got to get the feel for the bike until you are able to balance well and move forward independently. No one can do it for you no matter how much they love you and want to see you succeed.

If after your first fall on the bike you gave up, thinking you were a failure, you'd never have ended up joining your friends on the trails. If you have children and have tried to potty train them and they have accidents, would you say: "Oh I guess this one is just going to wear diapers all of her life?" Never! The thought is ridiculous.

When my grandma started having mini strokes in her 80s, she was placed in a home despite her desire for independence. Her room was in a wing with dementia patients, even though she appeared lucid with me. They seemed to feel she was no longer capable of caring for herself. She grew despondent and told me she was ready to give up on life. She was losing the very thing she had changed my life with: hope. Since she had been totally independent for decades, the thought of losing her freedom to come and go as she pleased and the ability to make her own decisions was mortifying to her. She'd rather be sick at home alone than have someone else in complete control of her life decisions, she said.

I prayed and fought with everything I had to allow her to keep the right to make her own decisions. Since the strokes had left her bedridden, the first task was to teach her how to walk again. I would visit, keeping her mind focused on the future and setting new goals, and not on the present. I would bring her favorite foods and take her to the patio

tion. She'd grown lazy, so it took quite a bit of persuasion on my part to do it. I would wheel her up to a hand rail out in the July heat, help her pull herself out of the chair, and then quickly wheel the chair down the rail about 10 feet. I told her that all she would have to do for the day was walk those 10 feet, but once I saw it was almost effortless for her to go that distance, I would wheel it further. She'd throw a fit but I think she knew at some level that

> *"I'm proud to say she fully recovered her ability to walk. The home moved her out of the dementia ward to a normal floor on their own volition after seeing her progress."*

I was doing it out of love. She would make it, wet with sweat, and collapse in the chair. She would swear never to let me do it to her again, only to be back at it the next day.

I'm proud to say she fully recovered her ability to walk. The home moved her out of the dementia ward to a normal floor after seeing her progress. Eventually a neuropsychologist was called in to see if she was capable of making her own decisions and looking after her

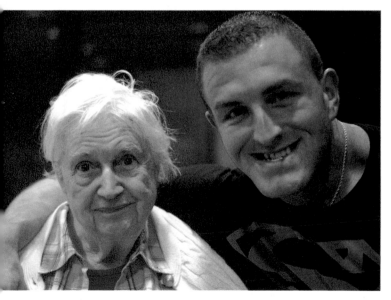

into the sun and cool breeze. Naysayers said she wouldn't make it six months, but I was determined to prove them wrong! That's the thing about achievers: when we are given a challenge, we work that much harder! Soon, I was going up to visit her every day and began the task of getting her out of the wheelchair despite the staff's pessimism at her condi-

daily self care. For her two-hour interview process, she was dressed to the nines in the finest clothes and jewelry that we'd picked out together at an expensive department store the day before. (She had always said clothes make the man, meaning the care you take in how you dress impacts how you feel about yourself.) We went to have her hair and nails done, to really help her self-confidence while being evaluated—a process anyone would find miserable. The morning came. I got up extra early to go help her get dressed and to take her out to breakfast at her favorite restaurant, McDonald's, of all places for me to be seen, to get her in the right frame of mind.

She passed the test with flying colors and was declared competent and able to make her own decisions. I am a firm believer that we each should always have the dignity of choice. She then decided to move out of the nursing home she had never wanted to be in in the first place. Selflessly, she worried about leaving wealth behind for those she cared about. I reassured her, reminding her it was hers in the first place and it best use was toward the highest quality life experience she'd enjoy! She moved to a faith-based assisted-living home in a much nicer part of town, where she would be able to go to mass each day—a routine that was very important to her. She got her own room that was nicer than most apartments! She lived out her years there, coming and going as she pleased. We would go out to dinner and the movies several nights a week. No

> *"I was able to complete the circle by giving her faith in something she didn't think possible, much like she did more than a decade earlier when I was an obese and underprivileged kid."*

longer did she feel like a prisoner. Sometimes we wouldn't get back until midnight, and she was 85! This all stemmed from my belief that she could get better. And guess what? She did! I was able to complete the circle by giving her faith in something she didn't think possible, much like she had done more than a decade earlier when I was an obese and underprivileged kid. God always gives us an opportunity to pay forward the good others do for us.

Those of us who succeed at what we want don't ever give up. Unfortunately, sometimes we are more patient with others than we are with ourselves. To be successful, you must learn to understand all goals have a gestation period, and then use everything at your disposal, including the opinions of others and what you may consider your negative experiences, to spur yourself ever onward, going that much harder in the direction of what may have once seemed impossible. Look at every adversity, every naysayer, every challenge as a practice run for the life you will be living at the top!

Following the rules of success leads to it. Adopting the notion that you are a perpetual beginner can help greatly. I don't know of any happy or successful people who believe they know it all. Over-preparation is rarely a bad thing. Over-prepare yourself for what you want by learning all you can from sources who obviously have what you want. The greatest teacher is experience, and it often comes at a high price. Speaking to people who have made the mistakes can help you know what to avoid.

Learn the game of life. People often have a backwards view of rules. Rules aren't meant to confine, but to liberate! You can learn in an

> *"Learn the game of life. People often have a backwards view of rules. Rules aren't meant to confine, but to liberate!"*

hour what might have taken another person 10 years to learn. This is how each generation learns some things faster than the generation before, and we progress. The Bible gives us a wonderful way to understand success when we look to what God designed. Look at nature. Think about planting. To grow a beautiful garden you have to know about seeds, soil, which nutrients the flowers need and how long it takes for them to bloom. You have to be patient. You have to have faith in the entire process. You have to be willing to work. You can buy the best seeds, plant them in fertile land, fertilize them, bury them at the proper depth, water the seeds and weed the garden each day, but if you plant in the winter, you'll be met with failure. In other words, you have to understand how things work before trying to make them happen.

You also might plant seeds in the right season, do all the right things and still find they don't take. If that's the case, search out another spot and start anew. Be persistent. Keep watering. While sometimes things don't work out despite your best efforts, most often they will, especially if you keep planting relentlessly. Don't spend time on what doesn't grow, wasting time wondering why or doubting yourself. Move on, plant more seeds in new areas and give your attention to the ones that do take root and blossom.

"Information isn't wisdom. Seek advice from trusted and reputable sources."

Whatever you are undertaking, do your homework so you're as well informed as you can possibly be. Books give you all the information you need, but now you have technology, giving us access to boundless libraries, and access to others' experiences and opinions. When I say to take action when you get excited about a goal, that may mean buying a book to begin

the educational process, not necessarily getting a seed and digging a hole before you've learned the right time to do so, to use my metaphor. Get ready, then aim, and finally fire.

Lastly, never assume you know everything. Make the process of learning enjoyable by inviting a diverse but integrity-filled stream of wisdom into your life. Information isn't wisdom. Seek advice from trusted and reputable sources. When you close your mind totally, you limit your future. Be flexible enough to recognize there is always opportunity to get even better and more skillful at what you are doing. If you act like a know-it-all to stroke your own ego, you're sealing off any opportunity that you'll ever achieve or have more than you do now. Your ego is preventing your success, by keeping you from finding out information you will need to get past a hurdle. Don't let a negative surprise rob you of what you deserve because you didn't take the time you should have to really think through what you're going for. When our ego gets involved, we become full of ourselves, over-inflating our own worth. This is when something we call "hubris" sets in—extreme or foolish pride—and catastrophe is not far behind. "Pride goeth before destruction, and a haughty spirit before a fall."

Your Choice: Excuses or Success

Anyone who has been through a transformation knows that you have to come to terms with your true place, without excuses, in order to take the steps necessary to get to the place you want to be. But there's another more profound reason to achieve this state. You need to get to the point where you will not accept anything less than the best for and from yourself.

When you reach this state, you come to find you won't settle for less from others, either. Your change in standard begins to raise theirs, and those who aren't ready for that kind of traumatic upward growth won't stay in your circle because it makes them uncomfortable. Some people may decide it's easier to stay in a bad group than have to step into new territory and try to improve.

I'm very particular about the people I work with. I won't work with those I feel are not ready to hear the truth I offer. The people I do choose to work with know that the only way to get to where they were born to be is confront the parts of themselves that aren't where they want them to be yet. They need to understand that we all can improve—myself included—and they understand that a good coach will help them see the reality and work from there to become better. People who aren't ready for change may hear my empowering messages as disempowering. Because they are not prepared to accept their own role in their circumstances, they get angry and defensive when I point it out. You may have had a terrible thing happen in your life that in your mind is the reason for your troubles, but my job is to convince you that it isn't. It may be an instigating factor in the decisions you've made, but it is not the reason.

Often people say they are coming to me for help but really they are seeking validation of their excuses. People who come to me looking for a shoulder to cry on, a hand to hold and the allowance of self pity to be perpetuated usually leave my office angry with me and externalize their responsibility by misconstruing my words.

Especially having been bullied myself, the last thing I would do is say something with the intent to hurt another. However, I learned a long time ago that regardless of our positive intentions, people hear what they want to hear; they hear what resonates with their own self-concept.

That's why it's important to open yourself up. Accept that we all have made decisions that are not in our best interest. When you learn to exchange pity for self-reliance and responsibility, your life immediately improves.

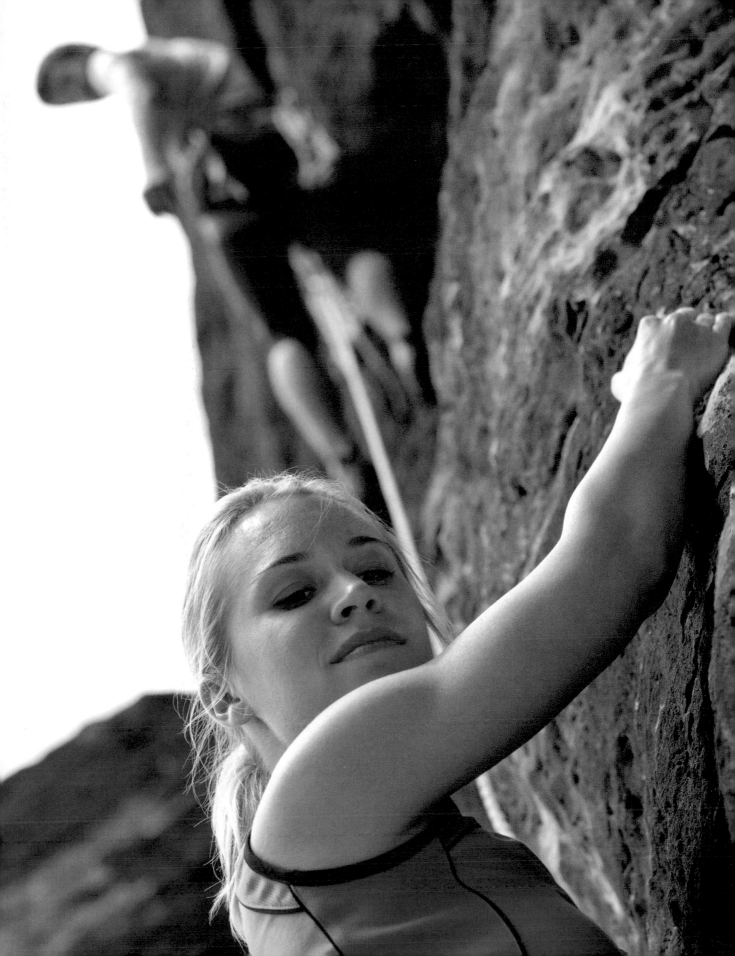

4 Ritualize Your Routine

Once you have thoroughly educated yourself and have a clear plan, take action. But keep in mind, while education is important and preparation is necessary, over-caution might rob you of your future. Caution can be another excuse, preventing you from fulfilling your goal. Simplify your plan and then ritualize it. Make it a routine. Make the action plan so easy a third-grader could follow along with you. Sometimes we make things seem far more challenging and complicated than they really are as a way to make ourselves feel better about our inaction or inconsistency. Replace the arrogance of complexity with automation and simplicity.

Success is simple, and results from making good choices consistently. Make your positive daily habits as basic as hygiene. The more mental space you make available by not having to think about trivial things like what you will wear each day, what time you're going to wake up and how you're going to fit in your healthy food and exercise to stay at your peak physically, the more energy and creativity you will have to help with your success. Have a daily ritual of your activities such as eating and exercise planned out before you get up each day. Set a consistent time to wake up and go to sleep. Schedule your meal times to be routine each day. If your goal is weight loss, set up a healthy and sound food plan and prepare your food for every meal of the week at the same time. This both makes your life easier and fortifies you against any issue that could compromise your efforts. It also helps to literally reprogram your brain, laying down new neurological pathways, so doing what's right becomes second nature. Use my Scary Easy guide in my book *Think*

"Arrange to do your exercise first thing, so it isn't lost in the inevitable unexpected demands later in the day."

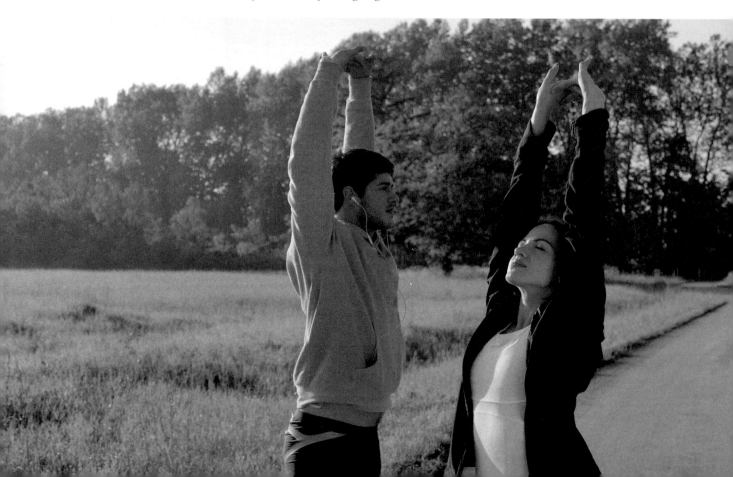

and Grow Thin and eat the same things each day for a while to disconnect the emotional attachment you have to food. Arrange to do your exercise first thing, so it isn't lost in the inevitable unexpected demands later in the day. In the same vein, if your goal is financial independence, set up a system that forces savings. There are apps for your phone that can aid in all of these processes, just like a good coach can in person.

True greatness leaves no room for excuses. Self-reliance and self-discipline are the keys to any achiever's philosophy, and they're the primary drivers of self-esteem and confidence. If you want to enjoy the pride in creating a legendary life, you must unlearn the habit of creating stories to excuse why you aren't there yet, and develop the patience in the process of getting yourself there. Be so focused on getting what and where you want you don't have the time to be aware of anyone else's opinion or awareness of your efforts. The less you feel you need the praise of others, the more you'll discover you get it!

Lots of people talk a good game and may even begin the process of learning, but then they let a story creep in that masks an underlying fear, and this stops them from taking action. Thinking, while important, isn't enough. Take action, choose the right course, and accept this reality: if it's going to be, it's up to me. Prepare for the inevitable hurdles while expecting the absolute best to occur in your life.

You are a growing person right up until the instant you pass on to whatever comes after this lifetime. That means you'll never be "perfect" and you'll never have achieved "enough." That's life's design. Don't make perfect the enemy of the good. Understanding greatness is a process centered around the acceptance of being perpetually incomplete. The more challenges you're having now, the more indication your life is really rocking and shaping you into someone great. When you're comfortable, you can be sure you are not in a growth cycle. It

might sound paradoxical, but a dynamic life means an ever-changing one. You will continually be upgrading both your hardware (your body and way of life) and your software (your emotions and thinking) throughout your life.

"The more challenges you're having now, the more indication your life is really rocking and shaping you into someone great."

Accept and embrace that process happily, and you will gain much from it. The greater you become, the more you realize just how little you know, and you will find yourself in complete awe of how blessed your life is despite it.

Once you have formulated your action plan, make it so simple anyone could clone your outcome. Reduce it down to a simple com-

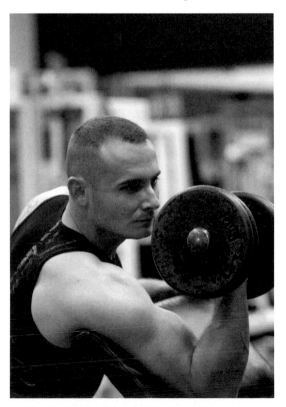

mon-sense set of actions and disciplines. Your head will try to stop you from doing this by telling you all sorts of stories. It will be very convincing! Your head might use math, statistics and science to justify continued paralysis and inaction in your life. Don't listen to it. You know the truth: if 1% make it, you will be in that 1%. Simplify the approach you're choosing by making it a routine like I've described, and commit fully to it, measuring your progress regularly so you can modify your actions should you need to. Don't look to others to validate what works for you. It was Einstein who said that if he couldn't simplify something, he didn't understand it well enough!

⑤ Partner With the Ultimate Venture Capitalist

"Decide your life will be created organically by your own vision and choices, not by comparing and contrasting yourself to "norms" of society or those in your circle."

Lastly, trust God, your Creator, to do what you can't. Get rid of internal conflict by stepping out in faith, knowing that your vision is divine. As we discussed above, your mind will try to convince you that what you want is not possible. So too will forces I believe are dark spiritually (some call it/them the devil), and even those you love. Note: they do this not because they're trying to hurt you but because they listen to their own dark voices of fear, scarcity and self doubt so they honestly think they are speaking truth.

If you're thinking like everyone else, then you really aren't thinking. Mark Twain said it well when he said, "Whenever you find yourself on the side of the majority, it's time to pause and reflect." The thinkers are the people who change our world. Become one. Accept that by being different you won't feel normal. Don't judge yourself or your potential by looking at what's "average." Remember, the extremes inform the mean (average). There is a funny parable Charles Wheehan uses, which I'll paraphrase to make the point, "Bill Gates walks into a bar. Suddenly, everyone is a millionaire." This is to illustrate that statistics can obscure quite a bit of important information, especially in extreme cases.

Decide your life will be created organically by your own vision and choices, not by comparing and contrasting yourself to "norms" of society or those in your circle. Replace all doubt with expectation that what you want wants you, and it's only a matter of time before it's yours. When you accept an assignment from God in co-creating for the betterment of all, you have unlimited resources at your disposal. Do you remember what Jesus said is possible with God? Did he say some things are possible?! NO! ALL things are possible. Your creator put you here for a purpose, and He wants you to fulfill your divine assignment that won't only make your life better, but it will make everyone else's better as well. Become enthusiastic and even obsessed with this process.

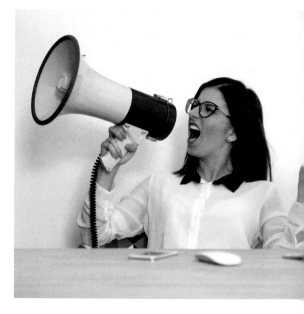

Many call me crazy when I'm really excited about some new project or endeavor. You must understand that when successful people get an idea, it dominates their existence. In order for you to have the type of life you've decided to embark on, you too must get engrossed and completely obsessed by your dream. Light fires of desire inside your heart so deep and so blazing hot that they get you out of bed early and keep you up long after your family has fallen asleep. Let it radiate so much positive energy it excites all those around you. When you align what you want with who you are and what you value, mountains will move at your will. The power you have will be inspiring to others, exciting them to similar action. Personal alignment allows for that type of transformation.

What you get is one thing, who you have to be to get it is that much more important. The investment you will be making in going for what you want ensures that you will increase your physical, mental, spiritual, and emotional equities—meaning you will reap far more than ever before, considering all you've sown into yourself. You'll never regret investing in your own personal education, whether you've gained it through formal or informal means. It is something no one can ever take from you, ever. As with everything, you've got to go through a little trial and error to uncover what will work with you personally. There isn't a cookie-cutter plan. We all have to take what works for each of us and discard the rest, respecting that what we discard may be what another feels saved their life! Respect differences.

When I say to get obsessed I do mean that, but you must ensure that you don't burn out. I suggest you find a happy balance between acting on your dream and resting. I recently encountered a young man in the gym who had lost over 100 pounds in only a few months. It was obvious to me that despite his success, fear of relapsing was now driving him. I could see the joy that had activated his transformation had long gone. Now he was fiercely and

"You'll never regret investing in your own personal education, whether you've gained it through formal or informal means."

intensely going through the motions, screaming at himself alone with the weights when
he couldn't get the number of pull-ups he'd
hoped he would in a set. I pulled him aside
and shared my story, wanting to see how
open he was to my suggestion. I offered him
the idea of being more patient and accepting
himself and his process. I could see his great
potential. but I could also see potential for
destruction. I suggested he slow down and be
a bit less aggressive in his efforts. I also said
I could tell that a lot of anger and fear was
behind his drive, saying that much like jet fuel,
it's effective in the moment but short lived.

I saw him again not three weeks later. It was
obvious he hadn't taken my advice. He was
limping around the gym, doing all he could
to get through a workout having torn a liga-
ment in his leg. Bruce Lee put it well when
he recommended we be like water, yielding to
life and not breaking: "You must be shapeless,
formless, like water. When you pour water in a
cup, it becomes the cup. When you pour water
in a bottle, it becomes the bottle. When you
pour water in a teapot, it becomes the teapot.
Water can drip and it can crash. Become like
water my friend." Sometimes it's best to listen
to your body, heart and mind, and go with
the flow.

In the Eastern spiritual tradition, there is
an ancient text called the Tao Te Ching. It
has been the source of spiritual guidance for
people in the Chinese culture for thousands of
years. It talks about understanding duality in
life, the idea that you can't have good without
bad, light without dark, joy without sadness—
that one seems to necessitate the other. In that
line of thinking, it teaches that as much as
we need to take action, we also need to rest,
knowing that all is working together for our
good. They call it "Wu Wei." This teaches that
often the smallest effort can bring about the
most amazing outcome. It's those times when
you find things just fall into place with little
or no obvious work on your part. It's when you
are in alignment with God and His will, in my

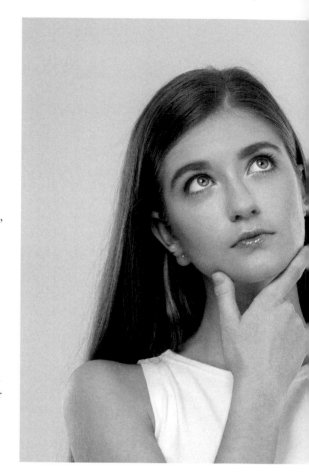

opinion. It's life balance. It's living on purpose.
Being yourself. It's grace. In Chapter 38 of the
book, it says:

A truly good man does nothing,
Yet nothing is left undone.
A foolish man is always doing,
Yet much remains to be done.

This step-by-step approach I'm briefly taking
you through here is the reason I'm a life consultant rather than a weight-loss coach, and
that's why my clients are so successful. While
the process in person is more immersive and

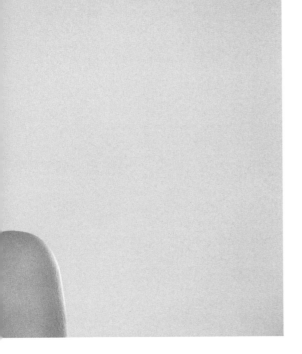

"When your thought processes change, how you feel changes in turn."

cess is contagious. The path to success in one area looks the same as the path to success in any other area, and once you get in the habit of following that path, it gets much easier to recognize and trust in it leading you to where you want to go.

Health and weight-loss goals are great examples for me to use. This is the main reason people come to me, but it's also something almost everyone can relate to, because almost everyone has experienced wanting to get healthier or lose weight at some time or another. During any given year, from 25 to 35 percent of Americans go on a diet to lose weight, and many more consider it. Right now, over 75% of the US population is overweight! Chances are you've wanted to lose weight

"The path to success in one area looks the same as the path to success in any other area, and once you get in the habit of following that path, it gets much easier to recognize and trust in it leading you to where you want to go."

directed when I work with someone one-on-one, the principles are the same as above. I don't just help them change on the outside; I help them change from the inside. It's not just their bodies that change; their thought processes and their emotions change, and it is the change in the thought process and emotions that results in the physical shifts. That is true transformation. When your thought processes change, how you feel changes in turn. Then what used to seem difficult to follow through with no longer does. This makes reaching your goal and staying there infinitely easier.

Once you master this, your life really does change. It's not difficult to see why so many of my clients who come to me for weight loss end up becoming successful in other areas of their life as well, just as it happened for me. Suc-

and if not, you've certainly seen it with others around you. I'll bet you've seen a friend or relative lose weight, look great, feel great, get all kinds of compliments, and the next thing you know they're back to their old size.

But weight loss is far from the only time we humans try to transform ourselves and fail. All kinds of people deal with addictions or with habits that act like addictions. There's a raging argument in the psychology and medical community about what constitutes an actual addiction. For our purposes, it really doesn't matter whether something is considered a clinical addiction or not. If you continue to do something despite knowing that it's detrimental to your life then it is enough of a habit to use the word "addiction" for our discussion. So you can see I'm not just talking about drugs, alcohol and cigarettes. We humans make many different void-filling choices and use many inefficient coping mechanisms like we spoke about earlier.

You've heard of retail therapy, no doubt. For some people, going shopping is an affordable and fun antidote to a rotten day but for others, shopping has a whole other meaning, and has become such an addiction that they're badly in debt, hiding their purchases from their partner because they know they'll get in trouble and may even lose their relationship. Half the time these shopping addicts don't even remember what they bought.

Gambling is another addiction that destroys people's lives. While the flashing lights, music, and lavish environment of a casino might seem appealing, watching someone pray they win big in order to buy their family dinner that night as they put their last five-dollar bill down on a bet is agonizing. I have seen people so addicted to gambling that they've lost everything they owned, lost successful businesses, had to move their families from beautiful luxurious houses to crappy little run-down apartments, developing lung cancer in the process from being around smokers for so long!

"Any of these behaviors and many more can cause you to be where you don't want to be, and if you continue with them, you will take up permanent residence there."

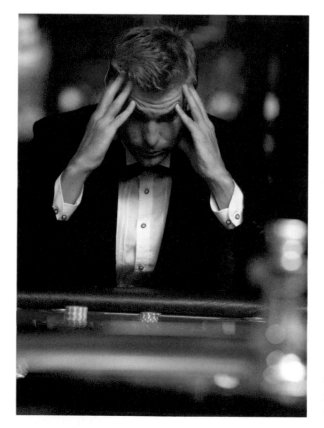

It's been said that the majority of people who play the lottery are underprivileged. The notion of putting in a little with a dream to get a lot says it all. I think it's a flawed philosophy, so I choose not to gamble at all. I think gambling says more about one's worldview than they may consider. People who fall victim to this habit usually have terrible credit, they're unable even to get a car, and what's their solution? Instead of rectifying the underlying issue, they find a way to borrow more money to gamble more, because they are convinced that one day they're going to win big and get everything back.

Casinos can be so luxurious because they almost always win! How do you think they can afford such extravagance? We blind ourselves to this instead of reasoning it out. The atmosphere seems extravagant and so convinces us we will win when in fact it's just the opposite. It's been said that casinos check their profit and loss statements several times an hour to be sure they are still raking it in, and you want to play that game?

Spending more than you earn, eating more than you need, letting porn or even general online surfing take the place of things you need to do in life to make it the way you once dreamed—these and many other habits I could name might not be addictions by the clinical sense of the word, but they definitely are detrimental to the person who is choosing to continue doing them.

Can you relate to any of these? Do you spend money you know you don't have, choosing to forget about the added debt and the fact that each month even more money will be going out to pay as interest to creditors? Do you say you just can't resist that new pair of shoes even though your spouse has made it clear he thinks it's a serious problem and will be very angry if you buy more? Do you work late, bring work home, work weekends and miss parts of your child's life because of work? Yes sure, periodically we must make sacrifices to succeed in the workplace or to graduate from school with a tough degree, for example, but occasional sacrifice is one thing and missing out on your life and your child's life is an entirely different story.

Any of these behaviors and many more can cause you to be where you don't want to be, and if you continue with them, you will take up permanent residence there. They cause financial problems and relationship problems and make it difficult to find joy. But it's not just what we do that can have this effect; what we don't do can also be detrimental. Neglecting to keep up on necessary maintenance and procrastinating can have the same effect. Not keeping up on your work can mean losing your job or not going as far in your career as you could. Not keeping up on schoolwork can mean failure, or not getting into the graduate program you would really like. Not keeping the house clean or the laundry and dishes done will create an unpleasant living environment that may include bugs and rodents—and eventually cost you money to eradicate. Not getting your bills paid on time will mean poor credit and extra payments, never getting your principal paid off. Not eating properly or getting enough exercise will cost you your health and lose you energy. If you don't take baby steps in dealing with these things one step at

a time, they will stack up, burying you in a situation you hate, making you feel powerless and helpless, and as if you're unable to change it—despite the fact that your choices brought you there in the first place!

"By not helping yourself to reach your own potential, you are indeed choosing to cause yourself harm."

These are very specific issues, but in life things are not always so cut and dry. How about something a bit more general, like not fulfilling your ambitions the way you could? Feeling purposeless? If you're choosing to live a life that is not as fulfilling or rewarding as it could be, if you're making choices each day that keep you in a place you are not happy with, even if you're not drinking or gambling, you are choosing activities each day that cause you harm. You are probably focusing on what's not right in your life yet instead of all the things that are. By not helping yourself to reach your own potential, you are indeed choosing to cause yourself harm.

What does this have to do with transformation? This: These intrinsic behavioral patterns are strong, whether or not they are true addictions. Changing your activities on the outside without changing the core of the thinking and feeling that's driving the behavior on the inside is not going to have a strong enough effect to create the lasting change you deserve. You think hiding credit cards is going to make you stop using them? Just about as much as hiding alcohol will make you quit drinking.

I remember when my mom became addicted to prescription drugs I risked my own future by taking her pills to school with me, thinking it would make her quit taking drugs. There is zero chance these things will work. Only a true transformation, one that changes the way a person sees and perceives themselves and the things in their lives—their past, present and future, can do that.

Have you ever bitten into an apple that looks beautiful but the inside is all brown and bruised or mealy and terrible tasting? That's us when we change the outside without transforming our outlook, perspective and perception, because we're focused on the wrong thing. Bishop Jakes uses a wonderful illustration when he talks about dating. He leaves the church to go out to the parking lot and shows a beautiful shiny new black Cadillac Escalade. At first glance, it certainly is attractive. He says many people choose their partners like choosing a new car, just by its appearance. He

accomplished something, but what then? How will you stay motivated enough to remain at your goal weight? You have a beautiful apple on the outside, but the inside is just the same.

I've always said success in weight loss is like a three-legged stool: You need diet, yes of course. You also need exercise. Those are two important legs of your success. But a two-legged stool is completely unstable! You may be able to balance on it for a short time, especially if you have something or someone to lean on, but move that support away and Bam! You fall.

The third leg and the one you absolutely cannot succeed without is your mindset. It's the glue that holds it all together. To truly be successful at achieving anything at all, you need to be in the right frame of mind. You need to train your mind like any other muscle: daily. You need to feed it and challenge it, and you also need to give it rest from time to time.

"To truly be successful at achieving anything at all, you need to be in the right frame of mind. You need to train your mind like any other muscle: daily."

goes on to open the rear hatch and a mountain of trash collapses out. He concludes his demonstration cautioning all of us to make sure that we're aware of the "junk in the trunk" before investing much of ourselves and our hearts into things that look good on the surface—very wise advice.

Don't get me wrong. I'm not saying thoughts are everything. The actions you take are necessary, but they're just part. If your goal is 150 pounds, you have that goal seared into your mind and then you reach it, you've really

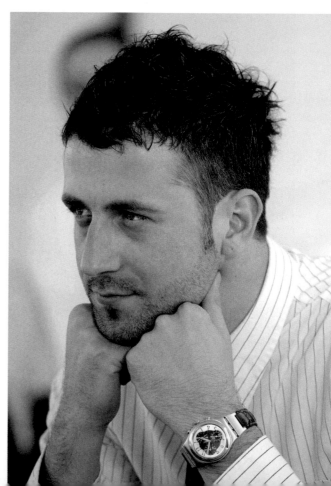

To truly transform, you need to change your mindset and condition the change through positively reinforcing it. Just as positivity is a greater indicator of success than intelligence, mindset is a greater indication of success than simply going through the motions.

Story after story exists about an underdog in sports or in the performing arts or in business being told they can't make it and ultimately outperforming everyone else. "Hard work beats genetics" is a term you often hear in the fitness world. Some people naturally develop an exceptional physique, building muscle easily and losing fat easily. Some of those same people have an especially aesthetically pleasing shape. But if you stack them up against the people who started further back but drive themselves day after day after day, it's the latter group who will come out ahead in competition, and often will look even better as they continue to age, unlike the former group who are taking it for granted. Sports fields are littered with the carcasses of people with a natural ability who did not work hard to make the most of it, long ago surpassed by the people with the drive and ambition to overcome their weaknesses.

This has certainly been the case with me. You couldn't find too many people in worse shape than I was as a 360-pound teen. You already know I had a hard time making it up the four steps to my classroom, but you may not know I had a hard time even doing nothing. Standing at a bank counter was mentally exhausting, as I felt all eyes were trained on me and how large I was. Physically, I would break out in a cold, clammy sweat for no apparent reason, even just sitting at my desk during a class. My life consisted of walking to my car and going through drive-thrus of fast-food establishments, before, during, and after school. There wasn't much further down I could go. Once I changed my mindset, however, I was unstoppable. Yes, I lost 160 pounds of pure fat, but I have also kept it off for well over a dozen years. Not only did I keep it off, I gained at least 25 pounds of muscle. I got an actual six-

"You make every single choice in your life and you create every outcome."

pack. And I became one of the fittest, healthiest people around on every level, from strength to cardiovascular fitness to the numbers I get at the doctor's office. Believe me, I'm not saying this for you to see how amazing I am. I'm saying this to tell you how far you can go!

Your mind is the strongest and most powerful muscle you have, if you train it properly. And it doesn't take a whole lot of work to train. This "muscle" is the true engine of your body and of your future, but it is also the conductor and the engineer. This muscle decides where you're going, figures out how to get there and powers the machinery that takes you there. Everything you are stems from your mind.

The first and most important step in training the mind is to see and accept that you are the one who calls all the shots. You've got to identify where you are to decide where you're going. You make every single choice in your life and you create every outcome. You may not like the choices you have to choose from at the start, but they are your choices, and they will ultimately bring you exactly where you choose to be. The quality of your choices will improve just as you do.

And don't think for a second this means you can just hand over the reins and all will be well. By not taking control, you become a pawn in another's person's chess game. Every single time you choose not to make the right decision, you are making the wrong decision. It's time for you to consider the choices continuously lain in front of you every second of every day, and take on the starring role in your life.

Once you do accept your starring role in your own life, you will see choices all around you every day. You always have Corn Flakes for breakfast? Why? Maybe today you should have eggs and slices of tomato instead. You always brush your teeth left to right? Why not brush them right to left? This might be a silly example but I use it to demonstrate your power. Every day has thousands of decisions that, once combined, add up to your life. At a deeper level, you'll start to notice meaning in life's occurrences where once you just labeled such events as "coincidence."

Now you have an opportunity to really take a look at where these daily decisions are bringing you. Whatever in your life you would like to change, you have been making choices every day that have brought you there. "No wait, Charles!" I hear you say. "But I didn't make these decisions. My husband did! It's his fault I'm here!" "My daughter has type 2 diabetes and is single with four kids. I didn't choose this!" No, no, no. Both your spouse and your daughter made their decisions and you made

yours. I'm not saying what you've experienced as a result of their choices wasn't painful or difficult for you. Nor am I saying that it had no effect at all on the choices you had on offer. I'm just saying neither they nor their choices are the reason you are where you are. Are your choices different than they otherwise would have been if they were not in your life? Sure. But your decisions were and are still yours, from being with them to staying with them to supporting them to whatever choices you made in response to the choices they made. There isn't a law that says you have to be involved—you have chosen to. Face that.

"If you want to see where you're going, look at where you've been."

You have the ability to leave a bad marriage. You have the ability to refuse to sign a loan you don't agree with. You have the ability to open your own bank account and take control when your spouse is not following the budget. You have the ability to eat what you want for dinner and not what you're expected to eat or what your family is eating. I can feel the resistance now, already hearing the arguments and excuses that are flooding your head. "But if I do that then they will get mad." That may be, and you may decide to follow their whims based on that, but you are still the one making that decision! And when you accept your position as the decision maker in your own life, then you will clearly see that your spouse will also end up making his/her own decisions, though they may be partly influenced by you. Because your spouse chooses to eat ice cream for dessert every day does not mean you have to do the same. While we cannot control others or life's circumstances, no one and nothing can ever take away your ability to choose how you feel or how you respond. Choose wisely.

So, where have these daily, weekly, monthly, yearly choices been taking you up to now? Where will they take you in future? Are you

"There's something you have to come to terms with about time. It passes, whether we like it or not."

where you thought you were going to be by this stage in your life? If you want to see where you're going, look at where you've been. Where were you one year ago? Two, five, 10 years ago? Were you healthy or not healthy? Were you lean or overweight? Were you in less debt or more debt? Were you thinking about a promotion you still haven't received? Were you thinking of taking a course or program that would have taken you in the career direction you want? Have you made progress or only gotten worse?

Have you gained 10 pounds each of the last three years? If so, by next year chances are you'll have another 10 added on, unless you change your daily choices.

Haven't had a promotion that you've been waiting for these past two years? You'll likely be complaining about this lack of recognition yet again over the next Christmas holidays unless you change your daily choices. Don't count on others to change for your life to improve.

I know a woman who wanted to go back to med school about 10 years ago and decided it would have been too financially difficult. Now she's still struggling financially in low-end jobs whereas if she'd bitten the bullet and gone back to school she'd be in far better financial shape now, and would have been for years. Was there validity to her choice? Sure! It would have been hard to spend a few years in school again.

But her choice to avoid that difficulty did not remove the difficulty—it extended it. The reality is, the time still passed. At the end of that time she would end up better off or worse off, and the choice she made ensured that she was worse off.

There's something you have to come to terms with about time. It passes, whether we like it or not. If you're like most people, you have

"What you can do now is start moving in the right direction."

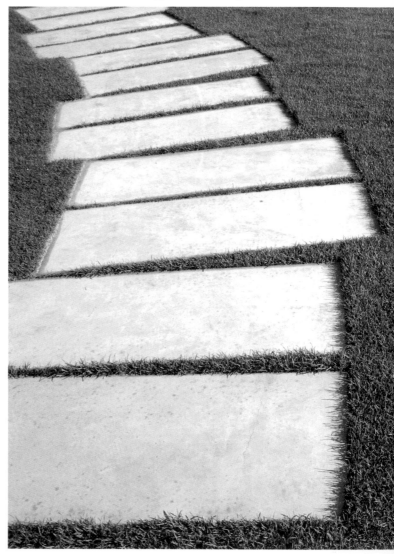

some arbitrary idea of where you want to be at some arbitrary later date, but you do not have a clear plan of how to get there and you are therefore not making the choices each day that will bring you there. There's no use in regretting or bemoaning the fact that you didn't start moving in the right direction last year, or two years ago or five years ago. You can't do anything about that aside from take a valuable lesson from it that you will use from now on. You can feel good with that. What you can do now is start moving in the right direction. The woman I know didn't make the right choice 10 years ago, but she can make it now. And then, a few years down the road, she'll be a doctor instead of working at a coffee shop, regardless of where she's been for the past 10 years.

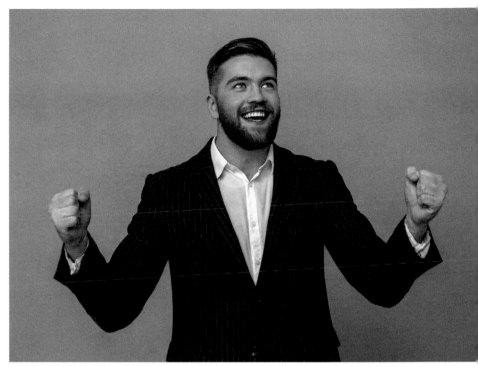

People are like this with weight loss all the time. Let's say last year at this time you felt you needed to lose 45 pounds and you were overwhelmed with the thought. It seemed like it would take such a long time. Now that time has passed. If you'd started then, those 45 pounds would be gone. Instead, you now have 50 pounds to lose. The next year will also pass, whether or not you are making the choices each day that bring you will bring you to your goals. So why not make those choices? Then one year from now you will not look back with regret and will instead look back with feelings of accomplishment!

Change your choices and you'll change your life. You may not have made the right choices in the past—heck, we all make bad choices!—but you can learn from them. If you don't start now, then one year from now you'll wish you had. Change your daily food plan and exercise habits. Call a meeting with your boss to find out what positions are available and what new skills you need to acquire to get the promotion. If you're not doing the things you need to get that promotion, then your boss might

"You don't have to settle because someone else won't change. You change and your life will change with you."

not even be aware you want it. If you've taken these steps and your employer is not open to paying you more despite your honest effort and willingness to bring more value to their company, perhaps it's time to start marketing your skills to other employers who can see your value. You don't have to settle because someone else won't change. You change and your life will change with you. Things you want to have happen in your life do not happen by themselves. You need to make them happen. Be proactive. The way to do that is to be conscientious, pay attention, and make the right choices to bring you there. Strengthen your weaknesses.

Do you watch the Olympics or professional sports? When you watch a professional or

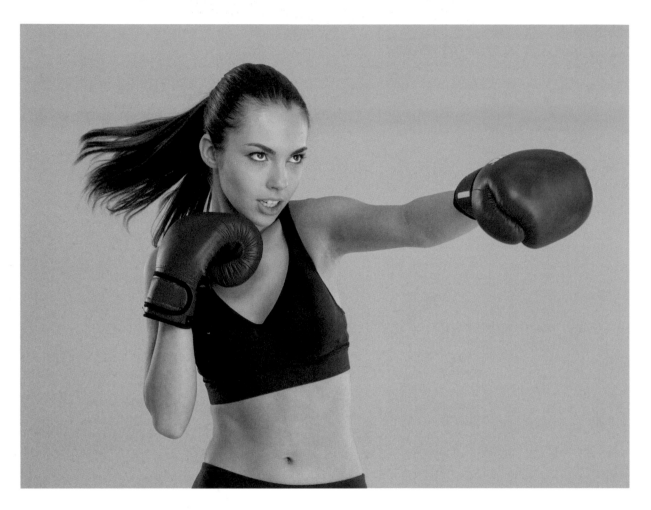

Olympic athlete, you are seeing how incredible their skills are. You are watching that gymnast doing flips in the air and landing on a tiny little place. You are watching a swimmer move at speeds unimaginable to you. You say how amazing they are, but you don't necessarily think about how each of these athletes began as a kid just like you did. What separates super-athletes from regular people is mostly not natural ability; it's a goal and a strong desire to reach that goal. The gymnast started as a kid just working on simple flips, working constantly on improving her weaknesses until she could perfect them, and then learning bigger, more complicated flips and working on her weaknesses until she could perfect *them*. Day after day after day, getting better and better and better, in tiny increments.

"Achievers make choices that will bring them right back on the path to success, instead of giving up."

Top athletes that you think are just naturally amazing are always trying to strengthen their weaknesses. They watch videos of themselves to see where they can improve. Wherever they see something that can improve, they practice all the time to improve it. Soccer players spend hours every day practicing their ball control. Tennis players spend hours every day hitting backhands. They may have natural ability, but the reason for their success is not their ability, it's their tenacity, and making the choice every day to improve.

Unless your goal is to be in the Olympics or compete at Wimbledon or in the World Cup, you don't have to spend hours every single day perfecting your technique or working on your weaknesses, but you do have to work toward your goals and keep them foremost in mind. Serena Williams did not choose to watch TV and eat bags of chips instead of practicing her backhand just because she didn't feel like practicing, and you will not reach your goal of getting the promotion you want unless you find what you need to work on, work on it and make it your strength.

Successful people make good choices every day, they look for ways to get around obstacles and they work to improve their weaknesses. But this does not mean they never make mistakes! Every single person makes mistakes and every person can improve. The big difference is they don't place blame or responsibility anywhere else but on themselves. If they did, they would feel like they were losing their own power to get better. So must you adopt this philosophy for improvement: Stop blaming your family, your trainer, your history—make today the start of an entirely new you!

Achievers make choices that will bring them right back on the path to success, instead of giving up. A great teacher once recommended we all take on the "ant philosophy." If you put your foot down in front of an ant, it doesn't stop and wait for you to move. It crawls over, under, around, whatever it takes to keep moving. Bees never question themselves. Theoretically, bees shouldn't be able to fly, but no one ever told them they can't, so they do! Their bodies are heavier than the weight their wings should support, but somehow they pull it off! Sometimes the only thing stopping you from doing the impossible is someone else's opinion!

Don't beat yourself up over the errors in judgment you've made early on, just educate yourself with them. Remember the different ways to look at experience? The woman who successfully quits smoking learns that she

can't hang around with all her friends drinking beer and smoking or she will have a cigarette. She does not look at her experience starting again after trying to quit as a sign that she is incapable of quitting. She doesn't ask why it seems so much easier for other people. She sees how things are for her and works with it.

The same goes for the man trying to lose weight, who finds after experience that he goes off his diet when he hasn't planned for being hungry at the morning meeting where there are often donuts. He learns that he must eat something healthy before the meeting, because having food in his belly and stable blood sugar will help give him the willpower to resist the temptation. The successful dieter is not one who has never eaten something that was not on the plan; the successful dieter is one who learns how to bounce back very quickly from these mistakes with little if any collateral damage and self doubt.

"Successful people make good choices every day, they look for ways to get around obstacles and they work to improve their weaknesses."

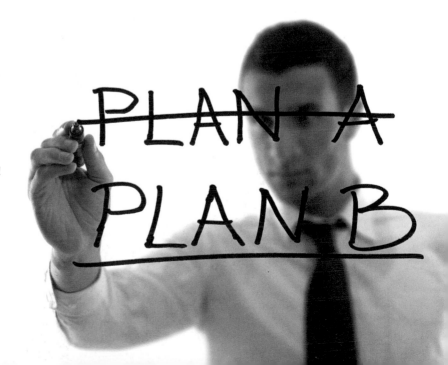

Finally, transformation requires consistent and committed action. People sit around dreaming about landing that great job or losing weight, but they often never fully go all out in getting the things they could. Lack of energy is a big part of this reality. You need energy to help you take the steps necessary to succeed. This energy comes from the way you think, from excitement about your goals, and also from what you're feeding yourself and what you're doing with your body physically. You will hear people recommend that you set "realistic" goals. I'm a little different in that way. I want you to set exciting goals that stretch you, but not break you! If you weigh 250 pounds and your optimal weight is 150 then you might come to me saying you will be happy to reach 180, but my response will be, go for 150! If reaching 180 is ok then reaching 150 is incredible! Get excited! If your goal is to get the promotion at work, then why not make it your goal to run the department? Stop limiting yourself. You are filled with greatness. Give yourself permission to be great! Live your real dreams, not the dreams some other person has told you it's ok to have so you fit in and don't rock the boat you've outgrown long ago!

When you are excited with your goal and you have the right mindset to make those daily choices that will bring you to your goal, you will find doing what is necessary is no longer difficult. Once I knew where I was meant to be and I made the decision to go there, then what had been so difficult to me before—resisting junk food—became easy. With a burning desire, clear vision, smart strategy, and measurable progress you will find yourself hooked! When you're passionate and excited, then that creates the energy that creates the motivation. Throw in the positive validation from a few people who really care about you and notice the change, bam, you're on fire! That is true transformation. Once you have the mindset that will lead you to transformation, you will probably find you do not have to think about these other steps, just like you no longer have to think about everything involved in riding a bike. You just do it, because all stems from that initial shift.

"You need energy to help you take the steps necessary to succeed."

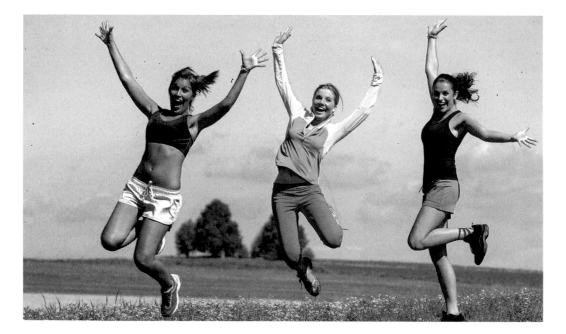

What You Can Be Sure Of...

• You have complete control over the rest of your life.

• You are the only person to congratulate or blame for the way things are right now for you.

• You must be patient with yourself in the process of making progress.

• You make thousands of choices every day. Start being conscious of those choices and their impact on your life.

• It's said we think 80,000 thoughts a day—the trouble is that most of them are the same as yesterday. Replace the disempowering thoughts you're giving energy and attention to with empowering ones. Consciously program your mind for success by only focusing yourself on possibility, opportunity, love, and promise—not limitation and fear.

• Hard work and good attitude beats good genes. You can be as smart, athletic and handsome as anyone, but if you aren't working hard and being pleasant to those around you, your success will last only so long. Substance will always win out over style.

• You will continue moving in the direction you have been unless you decide to take stock of where you really are, no matter how painful it might be to realize, and go in a new direction, taking the steps necessary to do so consistently – in other words, take action in the direction of your dream, now.

CHAPTER TEN

Clear Strategies to Start Living the Life You Desire

You've read the book, you're fired up to achieve your potential, you have a much clearer vision of the direction you're headed (at least at this stage!) and you are starting to understand what God wants for and from you. With this newfound clarity, you are beginning to see where some of your daily habits have brought you. During an examination such as the one we've been having throughout this book, we often begin to see which things we have been blindly doing each day that have been taking us in the opposite direction from where we truly want to go.

Now that you've taken off the blinders and have a clear vision of your true place in life, you might be wondering, 'Ok, so now that I

"Simply put, the key to achievement is desire + strategic, intelligent, proven action steps + consistent application of your chosen approach + flexibility."

know the habits I need to replace, what exactly am I to do to get the life I want?' You feel ready to take the next steps, but what are those steps? The path to progress will be similar regardless of which goal you're trying to reach. Primarily, you must keep your mind focused and energized by the grander vision of your life. This focus and energy will keep you moti-

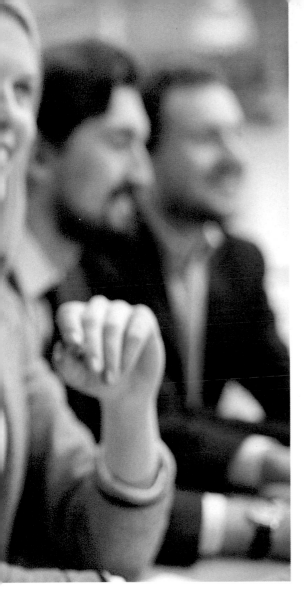

nation of what others may see about you that you don't, and a good guide.

Here are a few steps that everyone needs to take to reach their goals, whoever the person and whatever their goals may be.

Daily Infusions of Motivation

As we've discussed throughout this book, it's very common to get excited when you first attend a seminar, read a motivational book or meet someone inspiring, but staying motivated throughout the process of changing your daily habits over the long term can be considerably more difficult. Here are some tips to help you visualize, bringing your success to fruition.

Keep your goal in front of you, both figuratively and literally. Practice visualization every morning and every night. Don't just think abstractly about what you want. Know it wants you as much as you want it, even if your senses or situation seem to contradict this. Use all of your awareness to get every tiny detail down so you see, smell, feel and experience what it feels like to have what you're after. Feel as if you have already reached your goal. Speak in the present tense about what you want, as if it's already in your possession. In doing so, you are telling the universe there is no lack of this thing in your life. This sets in motion the invisible forces that bring what we desire most into our lives. If you feel, talk and act as if you lack it, whatever it is, then you will find you repel it, like chasing a butterfly. Success is attracted to those who are successful by their own internal definition of themselves. The combination of having this type of faith, accepting responsibility for doing all that you can and leaving the rest to God, stimulates great forces in the universe that none of us fully understand, but work.

vated to consistently take the necessary steps. While most of these steps are very simple, they are not all easy, and you do not want your motivation to wane.

Simply put, the key to achievement is desire + strategic, intelligent, proven action steps + consistent application of your chosen approach + flexibility. You will achieve your goals not only from recognizing which daily habits brought you where you don't want to be, but also by following the daily habits that *will* bring you where you *do* want to be. You need to begin to replace the negative habits with more positive habits, those that invest in your future rather than withdraw from it. This can take some work, recognition, an open exami-

Is your goal to lose weight? Then plaster pictures of those who have the physique you want all around you. See yourself looking into the mirror easily gliding into that brand-new outfit, your waist slim and lean, your legs not rubbing together. Be at the beach when you're looking super sexy in a swimsuit, feeling good and comfortable there no matter who's around! Smell the ocean. Squish the sand between your toes. Feel the warm rays of the sun cloaking your shoulders. Hear the waves. If your goal is to get out of debt and have an abundance of financial resources then imagine opening up your bank statement and seeing tens of thousands of dollars in your account. See the actual goal number. Is it $10,000? $15,000? More? Imagine hearing the phone ringing and feeling relaxed, knowing that all debts have been paid—you can answer it without any concern, because you know you no longer owe any money and don't need to fear the sound of a collection agent on the other end. Feel that wonderful sense of freedom. Make these visualizations as clear and detailed as you can. Crystalize them and increase the detail every single day. The more you are "in" this vision, the more you will see yourself as part of the life you want. Always remember there are millions of people who have achieved the goals you want and the only thing stopping you from achieving them is your thinking!

Vision boards can be very helpful. Again, put in as much detail as possible. Think of all the things you can't do now and would like to, and find something that represents that to you. Don't make it all physical. Maybe you want to be able to go on a roller coaster with your child, but can't physically fit at this time. Put a picture of a parent and child enjoying themselves on a roller coaster. Choose images and writings that bring about the feelings you want to have. Feelings of joy, energy, love and confidence.

In America, about 70% of people, the huge majority, want to lose weight, and about 35% are clinically obese. Meanwhile, 80% of Americans are in debt, and a recent study shows that about 37% have such bad debt that their future is threatened. While we're talking percentages, between 40 and 50% of marriages in the US end in divorce.

Porn addiction is rampant. Pornography is easily and readily available at no cost or shame to the consumer, although many suggest that it erodes the basis of a relationship founded in reality and true presence of the other. An estimated 40 million Americans watch porn regularly, and 18% of all men in the US believe they are or might be addicted to porn. Abuse of alcohol, drugs and gambling are all also prevalent, and a total of approximately 10-12% of the overall population having a serious problem considered addiction.

"Think of all the things you can't do now and would like to, and find something that represents that to you."

With numbers like these, it's a pretty safe bet that you might have a problem with at least one of these common concerns, and in fact if you have a problem in one area it's likely that you have a problem in multiple areas, because the way of thinking that brings about one is similar to the way of thinking that brings about all.

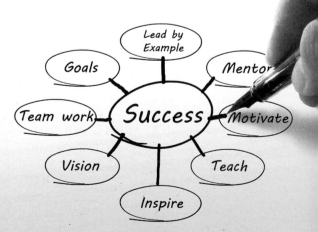

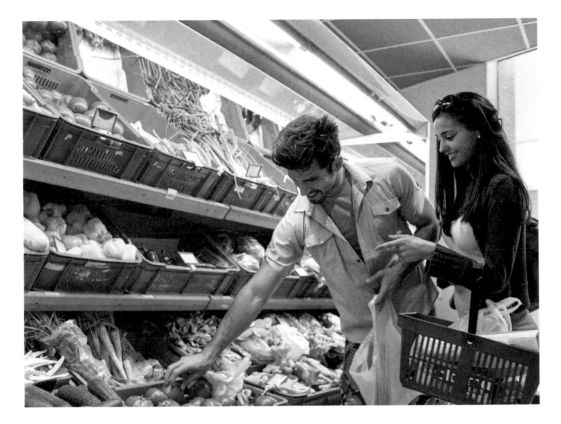

Weight Loss

A few years ago I wrote an entire guide on winning the battle of the bulge, called *Think and Grow Thin*. While the focus of this book is different, chances are you still want to lose weight. Any number of weight loss plans will have an effect and you don't need a degree in nutrition to know that eating more vegetables and lean meats and less fast food, potato chips and soda every day will certainly have some impact. Move more and eat less, or move more and eat less of certain foods and more of others in order to achieve your goal.

The main thing you need to get a handle on is the underlying driver of the choices you're making. The major operant mechanism in those who have not only lost their excess fat but also kept it off is absolute consistency and a sense of personal worth, and that is where

this upgrade in mindset becomes critical. You must challenge and change your daily habits, first by becoming aware, then by looking at why you are overeating and under-exercising. Get truly associated to the long-term consequences of continuing in that same disempowering pattern.

"You would set up a plan to eat the same healthy food for each meal at the same time every day, and you would also perform the exact same exercise at the same time every day."

If you were to start working with me, we would look at your ultimate goals, planning your strategy in 14-day intervals. You would set up a plan to eat the same healthy food for each meal at the same time every day, and you would also perform the exact same exercise at the same time every day. After 14 days we switch it up, increasing the exercise slightly and changing the foods if you desire, but that schedule/plan will then stick for another 14 days. This frees up your mental RAM since you don't have to think about what to eat, when to exercise or what you're going to do at the gym. It's all decided ahead of time, by you.

Some people think this sounds boring and it might be, but it works. Actually, the fact that it's boring is part of the reason it works, because it helps to sever your emotional cord to food. This allows your emotions that your dysfunctional food behavior has been masking to come to the surface to be resolved. If you've ever finished eating a very satisfying meal only to find yourself pacing the kitchen opening the fridge and cupboards 10 minutes later, you have to know this is not rational. Emotional attachments to food are a huge part of any weight problem. Simply put, if you use food only as nourishment, which is what it is intended for, instead of using it try to fill emotional and psychological voids or provide short-lived and short-sighted comfort, you will find it easy to maintain a healthy weight.

Another important way this system works is by creating an environment where your natural drive for variety and spontaneity in your life isn't serviced by overindulgence in food. If you know that every single day you are having a

turkey sandwich for lunch and you have that sandwich with you at work, for example, then when lunchtime comes and you're hungry you won't start wondering what you want, with this thought process leading you to make bad choices. Your focus becomes finding joy in connection and meaningful relationships, not the excitement of what the new drive-thru restaurant menu will have on it.

Similarly, my clients choose a time when they will exercise each day, unconsciously coming to value themselves enough to set aside time each day for just them. The exercise I recommend is modest, with just 30 minutes of walking on a treadmill, in order to keep a consistent pace and incline. Every 14 days that time increases five minutes until we hit a maximum of 60 minutes. Walking is a wonderful exercise and the treadmill is a great way to stay consistent with your efforts, but really any exercise performed every day at the same time for 30 minutes (increasing 5 minutes every 14 days) with a consistent level of difficulty will do just fine.

Again, if you feel you need more guidance, you can read more about the specific program I offer coaching clients in my book, but here in the chart to the right are some golden nuggets to get you moving in the right direction.

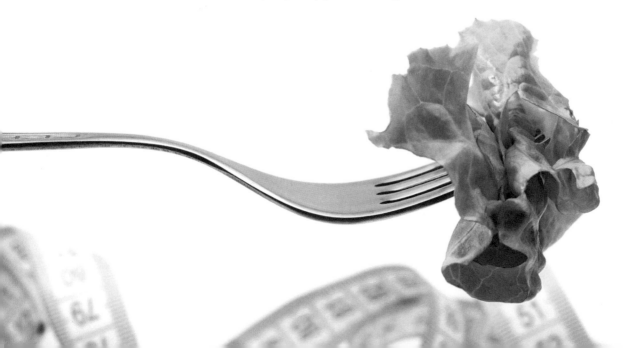

• Choose a time to exercise and a type of exercise that you will be able to do at a slightly challenging level for 30 minutes, connecting it with a joyful activity. Get an iPad, iPod or similar entertainment device that will allow you to enjoy your favorite music or lectures—feeding your mind and soul while working your body.

• Choose the times each day you will eat three meals and two or three snacks, making sure you eat something every three hours. Nutrient timing is important. You want to get to the point where your body knows what time it is without you needing to check a clock. Here's an example:

Breakfast: 7am	**Snack: 10am**	**Lunch: 12:30pm**
Snack: 3pm	**Dinner: 6pm**	**Snack: 9pm**

• Plan ahead which foods you will eat at each of these times, giving yourself an adequate and nutritious diet. My specific recommendations are in the book *Think and Grow Thin*.

• Prepare them ahead of time or know exactly how you will get them so you buffer yourself against the inevitability of unexpected circumstances that could derail your efforts.

• Eliminate all empty calories from your day, starting with beverages. Say goodbye to soda, fruit juices, yes, even milk. We want to be sure all calories and all actions are purposeful and strategic.

• Eliminate white from your diet—white bread, white rice, refined sugar and salt.

• When in doubt or in a bind, choose lean protein and green veggies as a meal. They're the most nutrient dense, satiating and clean. Feed your muscle, not your fat.

• Sugar is either a cause or strong contributing factor to a number of serious diseases, including heart disease, stroke and diabetes. While hydrogenated oils are certainly harmful on multiple levels, some of the excess fats in blood, which help bring about heart disease, are actually caused by excess sugar in the liver. Avoid sugar.

Debt

As with any goal, to get to where you are going you must confront the reality of where you're starting from. The very first step in freeing yourself from debt, then, is being honest about where you are right now. Feelings of terror and being overwhelmed aren't uncommon when you begin to face this reality, but as we discussed in the last chapter, avoiding or ignoring the reality doesn't make it any less real; it just buries you deeper and deeper in the hole you've been digging yourself until one day you are truly buried too deep to escape without bankruptcy. With this awareness you can begin the gradual and steady process of digging yourself out, gaining your freedom.

A man I know recently went through this exercise. He and his partner owed $90,000 in consumer debt. At the end of one year, they'd reduced that to $50,000 and were on course toward being completely debt free within only about two short years. He said he couldn't believe how liberated he felt, and how easy it was once he changed his thinking. Depending on your income and your debts this freedom might take you more time or less time, but the exact time it takes isn't nearly as important as getting started with it now. Your freedom from the heavy burden of debt is on the horizon as you commit to change.

"If you don't prepare for this inevitability then you are at serious risk of homelessness, and that is not an extreme statement."

The first step: Write down how much after-tax income you make monthly. Write down all sources. Now, take 10% right off the top of that number. That is going to be your savings. Not possible, you think? It has to be possible and you have to make it possible. You need to have savings. All of us encounter points in our life where we have extra expenses for some reason, either planned or unplanned. Will you be having children? Will you need to take time off work to do so? Will you want to help your children attend college down the road? What if you, your partner or child becomes ill and needs care? What if damage occurs to your house or car that your insurance won't cover? Or your insurance covers it but you have a huge deductible?

Every single person will encounter incidents such as these in their lives. If you don't prepare for this inevitability then you are at serious risk of homelessness, and that is not an extreme statement. The majority of homeless are not those you see sleeping in doorways.

They are the hidden homeless, seeking the generosity of friends and family, sleeping in spare bedrooms or on couches while they try to get back on their feet. Between 60% and 90% of homeless people fall into this category, and about half of these people are families. Every year 600,000 families with 1.35 million children experience homelessness in the United States.

So, start with your take-home income minus 10% as your actual income in one column. When something becomes necessary, we always find a way. Make a savings plan happen today.

The second step is to write down every single expense you have in another column. This can be tough, because people tend to forget about certain expenses they have through the year—for example, if you're reading this in June you might not be thinking about how much you'll be spending on Christmas presents. Also, think of birthday presents, baby showers, wedding gifts, etc. You need to take into account all your expenses, including potential expenses such as car repair. I've included a list, and you can find templates online to download. Pay close attention to be sure you're not leaving anything off your list. The goal here is to leave nothing unaccounted for. If even 50 cents is going to be leaving your hands, you need to know where it will be coming from and where it will be going. Being unconscious financially is calamitous. Seeing everything that was once in the catacombs of your mind in black and white will allow you to see where you need to taper back.

In your expense column, first write down all your necessary fixed expenses: Rent, medical insurance, house and car insurance, property taxes, bank fees, utility bills and anything you have a contract for, such as your phone, will be included in this column. You should also include repair and maintenance of your house and vehicle in this column, because those are expenses you will incur. At some point you will

need to get your brakes fixed, you will need new tires, you will have to change your oil, and you will have unexpected breakdowns that require a new starter, battery or alternator, for example. You may go for a year without needing most of these things and then you may need them all at once. If you own your house, you will have to fix issues with your furnace, or you'll have a flood, or you'll need to repair your siding or your plumbing. If you plan for these expenses, they will never put you behind the 8-ball. If it happens that you don't have any of these "unexpected" expenses for a long period of time, then that's great! Keep enough on hand to deal with them and use the extra to pay down some other debts or invest. It's helpful with these irregular but inevitable expenses to look at an average yearly total and divide by 12. Your debt repayment will also go in this column once we get to that.

After you've covered all your fixed expenses, write down your variable expenses. Variable expenses include food, clothing, household goods, entertainment, gifts, vacations, restaurants, gas, daycare, parking, hairdresser, sports, recreation, lessons, newspapers/magazines/books, and tobacco and alcohol if you use them.

Many of these expenses will not be paid monthly. If that's the case, look at what you pay over the course of the year and divide by 12, as with the car and house expense example above. For example, let's say you pay baseball and basketball and dance fees for your kids. Combined, they come to $1500 per year. In that case the monthly amount is $125.

NOTE: Multiplying weekly amounts by four for the month's total is not accurate. Instead, take the weekly number, multiply by 52 and then divide by 12. For biweekly payments, multiply by 26 and divide by 12. So for example if you pay $150 per week for groceries, then the monthly total is $150 x 52 ÷ 12 = $650.

Expense Sheets

Monthly fixed expenses

Rent or mortgage	
Property taxes	
Utilities	
Internet	
Phone	
Vet bills (expected and potential)	
Medical insurance	
Dental insurance/payments	
Car insurance	
House insurance	
Car repair and maintenance	
House repair and maintenance	

Total:

Monthly variable expenses

Groceries	
Restaurants	
Fast food, vending machines, soda, candy etc	
Cable/Netflix/Spotify	
Other entertainment: concerts, dancing, etc	
Recreation fees, including any tournament/competition fees	
Lessons	
Vacation (Not just resorts. Do you go camping, for example?)	
Clothing and shoes	
Gifts	
Personal care, including hairdresser, manicure, skin and haircare and makeup	
Daycare and babysitting	
Tobacco and alcohol	
Gambling (including lottery tickets, fantasy football, workplace pools, etc)	

Total:

At this point you should be able to see where you're overspending or which expenses you're forgetting to take into account. Many people are surprised to realize how much they spend on fast food plus snacks and drinks at convenience stores. When they mentally consider their expenses, these purchases often do not fall into the categories of either groceries or restaurants, and so they often unconsciously delete them from their memory. But a few dollars here or there spent on these useless extras can add up to huge amounts over the course of the month and are entirely (and easily) avoidable.

Another way we get into the trap of overspending is in using things that withdraw from our own vitality and power—throwing money away on things like tobacco, alcohol and lottery tickets. If you smoke regularly, drink just one beer with your coworkers after work and buy a couple of lottery tickets each week, you can

"It should be very apparent to you that if you don't take control of your situation, you may soon start losing anything of value you have— including your mind!"

easily spend $400 per month, or $4,800 per year and possibly much more than that. Now consider that you might need to make $6,000 or more before tax to spend that much on your bad habits!

Now it's time to write down all of your debt. Write how much you owe, what the interest rate is and how much your minimum payment is each month. Mortgage payments are included in your fixed expense and are likely non-negotiable, so while a mortgage is a debt, we won't include it here.

The total of these minimum payments need to go on your fixed expense list, but keep in mind that by paying just the minimum payment you will never pay your debt down. Compounding can work for you if you're earning interest, or against you if you're borrowing. If you have a high interest rate, you may never end up paying against your principal (the actual money you borrowed)!

It should be very apparent to you right now why you are having debt problems. It should also be very apparent to you that if you don't take control of your situation, you may soon start losing anything of value you have—including your mind!

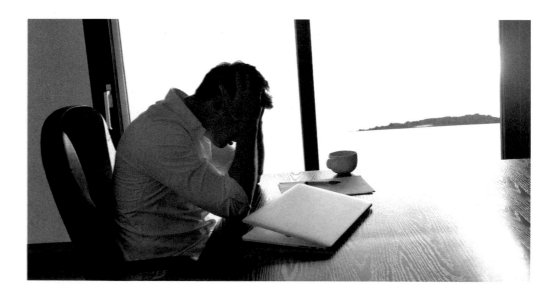

Debt Sheet

Creditor	Owing	Interest Rate	Minimum Payment
Car Payment			
Bank Loan			
Student Loan			
Visa 1			
Visa 2			
Mastercard 1			
Mastercard 2			
Store Card 1			
Store Card 2			

Total:

Note: Think of all you own that you don't need. You can start paying off debts by selling off much of what you have in your home that you're not using or could easily live without. Have a yard sale or sell your items on local buy-and-sell sites. Use that money to pay down your debt with the highest interest rate.

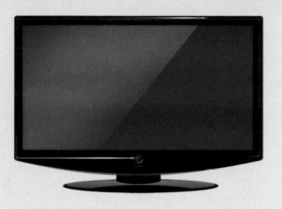

People with debt problems often fall into this specific trap. They see something on sale and don't want to pass up a deal.

They buy it with a credit card, not taking into account how much it will actually cost over the long run. It's alluring to be able to buy something with no money down, but understand those retailers are making that money from somewhere. If you're buying it with no money down then chances are you can't actually afford it.

If you are in the habit of just making minimum payments, you will be blown away by how much these items end up costing you in the long run, especially if you are using store credit cards with high interest rates. If you are not making your minimum payments or make late payments, then you will end up paying even more.

Let's say you buy a beautiful 60" HD TV for $1,000 and put it on a credit card with 19.99% interest. (For the record, most store cards are actually about 28% interest.) You are making just the minimum payment each month, with the minimum set at 2.5% of total. Are you ready for the truth? It will take you 176 months (that's over 14 years!!) to pay for this TV, and you will have paid $2,462.56 for it. That's more than double for a piece of technology that will be long outdated by the time it's paid off! If you were to use a store credit card at 28% to buy the TV and pay minimum payments, it would take you over 300 months to pay it off, and that $1,000 TV would end up costing you around $6,500! Doesn't sound like much of a deal now, does it?

The good news is, you can take control. Here are the steps you need to take in order to do so.

1 Live BELOW your means

I like Dave Ramsey's quote: "Live like no one else does now, so you can live like no one else does later!" In other words, pay the price of discipline now to enjoy a very fulfilling future. Some changes will be relatively easy—stop buying fast food and other junk from the convenience stores, for example. Cutting down on expenses for clothing, shoes and groceries is usually not too tough either. But you may have to make some really tough decisions like telling your kids they can't play soccer this year. Understand that they will much prefer the short-term pain of giving up a year of soccer this year to losing their home next year. If you find there are some things you're really not willing to give up, like your daughter's riding lessons, for example, then you'll need to figure out a way to make more income and pay for those lessons instead of continuing to pretend you have enough income while sinking further into debt. It's not that what you want is too expensive, it's that you have yet to create the income to deserve it. Now's the time to start.

2 Stop buying on credit, period

With the possible exception of large purchases such as a house or vehicle, or unexpected repairs before you've saved enough using your new plan, then if you can't pay cash for it, then you can't afford it. You should keep one low-interest credit card with a low limit for absolute emergencies and for when you need a credit card, such as when you register at a hotel. Decide to shred the rest of the cards. Call and cancel them today.

3 Negotiate lower interest rates

First, the very best way to negotiate is to have relatively good credit, so make your minimum payments. Second, despite their reputation as being inhumane, credit companies would rather get some of their money back from you than none of it. They will sometimes take into account that you've had personal troubles that led to problems with debt. This might be a loss of job, sickness in your family or other reasonable unexpected issue. Explain this to every individual you're speaking with during the process, as this type of human disclosure can help greatly in your negotiations. Most people sincerely want to help those who are really making an effort to help themselves (even people who work for creditors), and most companies will allow for this help, but it can definitely take some effort on your part.

If you've always made your minimum payments, then ask to have your interest rate reduced. Sometimes, it can be this simple. If this is not possible, you might be able to just switch your high-interest cards to lower-interest ones. Phone your credit card companies to ask if they have a card with a lower rate. You might be able to simply transfer your balance over. Always phone instead of using another method of contact.

With the credit cards you are giving up, explain that you are working to avoid bankruptcy. As I mentioned earlier, they would rather get something than nothing. It is important for you to know that any of the following methods will affect your credit rating, but right now your concern is climbing out from under massive debt; you can worry about improving your credit rating again later on. Often, companies will accept 50% of what you owe them and close the account. If this is not possible, then ask them to give you a lower interest rate and set a payment plan with them that you can manage. While you are paying this off you will not be able to use these cards. Your credit limit

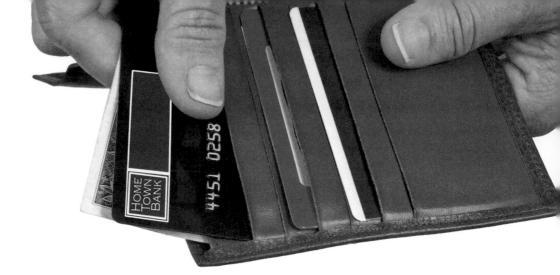

will decrease as you pay it off. But that's fine—you don't want to use credit anymore anyway.

4 Get a consolidated loan or line of credit

The better your payment history, the more stable your job and the more value (equity) you have in your home, the easier this will be. Imagine if you have five credit cards that average 16% and you can pay them all off at prime plus 1% with a low monthly payment! You have a massive caveat with this one though. You must close off your credit cards as you pay them off, with the exception of the one you will keep for necessity. Otherwise it's very easy to suddenly have all your debt back PLUS the consolidation loan.

5 Make it a must to pay more than the minimum

If you can't get a loan or line of credit, don't want to destroy the credit you've built up and also have a decent income-expense ratio, you can simply pay off more, and get out of debt more quickly than you otherwise would have. Try for at least double the minimum payment, but make sure to focus a little more on the higher-interest cards. It doesn't really make sense to put as much effort into paying off your 11.99% credit card as your 28% store card. (Although make sure you make payments on those ones too!) Once your high-interest cards are paid off, you can take the money you were putting toward their payment and add it to the payment of your lower-rate cards. You might be able to pay extra on your mortgage, too—just be sure there isn't any prepayment penalty you'll incur by doing so. In some jurisdictions the law states that lenders must allow a certain amount of extra payment each year, but not all. If you're not allowed this extra payment, then see if you can change your payment plan to an accelerated weekly or biweekly.

Keys to Lasting Relationships

The key to any lasting and significant relationship is trust. Without it, there is no hope for lasting connection. And the first place for honesty is with yourself. If you aren't honest with yourself, you won't find it easy to be so with others. Work to be the person you desire in a partner. We attract those to us who are often most like us, or who possess aspects of personality we've divorced ourselves from acknowledging. For example, a strong attraction might develop between an organized, take-charge woman who plans every moment with a man who is spontaneous, fun loving and random. This dynamic can be wonderful at first, but must result in a merging of sorts, where the woman develops her spontaneous side and the man develops his structured side, or resentment will eventually result. Attraction forms from what we find unique and different about one another but love comes from what we share in common.

Just as with amassing financial wealth, building health or any other aspect of life where we can find ourselves in a tough spot after years of neglect, relationship problems are often caused by failing to routinely invest in them. It's easy to slip into bad habits that can be resolved by deciding to do better and making the daily choices that follow that decision.

The most important thing is to look at the relationship, whether personal, professional or intimate, from the perspective of giving to something greater than yourself for the benefit of all. You don't simply stay married because you're committed to your partner; you are committed to the concept of marriage and the promise you've made and hold yourself to. Now, the hard part is that if you weren't thoughtful in who you've selected as a partner in the first place, you might have chosen a "taker." Sometimes "givers" end up being taken advantage of by "takers." Remember, it's not your job to make your partner happy; your job is to be loving and compassionate, to walk through life by that person's side and bring joy.

To prevent an unhealthy dynamic from developing, be sure to take time to think strongly before entering into a relationship of any kind. All too often, we allow our biochemistry to drive us in making irrational decisions based on our hormones or history. We make decisions based on what we wish were true instead of what is, not allowing ourselves to see the reality. Maybe you start dating someone with a drug problem. You know it's not healthy for you, but you discount this knowing, and stay in the relationship anyway. Perhaps upon reflection you integrate the truth that you lost someone to that pattern who you loved but couldn't save in the past. Now, you blindly stay in a disempowering relationship trying to unconsciously undo that with someone who may have no interest in playing the part you want them to play. Don't let another's problem be your excuse for being absent in designing your own life and fulfilling your destiny. I don't believe it is God's will to avoid your own growth and the responsibility to find meaning in your life by choosing to be a martyr—constantly giving at the expense of your own fulfillment and future.

I must raise my own hand that I was once the person using others' problems to keep me from my own, so don't feel you're alone

"Don't let another's problem be your excuse for being absent in designing your own life and fulfilling your destiny."

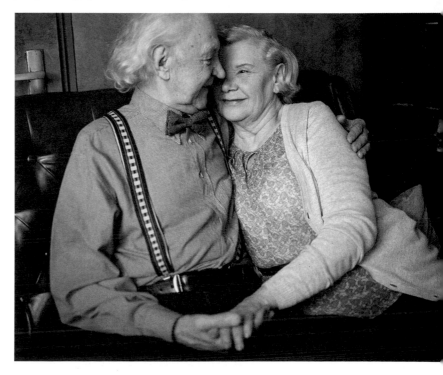

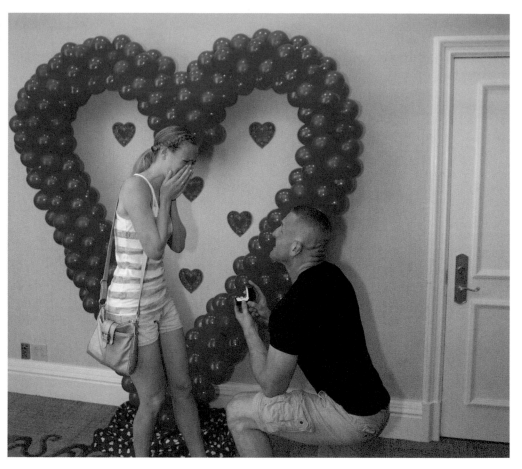

if you find yourself in this very place as you read these words. I can't begin to convey the number of clients I've seen who have let guilt and shame over their past or fear about their future shackle them to an unhealthy relationship that's only enabling a taker. In psychology, we call this co-dependency. It's not healthy for either party involved and is to be avoided at all costs. Such a malignant relationship can begin to rob every other area of your life if it goes untreated. See and understand where your responsibility begins and ends. Work on setting boundaries. As with many of the things we discuss in this book, this involves taming your ego in the situation.

When you do choose an appropriate person to spend your time or even your life with, look at what is actually important to that individual.

> *"The first idea would have fed my own ego, the second created an experience that Crystal will treasure forever."*

What are your partner's needs? How does he/she feel loved? Is it hearing the words? Being touched by you? Spending time together doing something fun or maybe doing nothing at all? We all have our own interpretation of how we feel loved and wanted. Your task in all of your meaningful relationships—intimate and otherwise—is to decode your partners. Meet them where they are with what they need most from you, not what you would want to be given.

One example I can offer about this from my own life is my marriage proposal to the greatest expression of God's love in my life, Crystal. I had originally planned to do a very public proposal onstage at a concert where nearly 20,000 people would be in attendance. I wanted to tell the world, how much she means to me and how grateful I was to have her in my life. I meticulously put the whole plan together, flew a videographer out to the city where it would take place and paid all the airfare. I soon realized in honest reflection, however, that this was *my* idea of what a wonderful proposal would be. It's what I would want, but was this supposed to be about me, or about the woman I love? Crystal is far more introverted than I, and the more I thought about it the more I realized she'd be uncomfortable with my grandiose plan. God would have it my plan wouldn't work out, fortunately! I took it as a clear sign that my hunch was right. I went back to the drawing board with a focus on what it would take to make her feel the most loved, appreciated and understood—signs she was making the right choice in marriage—from the man who's about to ask for her hand for life.

With my focus on what really mattered this time, I secretly flew all of her closest friends and family from across the country. I told her we were going for brunch, but really I'd booked a conference room at a luxurious hotel. The room was decorated with a romantic theme, I had place settings created that tied to our relationship history, and hired a violinist to play the theme from *Titanic*. In front of all the most important people in her life, I got down on one knee and asked if she would make me the luckiest man on the planet and marry me. She said yes. It was one of the most magical moments of both of our lives. The first idea would have fed my own ego, the second created an experience that Crystal will treasure forever.

That's a big example but this is the same case throughout everyday life. Thoughtfulness

doesn't need to be massive. Do you know your wife loves when you leave a cute loving note in a secret place for her to find? Then why not make a practice of it? Does your husband love when you set up a date night so he doesn't have to think about it? Then set up the date! All too often, people start saying something along the lines of: "Why should I do X when he won't even do Y?" This just sets the stage for a vortex of unhappiness. It makes the relationship like a business deal rather than a selfless partnership.

Each day, think of a few things you can easily do for your partner that he/she appreciates, and do them. You don't have to spend a penny. Time is far more precious than money or gifts, because it truly is limited. You can never buy or create more of it.

Chances are, with this new approach, your partner will begin trying to do more things that please you as well. And if not, don't stop! Giving induces reciprocation automatically. If you find after a few weeks or months that your partner has not begun to reciprocate, then you'll have material to work on and discuss together. That honest and real conversation may be all that it takes to get things moving in a better more invigorated direction.

It's important to note here that there are narcissistic and manipulative people who will use your own efforts against you. But the majority of people are good people who want to have a good relationship. They sometimes just don't know how or are too afraid to try because of past hurts.

Other Relationships

We usually focus on marriage or partner relationships in discussions such as these, but we are having a relationship with every person in our life, from our parents to our siblings to our children, and beyond to friends, coworkers and even the people who serve us at restaurants and in stores. We want others to behave as we want them to behave, and when they don't, instead of allowing them to be themselves or accepting it might not be the right fit for us, we try to force our ideas on them. Again, this usually comes from ego.

The way to have the best relationships with everyone is to take yourself out of it! Truly listen to them. Understand their perspective. Understand that their ego or their perspective may be causing them to be in a place where they are having a hard time dealing with others too. Because they have not found the emotional maturity to deal with these issues does not mean you need to act in an emotionally immature manner. Go into every encounter with every person with the same ambition of giving, of making their day better, and you will be amazed at how they make your day—and ultimately your life—unbelievably wonderful.

Connected to Disconnection

Technology has replaced so many activities in our lives. The last thing you want it to replace is true intimacy. As I said earlier, internet porn is becoming a huge problem as men in particular watch hour upon hour upon hour. While this point is debated, many studies point to this being detrimental to healthy sexual relationships. To me this seems sensible, but whether or not that is the case, spending too much time surfing the Internet, whether your focus is porn, funny videos, social networks, or the latest YouTube singing star, means you are living in distraction from the present moment.

Have you ever seen couples sitting across from one another, each on their phone even though there is a human being to truly connect with right in front of them? Maybe you are half of one such couple! Spending your time and energy doing something that does not benefit you or bring you where you want to be in life is a setup for regret. Go ahead and check out Facebook as a break after you've accomplished all you want to do in the day, but if you're wasting three or four hours a day scrolling down your timeline aimlessly, or at risk of losing your job because you're hanging out on forums or forwarding cat videos to your coworkers, then you really have to consider what's underlying your choices here.

The difficulty with inappropriate and excessive use of the Internet is that, for most of us, we can't avoid it. The Internet is a tool we all rely on for work and study, and it's very easy to get distracted. If you need to give up certain aspects and can't give up others, then the key is to lay out very strict rules and make it difficult not to follow through on them. Reward yourself for adhering to this new agreement, and punish yourself when you fail to remain steadfast to it.

If you really feel stuck in a bad pattern, then set your computer with strict parental controls, or even better, have your partner do it. This will not make it impossible for you to find porn, but it will make doing so far more difficult. Those extra steps will help deter you. Take a dedicated period of time off of social networks. Have a trial separation. Stop using social networking altogether if you don't need it for your role at work. If you do, then be sure to log out after every time you use it. Give yourself strict time limits and set your alarm. The extra step of having to log in will help you stick to your set times by making you aware of what you're doing.

> *"Each time you want to turn on whatever site you're drawn to, instead go for a walk, toss the ball around with your kid, clean the house, or call a friend, meet up and truly engage with another person in the flesh!"*

Replace this activity with a more beneficial one. Each time you want to turn on whatever site you're drawn to, instead go for a walk, toss the ball around with your kid, clean the house, or how about calling up a friend? Meet somewhere and truly engage with another person in the flesh!

I've discovered we usually don't break habits. Rather, we can get rid of bad habits by replacing them with ones that serve both the present and future. A good friend of mine quit smoking by exercising every time she wanted a cigarette. Not only did she quit smoking, she ended up getting in great shape!

Most important, understand that the Internet is yet another escape from being in the moment, just like junk food, drugs, alcohol, and so many other things. You are using the Internet to try to fill a void that it cannot fill. If you're having a hard time with a relationship, for example, then watching porn will not resolve it. Get to work on what your underlying needs and issues are. Seeing a coach or therapist who can be totally nonjudgmental, confidential, supportive and understanding often proves to be the most effective thing you do in your lifetime. A good coach doesn't give you anything you don't already have; he or she simply helps you become aware of obstacles that you alone can't see. I'm sure you've heard the saying, "Love is blind but the neighbors aren't." Once the obstacle becomes clear as you speak to a coach or therapist who sees him or herself as no better than you, but as a fellow traveler on life's road, someone you like, trust, and can be real with, leaving all drama at the door, you can begin to remove the obstacle or find your way around it.

CHAPTER ELEVEN

The Incredible Successes of Charles' Clients

"I've never achieved this kind of success before. You see people losing a lot of weight, but Charles made it a reality for me. Get in the right mindset, and you can do anything."

– Troy Schob

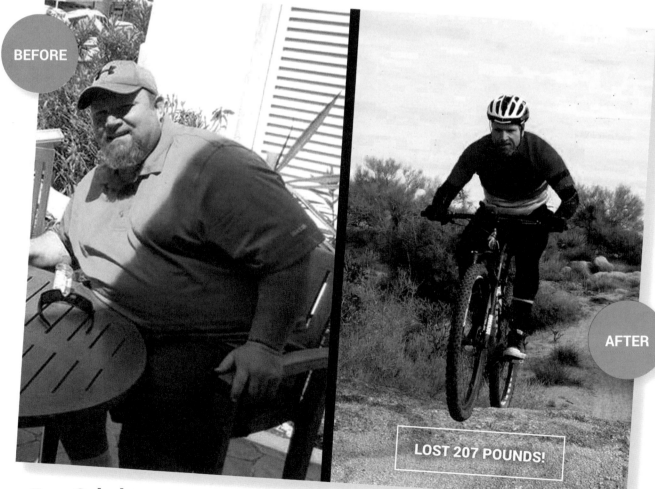

BEFORE

AFTER

LOST 207 POUNDS!

Troy Schob

Most people come to me thinking they want to lose weight, and that is part of what they're after. But when you look a little deeper they find they really are looking to change how they feel about themselves, their life, their relationships, their career or their spirituality. Weight is only part of that picture.

The first step no matter what you are seeking to change about yourself or your life is getting your health in order. Without the energy that comes from good health, you cannot truly invest all you're capable of into examining the way you think and the way you relate. If you are relying on stimulants or other substances to get through the day, it's easy to see that you're not going to be thinking or feeling as well as you could.

Often, the people who come to me start out thinking they know what their problem is, but end up being surprised by what they discover. They are aware that they don't have a healthy relationship with food, but come to discover the reason for this unhealthy relationship has more to do with the way they perceive themselves and perceive life in general than anything to do with food itself. Once their vision is clear about who they are, what they deserve, and who they must be to achieve their goals, when they are more focused on the present and future than they have previously been on the past, then embracing a simple and fundamental strategy to free themselves of fat becomes almost effortless.

A woman once came to me saying she wanted to lose 60 pounds, but every time she would make progress, losing 30 or more pounds, she found herself sabotaging her efforts—knowingly! After a little digging, she shared that she believed her husband would become jealous when she was getting attention from other men with her newfound health and confidence. With that insight, she was able to talk to her husband from a place of love and ask him to be her ally, giving him the reassurance she wanted to become the healthiest version

Lacey Ebert

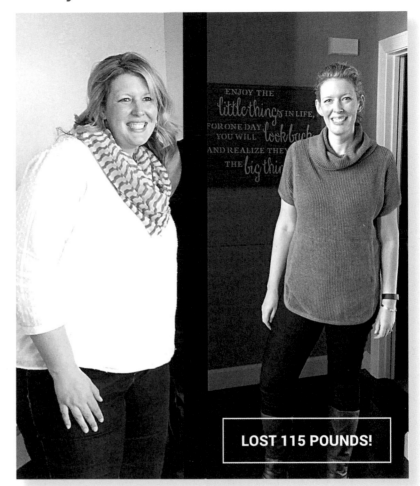

LOST 115 POUNDS!

of herself not for selfish reasons, but rather for very selfless reasons—wanting to be the woman she felt he and the children deserved.

While I help people resolve the challenge they come into my office with, we dig in deeper to resolve the real mindset issue that usually is having a pervasive effect in not just the area of their health, but other areas of life as well. If you're not disciplined with how you treat the vessel that carries you around each day—your body—it's not hard to imagine you're probably not as disciplined and tuned in to one or more of these: your relationships, your environment, your workplace, your finances, or other areas

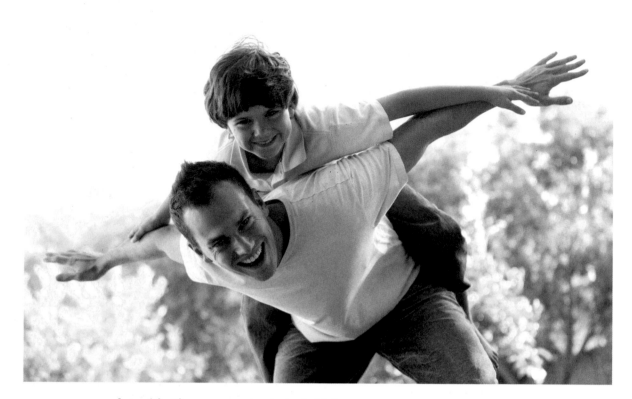

of your life. If you unconsciously don't think you're worthy of being fit and healthy, your mindset has to be worked on before lasting change can take effect. Without that work, change will be temporary at best.

"My health has vastly improved. I was borderline diabetic, was taking several medications and had a heart attack in April, 2015. Since I first decided to take control with Charles in September, 2015 I have been taken off all medications but one, and no longer worry about diabetes."

– Dan Farner

The Meaning of Success

At this point I think it's important to point out that each person must define success on his or her own terms. While we set clear goals and certainly take "before" and "after" pictures, as long as a person is making progress toward the goals they've outlined, I categorize them as successful. This is even the case with set-backs. If they learn and grow from them and don't throw in the towel, I believe them to be successful. Success is sticking with something even in the face of disappointment, frustration and what may sometimes feel like fruitless efforts. Staying on course and having faith that you will get what you've long hoped and worked for even when the circumstances look grim, that is success.

Those who are successful with me have a willingness to shift their philosophy from the one most of us are raised with—one of scarcity and lack—to one of possibility and abundance. They don't think only about what achieving their goals will mean for them, but what it will mean for all those they love, those before them who sacrificed so much, those after them who will look at their life with gratitude or disgust, and those who will benefit from their contributions to their community.

Spirituality

In my own development, there was a time where I felt psychology/science and spirituality/faith diverged. You might feel that way right now. As I've grown in maturity and experience, having a privileged coaching position in the lives of so many different people from so many different walks of life, I find that science and psychology actually serve to prove what teachings from all faiths have been putting forth for millennia. It seems to me that science is working hard to try to catch up to where faith is, and hopefully one day it will help us to understand just how present our God/Higher Power really is.

I don't think our minds will ever fully grasp it, but we can get closer than we are now if we can still ourselves and our minds to find eternal truths and feelings of love for all, even those who seek to harm us. The greatest enemy on the planet is the one that we each carry within ourselves telling us we have to get more, have more, and do more to be loved

"I feel that I really do have an impact on others by my actions. People watch me and I have a responsibility to behave in a way I want them to emulate."

– Dan Farner

SUCCESS STORY

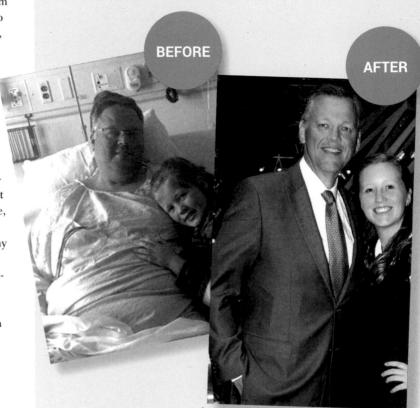

BEFORE

AFTER

Dan Farner

AGE: 49
STARTING WEIGHT: 370 POUNDS
END WEIGHT: 220 POUNDS

"These health successes have led to other successes. I 'led by example' with my family, so my wife and son have also lost weight. We are running 5k races and plan to do a marathon relay."

SUCCESS STORY

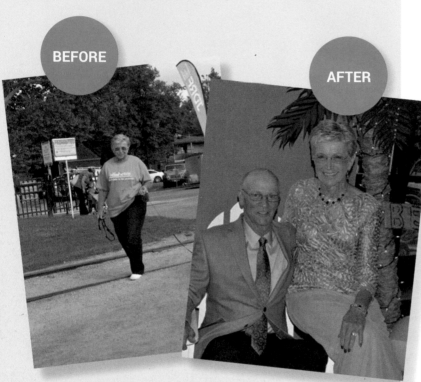

BEFORE

AFTER

Jeanette Koechner

AGE: 72
STARTING WEIGHT: 197 POUNDS
END WEIGHT: 146 POUNDS

"It has been a good journey and one that I know I will continue for the rest of my life. Charles helped me get to a place where I feel better. I know I am healthier and enjoy getting out and doing things."

or deserving. That simply isn't true. When you free yourself of this myth, you release a torrent of energy that can be shuttled to creative and positive ends to move humanity forward, starting with getting your own life in order. While we can't always explain the "miracles" our personal theologies offer, we can witness them, and I think sometimes that needs to be enough.

It is our ego and our mind that yearns to make things more complicated than they really are. Asking "why" is something I recommend, but only when it leads to positive outcomes. When it gets used as a weapon against oneself, leading down the road to more and more confusion, you have to break out of that cycle and hand it over to something bigger than yourself and your own thinking. It's called humility.

When you come to terms with your own mortality—something we call dealing with "death anxiety" in psychology—you begin to really think about what matters in life. You realize all the trappings of success don't matter when you lose a dear friend or family member, hear of a life-shaking tragedy or find the end has come for you. There is an old adage that says: "There are no atheists in a fox hole."

I think that faith, love and hope are truths we can all agree are crucial for our psychological, physical, emotional and spiritual health. I also know we are each on the path of our own life journey and none of us have the right to make another feel wrong who isn't harming anyone else. I have found that the more empathy you develop, the more love you have for your

"The fact of feeling better, of having more energy is success in itself."

– Jeanette Koechner

> "I could easily see, from the first time I met Charles, his devotion to his faith. It showed by his kindness, his concern, demeanor and conversation. I sometimes wondered if it was because of my age, but I don't think so. Kindness and compassion is just his nature."

– Jeanette Koechner

fellow human being, the less black and white your thinking becomes, the ultimate byproduct is a rich, meaningful, fulfilling life experience. I think that to become your best you have to have very strong drive and ambition. Those who have a sense of mission, of belonging to something bigger than themselves, whether that be family, peer group, church, temple, neighborhood or something else, fare much better in overcoming the inevitable adversities that we all encounter at some point when we choose to raise our standards and pursue more from life. When you're doing things not just for yourself but for a greater purpose, it pulls you through the times you might otherwise get stuck and caught in, filled with self-pity, doubt, fear and anger.

What Prevents Success?

I would say the number one thing stopping people from designing and creating the life they deserve is fear. Fear of failing, of not following through, of being derailed, fear of giving up, repeating their history, giving their goals all they've got only to be disappointed again. These are all experiences you can indeed have when creating a magical life, but much like the seasons these hard times are transient and temporary. They are opportunities to grow from if you will stay consistent and most importantly learn to interpret experiences that we all must endure in ways that serve and empower you to become more. All too often

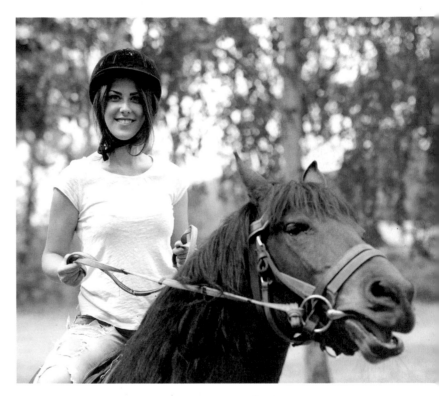

> "Charles understands us overweight folks' issues. He had them. He experienced the thoughts like 'I wish I were that size. I would like to take that walk, but I am already tired. My clothes are getting tighter but I will not buy a bigger size. I guess I need to settle for the dark colored clothes.'"

– Jeanette Koechner

Sarah Anglin

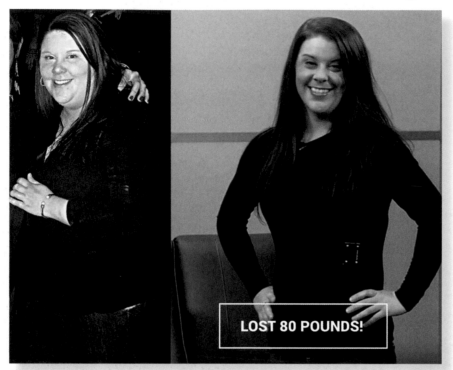

LOST 80 POUNDS!

improving another area of their life they're unhappy with.

Maybe they think losing weight will restore intimacy in their relationships or give them the confidence to do better and achieve more in their professional role. In general, most people I work with want to feel more certain about their lives and the direction they're headed in. Together we design a food and exercise program they don't have to think about, so they can use all their energy to begin to shape their life in a way they often are in awe of as the pieces come together! Couples who hadn't slept together for years suddenly are making love a few times a week, and people in sales slumps have their best months ever—as people begin to change the way they see themselves, their performance also changes.

One woman I worked with was in the restaurant business for years. Before starting in that business she had pursued a nursing degree, but was overweight and didn't feel she fit in. The anxious feelings eroded her capability in the classroom and, despite being very bright, she found herself underperforming—the idea that she didn't belong was starting to manifest itself in failure, since she gave so much energy and attention to that disempowering mode of thinking. She came up with a story to support her choice to leave the field. She told herself she obviously didn't

people assign to things outside of themselves the title of major obstacle to their happiness or achievement when in truth, the only thing that needs to change is the way you're looking at what you think is the biggest problem. What you call your biggest problem might be the greatest gift in teaching that you can overcome what you think is insurmountable.

Accidental Achievements

It always starts with wanting to lose weight, and that's a niche I love and feel passionate about. There is no better way in my experience to demonstrate to someone the power of their own mind than to help them transform physically. When a person goes from barely wanting to get out of bed each day to losing over 100 pounds and inspiring a dozen of their friends to do the same, it is radical! But for most people, losing weight really means

"What I have learned first and foremost is to act in the moment, before thinking could lead to negative effects on the future."

– JR Zachary

> "I think anything is possible at this point. I have nothing holding me back from achieving my dreams and goals."
>
> **– JR Zachary**

belong, citing her grades as the reason, and settled into the restaurant industry. At her core she was an achiever, despite her experience in nursing, so she quickly ascended the ladder, jumping the ranks and ultimately becoming a restaurant owner. She got what she wanted, the title of owner, but found herself feeling unhappy and physically unhealthy. She had gained much more weight after leaving nursing, so reached out to me. We talked at length about why she left the field she felt so passionate about, and I helped her see the story she was telling herself short-circuited her true potential. She embraced a disciplined pattern of healthy eating, daily exercise and, most importantly, gave much more attention to her mind's focus and thinking. In short order she lost over 80 pounds! Super motivated, she put in her letter of resignation with the restaurant and re-entered nursing school. This time, her physical health supported her as she felt congruent—modeling the example she hoped her patients would follow and taking better care of herself so she could better take care of others!

The Sky is the Limit

Once their physical limitations are overcome and people look in the mirror to see the person they've always dreamed of being, it's as if a rock has been moved out of the way of a burgeoning plant. Growth is inevitable in life and my role is to help people remove the obstacles

SUCCESS STORY

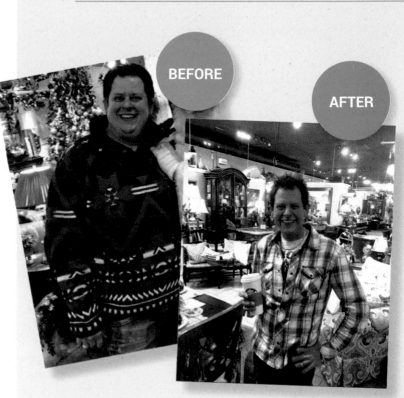

JR Zachary

AGE: 39
STARTING WEIGHT: 266 POUNDS
END WEIGHT: 165 POUNDS

"Taking a moment to think before reacting has made a profound difference in my day-to-day life. I have been able to overcome insecurities, my relationship is stronger, I no longer battle with food, and my career has never been better."

A DECADE OF DISCIPLINE

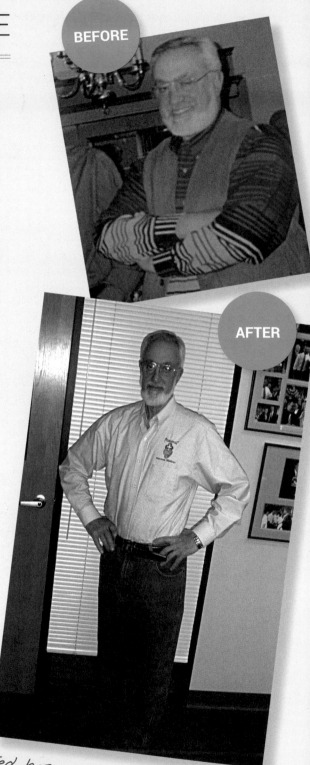

BEFORE

AFTER

Ted Vitali

AGE: 75
STARTING WEIGHT: 240 POUNDS
END WEIGHT: 165 POUNDS

"Charles taught me how to think about a lifestyle change, a much more disciplined lifestyle that led to a healthier way of life. He made use of the psychology of health, not just the mechanics of weight reduction. As the title of his original book signalled: *'Think and Grow Thin.'* Thinking and informed attitude was and remains the key to not only weight reduction but proper weight sustaining."

"I always had and still have a sense of purpose. That goes with my vocation and my profession. I just believe that I have a better chance now of living longer and thus doing more of what I am already doing."

Ted has now kept the weight off for nearly ten years!

that get in the way of that process, the things keeping them from growing into all they can be. So long as we identify and remove or grow around the obstacles, achieving other goals becomes inevitable whether that means other physical goals like weight training or running a marathon, relationship goals like finding a partner, career goals or anything else.

Strategies for Improving in Other Areas

Humans tend to learn very well, but are not necessarily aware of that learning. We function through identifying patterns. Just as Steve Jobs dressed the same way each day, finding that not thinking about what he had to wear streamlined his day and made him better able to focus on more important things, people often start to streamline other areas of their life once they've taken charge of their food and exercise plans. Mental energy is freed up once worrying about the future stops and excitement replaces it. Once this occurs, people start to do all sorts of wonderful things in their lives and in the lives of those they care about. Worry, self-consciousness and anxiety are drains on creativity. And once we stop the leaks by gaining momentum through a disciplined strategic approach to living, other areas really start to get charged up.

Many of my clients have reported that as they think more about their thinking and focus on things they're grateful for, they treat others better. Reciprocally, they experience much more joy in their relationships as their friends, family members and partners respond to this better treatment. Additionally, they start to reach beyond the self-imposed limits they once lived their life by. This can often translate to a higher position in the workplace and ultimately more disposable income! And they even get better control of their finances, often saving more or even starting to save. Once you train yourself to be in the here and now and not either the past or a nightmarish future, you design the future with joy instead of fear, and saving becomes something exciting, not dreadful.

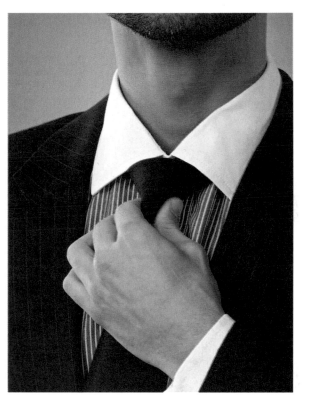

"I am still fully active in my career with no intention of retiring anywhere in the near future. I am as committed to my work and lifestyle as I have ever been, though I am stepping now from an administrative position (after 37 years) because I want to be free of the obligations and stress that go with administration, not because I haven't got the ability or energy."

– Ted Vitali

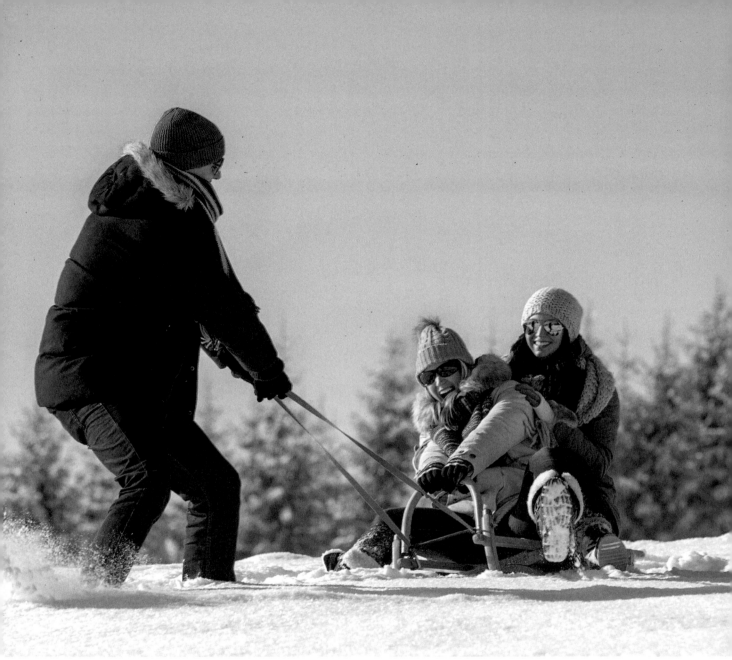

"When I weighed around 230, I was on blood pressure medication, my knees and joints ached, I felt sluggish. Now I am on no medication except for thyroid and I have no aches or pains. My joints are fine and I have the kind of normal energy of someone 20 years younger than I am. That says a lot."

– Ted Vitali

A New Chance

Parents often ask me if I will coach their children, because they interpret their own experiences as a child in a way that has disempowered them. Because of incredibly difficult situations they have had to divorce themselves from the uninhibited, curious, trusting, childlike part of their personality, simply to survive the environment and relationships they depended on. I've felt a lot of anger come from those who feel like they were denied a childhood and frankly, I probably had some of that myself looking back. When a person in that position finds someone to model themselves after, a person who was in as bad a situation as they might have been, but used it to both improve their own life and for the greater good, it becomes easier through that alliance to see the possibility of forgiving themselves and those who caused them pain. Once you are at that point of forgiveness, you can let go of the rigid adult stance that may drive you to abuse food or other substances.

You have to honor and love all parts of yourself and acknowledge them all to be healthy. We are not just one way all the time. I can be goofy and silly but also very serious and passionate, and we learn to do that through self-acceptance, learning what mode is appropriate and not pigeonholing ourselves into being one way all the time. Most of my work with young people, especially those who've chosen substances to deal with pain and fear, is to help them embrace the inner strength and warrior traits they carry, so they can replace the disempowering habits that certainly change how they feel in the moment at a huge cost and unimaginable life risk, with positive choices that may also change how they feel in the moment, but with a tremendous reward and opportunity for their future instead.

Karen Harris

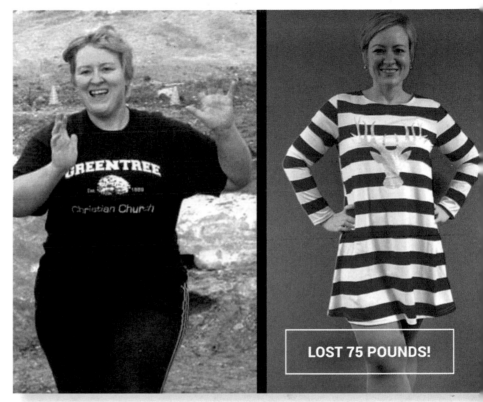

LOST 75 POUNDS!

Your Relationship with God

I have found that you can't accomplish success *just* with faith, but you certainly can't accomplish it *without* it. I think that most of us, including those who seek my coaching, have had some sense of a higher power at work in our lives. But life's disappointments combined with the pursuit of knowledge and certainty can all but extinguish the flame of faith in a person. The definition of "God" we may have been given when we were younger may not have meshed with what we thought of as that higher power. Coming to terms with our beliefs that could have been flawed or inappropriate for who we were at the time, or are even now, is an important step. I think

SUCCESS STORY

BEFORE

Tim Buchanan

AGE: 40
STARTING WEIGHT: 420 POUNDS
END WEIGHT: 210 POUNDS

"Today there are things I could do that before I would stress out over. Now I would have no problem with public speaking or walking into a job interview. I had anxiety about talking to people that did not know me, but now I have no issues with any public communication."

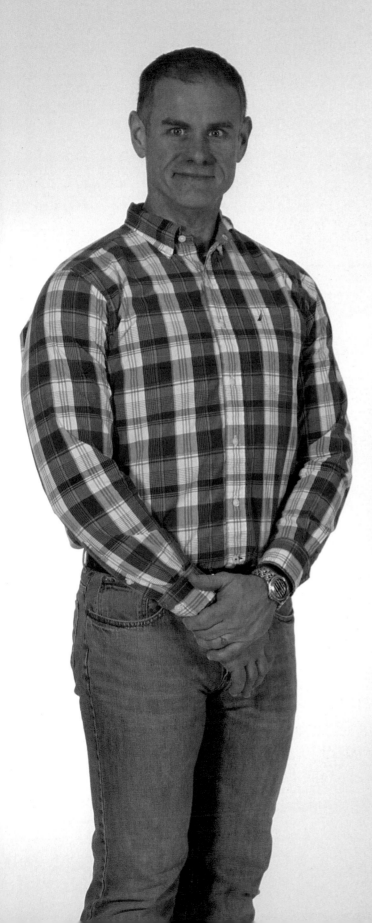

AFTER

"I have changed my future. I was borderline diabetic, had sleep apnea, high blood pressure and cholesterol, and I was diagnosed with fatty liver. I no longer have sugar issues. I haven't used a machine to sleep since my weight dropped below 275 pounds. My heart rate and blood pressure are at normal numbers every time I get them checked. My cholesterol and liver are both improving. These health improvements are directly tied to my weight loss. I know anything can happen and my time to go with Christ will be non-negotiable, but I believe I am no longer speeding that process up."

– Tim Buchanan

CHARLES' CLIENT FEATURED IN PEOPLE MAGAZINE'S *HALF THEIR SIZE* **2017 EDITION**

God is personal for each of us and meets us where we are in ways that we each personally can understand. That certainly has been my experience. If you find having faith difficult, you might consider what your understanding and definition of God really is, and consider upgrading it to a more appropriate one for yourself. Just because your definition and experience or lack thereof doesn't match the understanding of your family, or doesn't fit their mold and belief system, doesn't mean there is no God—it could mean your relationship with God is simply unique!

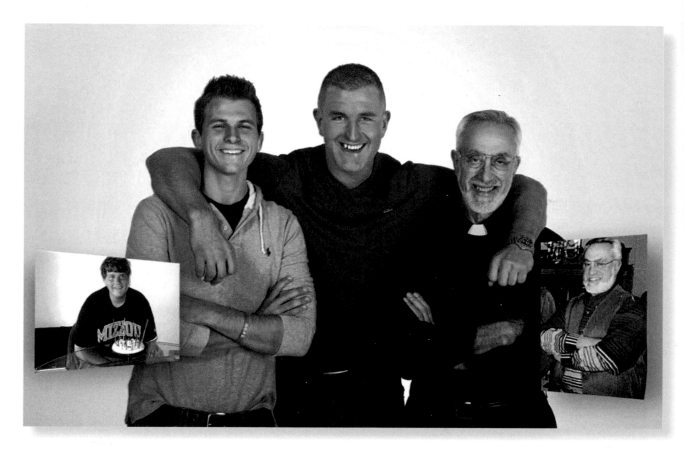

"You get two choices. Follow the plan or don't. [Charles'] plan works 100%. Not following the plan might work sometimes but the discipline created following the plan makes a relationship change with food. Now I consider the nutritional value and impact of food on my life instead of how it will affect my emotions."

– Tim Buchanan

A Final Note:

I want to say that while you long may have felt alone in whatever struggles you've been wrestling with, I hope you now know and feel you are not. We all have closets filled with complicated issues we need to resolve. Often they are cloaked in shame. I challenge you to get to work on leaving the light we now have turned on in the closet of your mind, and get to work on continuing to clean it out. Realize that in the mess and pile of what may seem massive and overwhelming are articles of beautiful clothing, tools, gifts from past family and friends and mementos. Once really looked at in the light, they can be appreciated for all that they are. The things you now can do without because they do not serve your purpose can simply be discarded. Now is the time to fully release any disempowering labels or judgments placed on you by anyone, authority figure or otherwise, who you subjugated your own God-given authority to. Now is the time to build the person you have decided to become.

While you may have long felt you didn't belong, as I once did, let me tell you, you do. You are a member of the human race. I challenge you to become the best member of it you can. God's blessings and grace on you as you continue onward in the journey.

Until the next time our paths should cross,

Charle

IT'S NOT HOW YOU START...

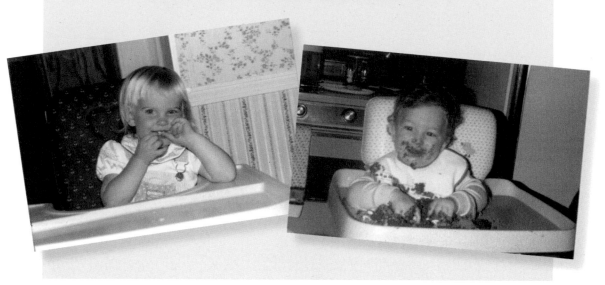

BUT HOW YOU FINISH THAT COUNTS!

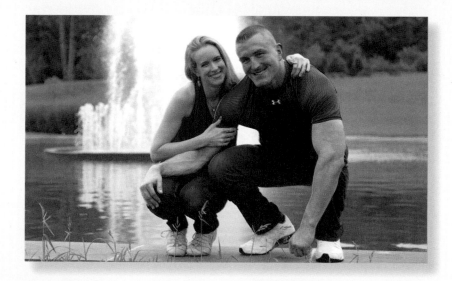

YOU CAN DO IT!

INDEX

BIOGRAPHY

Charles D'Angelo knows all about overcoming perceived difficulties and limitations – including those we put on ourselves – and finding the way to success.

By anyone's standard and in every area of life, Charles is a success. He has a flourishing business. He's financially secure. He has found the love of his life. He's tall, lean, attractive and incredibly fit. He's confident and self-assured. He's an accomplished author, and he has earned endorsements from such luminaries as President Bill Clinton, Anthony Robbins, Mark Hyman and more. Most important, he is happy.

But at one time, Charles was miserable. He was morbidly obese, weighing 360 pounds by the time he was a teen. He was bullied and emotionally abused by his peers. His family was poor. His mother got hooked on prescription drugs and alcohol, and his father was a hard laborer, working round the clock. Finally making the choice to take control of his life, he lost 160 pounds of pure fat and discovered a world of health and vitality. He learned to listen to and trust in God, and in doing so developed a life far beyond his wildest dreams.

Charles became the first in his family to get a college degree, and while still in school, he began teaching others how to reach their weight-loss goals by tapping into their inner power. Before long his name spread, and he was helping everyone from CEOs, Hollywood stars and Washington bigwigs to teenagers and stay-at-home moms in applying the disciplines of weight-loss success to all areas of life.

Now Charles can look back and see how God has continually put everything in his path to make his dreams come true and fulfill his mission to help others, but it was not always so obvious. He could easily have been controlled by his own fears and self-doubt, and at one time he was. Charles understands how our own perception can prevent us from seeing what's right in front of us. Nothing is more important to him than helping as many people as he possibly can to listen to the voice of God within themselves, develop their mindset and do as he did, create a phenomenal life.

Charles lives in St. Louis, Missouri with his soul mate, Crystal, and their adopted cat Leo.

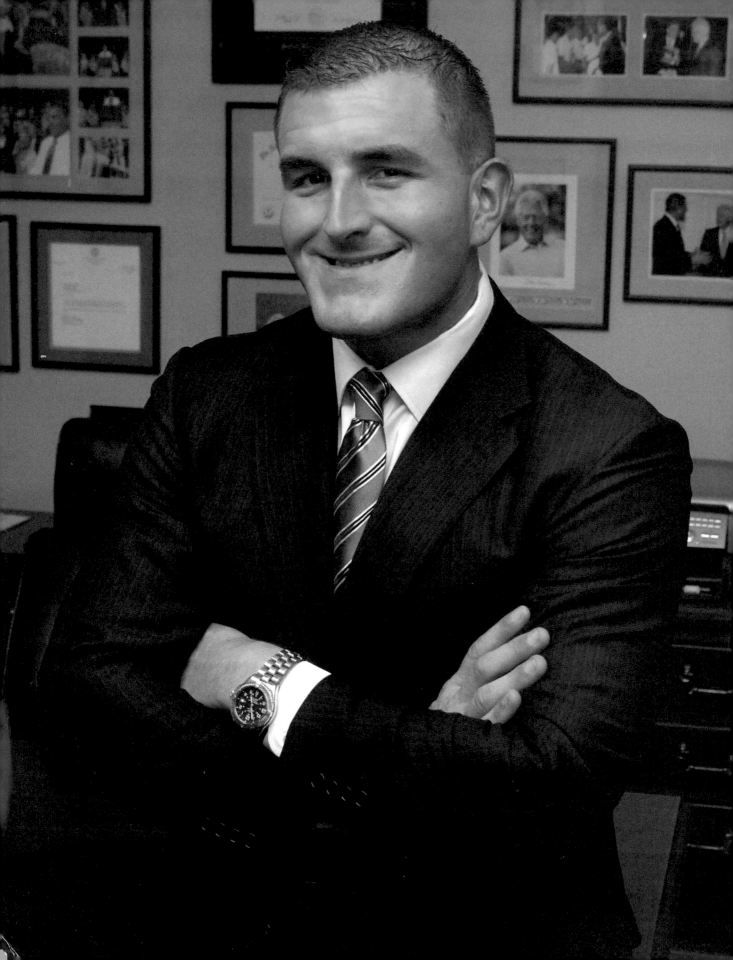